Hospital Patient Care Relationship Coordinator

Hospital Patient Care Relationship Coordinator

GD Mogli
PhD MBA FHRIM (UK) FAHIMA (USA)
Visiting Professor (Medical Informatics)
Mahatma Gandhi Institute of Medical Sciences
Wardha, Maharashtra, India
Dean, Health Information Management (HIM) Program
Ministry of Health (MOH), Oman
Associate Professor
HIM Degree Program, King Faisal University, Saudi Arabia
Head, Department of HIM Diploma Program
Kuwait Institute of Health Sciences, Kuwait
Head, Department of Bachelor of Medical Record Science
JIPMER, University of Madras, Chennai, Tamil Nadu, India
Senior Consultant/Adviser to the Ministries of Health
India, Afghanistan, Iran, Kuwait, Saudi Arabia
Oman, Bahrain, Qatar and United Arab Emirates
Ex-WHO Consultant and Senior Consultant (eHealth Management)
HEARTCOM, USA

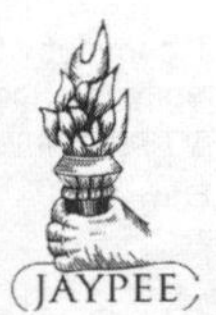

The Health Sciences Publisher
New Delhi | London | Panama

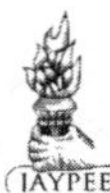

Jaypee Brothers Medical Publishers (P) Ltd

Headquarters
Jaypee Brothers Medical Publishers (P) Ltd.
4838/24, Ansari Road, Daryaganj
New Delhi 110 002, India
Phone: +91-11-43574357
Fax: +91-11-43574314
E-mail: jaypee@jaypeebrothers.com

Overseas Offices
J.P. Medical Ltd.
83, Victoria Street, London
SW1H 0HW (UK)
Phone: +44-20 3170 8910
Fax: +44(0) 20 3008 6180
E-mail: info@jpmedpub.com

Jaypee-Highlights Medical Publishers Inc.
City of Knowledge, Bld. 235, 2nd Floor, Clayton
Panama City, Panama
Phone: +1 507-301-0496
Fax: +1 507-301-0499
E-mail: cservice@jphmedical.com

Jaypee Brothers Medical Publishers (P) Ltd.
17/1-B, Babar Road, Block-B, Shaymali
Mohammadpur, Dhaka-1207
Bangladesh
Mobile: +08801912003485
E-mail: jaypeedhaka@gmail.com

Jaypee Brothers Medical Publishers (P) Ltd.
Bhotahity, Kathmandu, Nepal
Phone: +977-9741283608
E-mail: kathmandu@jaypeebrothers.com

Website: www.jaypeebrothers.com
Website: www.jaypeedigital.com

Inquiries for bulk sales may be solicited at: jaypee@jaypeebrothers.com

Hospital Patient Care Relationship Coordinator

First Edition: **2017**

ISBN: 978-93-5270-068-4

Printed at Rajkamal Electric Press, Plot No. 2, Phase-IV, Kundli, Haryana.

Dedicated to

Healthcare Providers

In the course of my four-decade career as Medical Record Administrator, educator, consultant and adviser, dealing with healthcare professionals in diverse organizations, in nine different countries, I felt the need for such concise book. Without losing the main information to develop a simple, tractable, handbook for the present users, who with too many subjects to learn, hardly find time to scan a variety of books on single subject available in the market. With this objective, a considerable time and effort have gone in preparing this book.

I have realized the need of participation of Hospital Patient Care Relationship Coordinator (HPCRC); is one of allied healthcare professionals with the similar educational background to coordinate and liaise between the medical, nursing, other allied healthcare services, administration, finance, transportation, etc. related to the patient care, and the patient, relatives or attendants of patients, referred institution and public. To ensure that patient healthcare issues are dealt with promptly and judiciously to the utmost satisfaction of all.

Having realized the importance of such position in the hospital, has synthesized the subject, prepared this unique book *Hospital Patient Care Relationship Coordinator*. It is the ultimate book for understanding how HPCRC work and to meet the facets of the requirement of the allied healthcare professionals such as students of paramedics including nurses, to serve as textbook in their academic programs, professional career building, besides reference guide throughout. Thus, this book is dedicated to the healthcare providers.

Preface

In the study and practice of paramedics, there is constant need for guiding principles, brief summaries of subjects related to the allied medical sciences, and explanations of techniques and procedures. It is evident that any medical, nursing and paramedics cannot become proficient in their respective fields without having a teamwork among all the medical, nursing and other allied health science professionals. A new concept of profession "Hospital Patient Care Relationship Coordinator (HPCRC) is going to play a vital role to oversee the comprehensive patient care in the health institutions, especially in hospitals.

The book deals with Hospital Patient Care Relationship Coordinator (HPCRC), one of allied healthcare professionals with paramedics-related educational background, to coordinate and liaison between the medical, nursing, and other allied healthcare services, administration, finance, transportation, etc. related to the patient care, and the patient, relatives or attendants of patients, referred institution and public. To ensure that patient healthcare issues are dealt with promptly and judiciously to the utmost satisfaction of all. HPCRC job is to oversee the patient care services from the time of patient's registration or even earlier from the date of booking, during patient's journey in the hospital as an emergency, outpatient or inpatient till his/her discharge from the hospital. During the patient's voyage, the HPCRC has to deal with the medical, nursing, other allied health professionals, laboratory, radiology, pharmacy, wards, operation theaters, intensive coronary care unit (ICCU)/critical care unit (CCU), insurance, billing, administration and many things which, depend on the type of care needed by patient. He has to ensure that the patient's medical record is complete in all respects by arranging that related documents are promptly placed in the main patient's record to facilitate the healthcare providers to render their services efficiently. Even after discharge, for some cases, there are many other issues to be settled. He has to maintain intra-, inter-relationship within the hospital, and with the outside healthcare institutions related to continued patient care, insurance, legal and other matters to facilitate the patient or his relatives and the institution for smooth functioning of the system. Precisely, HPCRC is the envoy of patient as well as the hospital.

I realized the need for the comprehensive HPCRC book, including fundamentals of anatomy, physiology, medical terminology, pathology, laboratory, radiology, radiation therapy, pharmacology, pharmacy, oncology, psychiatry, medical psychology, nursing, nutrition, physical and occupational therapy, medical social, medical records, public relations, medical secretarial profession, communication skills, leadership, and motivation coupled with medical terms and definitions and abbreviations. The book would be of immense value to the hospitals, hospital patient care coordinators, medical social workers, medical record-keepers, medical secretaries, law professionals, medical representatives, insurance companies, and healthcare software developers to serve as textbook in their academic programs, professional career building, besides reference guide throughout. The special feature is when too many divergent people and departments in a healthcare organization are playing the role of patient care, it would be hard to locate real setback, while the HPCRC can be handy acting as a single "window" system concept to clarify and deal with the issue promptly.

The book has 27 chapters; encompassing vital topics related to concerned paramedics services that will be grasped by the learners' mind much faster to enable him/her to coordinate with the medical and other related professionals that will lead to the diagnosis or to the treatment and its related issues. Precisely, this is a concise handbook for *Hospital Patient Care Relationship Coordinator*, and all allied healthcare professionals besides other professionals who deal with medical and healthcare issues.

GD Mogli

Acknowledgments

At the outset, my grateful thanks to Shri Jitendar P Vij (Group Chairman) and Mr Ankit Vij (Group President) of M/s Jaypee Brothers Medical Publishers (P) Ltd, New Delhi, India, for bringing out this invaluable book.

My sincere gratitude to State Health Ministers and Deputy Ministers of Gulf Cooperation Council (GCC) Countries and other administrators, and professional colleagues of India, Afghanistan, Iran, Kuwait, Kingdom of Saudi Arabia, Oman, Bahrain, Qatar, and United Arab Emirates (UAE), for their support, encouragement and cooperation.

My special thanks to Narendar Sampath Kumar [MA BMRSc PGDCS CHRIM (UK)], Medical Record Manager, Mediclinic Welcare Hospital, Dubai, UAE.

Mr Ramalingam Selva Kumar [MA MS BMRSc PGDHM AHRIM (UK)], Clinical Coder, Aberdeen Royal Infirmary Hospital, Aberdeen, Scotland, UK.

Mrs Mary Stella Alexander [BSc BMRSc CHRIM (UK)], Medical Record Manager, Hamad General Hospital, Doha, Qatar.

And lastly, I owe my sincere gratitude to my family for their unconditional support.

Contents

Abbreviations and Symbols

ABBREVIATIONS

Abbreviations	*Expansion*
A	Adult
AAA	Abdominal Aortic Aneurysm
AAR	Antigen Anti-globulin Reaction
AAS	Aortic Arch Syndrome
Ab	Antibody
AB	Asthmatic Bronchitis
A/B	Acid-base Ratio
Abd hyst	Abdomen Hysterectomy
ABE	Acute Bacterial Endocarditis
ABG	Arterial Blood Gas
ABO	Blood Group System of Groups (A, AB, B & O)
ABP	Arterial Blood Pressure
ABS	Anti-B Serum
AC	Abdominal Circumstances
ACC	Adenoid Cystic Carcinoma
ACE	Adrenocortical Extract
ACM	Albumin-calcium Magnesium
ACS	Antireticular Cytotoxic Serum
ACT	Activated Coagulation Time
ACTH	Adrenocorticotropic Hormone
ACVD	Acute Cardiovascular Disease
AD	Right Ear (Auris Dextra)
ADA	Anterior Descending Artery
ADH	Antidiuretic Hormone
ad lib	As Desired
ADS	Antibody Deficiency Syndrome
AEG	Air Encephalogram
AF	Amniotic Fluid
AFB	Acid-fast Bacillus
AFP	Alpha-fetoprotein
Ag	Antigen
A/G	Albumin/Globulin (Ratio)
AGA	Appropriate for Gestational Age
AGL	Acute Granulocytic Leukemia
AGN	Acute Glomerulonephritis
AH	Arterial Hypertension
AHA	Acquired Hemolytic Anemia
AHD	Arteriosclerosis Heart Disease
AHF	Acute Heart Failure

AHG	Antihemolytic Globulin
AHT	Augmented Histamine Test
AI	Aortic Incompetence
AIDS	Acquired Immune Deficiency Syndrome
AIH	Artificial Insemination by Husband
AIHA	Autoimmune Hemolytic Anemia
A/J	Ankle Jerk
AK	Above Knee
AKA	Above Knee Amputation
ALK-P	Alkaline Phosphate
ALL	Acute Lymphatic Leukemia
ALP	Alkaline Phosphate
ALS	Amyotrophic Lateral Sclerosis
ALT. dieb	Every Other Day (alternis diebus)
ALT. hor	Every Other Hour (alternis horis)
ALT. noct	Every Other Night (alternis nocta)
ALT	Alanine Aminotransferase
AMA	Against Medical Advice
AMI	Acute Myocardial Infarction
AML	Acute Myelogenous Leukemia
AMoL	Acute Monocytic Leukemia
An	Anatomical
ANA	Antinuclear Antibody
ANCA	Antineutrophil Cytoplasmic Antibody
AOM	Acute Otitis Media
AP	Anterior Pituitary
A-P	Anteroposterior
APC	Aspirin-phenacetin-caffeine
APH	Antepartum Hemorrhage
APO	Apolipoprotein
aPTT	Activated Partial Thromboplastin Time
AR	Aortic Regurgitation
ARC	AIDS-related Complex
ARD	Acute Respiratory Disease
ARDS	Adult Respiratory Distress Syndrome
ARF	Acute Respiratory Failure
ARM	Artificial Rupture of Membrane
AS	Aortic Stenosis
ASD	Arterial Septal Defect
ASHD	Arteriosclerotic Heart Disease
ASMA	Antismooth Muscle Antibody
ASO	Arteriosclerotic Obliterans
AST	Aspartate Transaminase
AT III	Antithrombin III
ATD	Asphyxiating Thoracic Dystrophy
ATS	Antitetanic Serum
AV	Anteverted

AVF	Arteriovenous Fistula
AVH	Acute Viral hepatitis
AVM	Arteriovenous Malformation
Ba	Barium
BB	Blood Bank
BBA	Born Before Arrival
BBB	Bundle Branch Block
BCG	Bacille Calmette-Guérin (Vaccine)
BF	Breastfeeding
BFH	Baby-friendly Hospital
BGTT	Borderline Glucose Tolerance Test
bhCG	Beta-human Chorionic Gonadotropin
Biochem	Biochemistry (Biochemical)
BID	Brought in Dead
b.i.d.	Twice a Day (bis in die)
BIH	Benign Intracranial Hypertension
BJM	Bones, Joints and Muscles
BKA	Below Knee Amputation
BMR	Basal Metabolic Rate
BO	Bowels Open
BOM	Bilateral Otitis Media
B/P	Blood Pressure
BPD	Bi-parietal Diameter
BPH	Benign Prostatic Hypotrophy
Br	Breech
BR	Bronchitis
BS	Bowel Sound
BSO	Bilateral Salpingo-oophorectomy
BSOM	Bilateral Serous Otitis Media
BSR	Blood Sedimentation Rate
BT	Bleeding Time
BUN	Blood Urine Nitrogen
BW	Birth Weight
Bx	Biopsy
C	Cardiac
CA	Cancer Antigen
CA 125	Cancer Antigen 125
Ca	Carcinoma
C_1,C_2	First, Second Cervical Vertebra
CABG	Coronary Artery Bypass Graft
CAD	Coronary Artery Disease
CAHD	Coronary Atherosclerotic Heart Disease
card	Cardiology
cath	Catheterization
CBC	Complete Blood Count
CBD	Common Bile Duct
CBGM	Capillary Blood Glucose Monitoring

CCF	Congestive Cardiac Failure
CDH	Congenital Dislocation of Hip
CEA	Carcinoembryonic Antigen
CF	Cup Feeding
CHA	Congenital Hypoplastic Anemia
CHB	Complete Heart Block
CHD	Congenital Heart Disease
chem.	Chemistry
CHF	Congestive Heart Failure
CK	Creatine Kinase
CLBBB	Complete Left Bundle Branch Block
CL	Clinic
cl	Clinical
CLL	Chronic Lymphocytic Leukemia
CML	Chronic Myelocytic Leukemia
CMR	Cerebral Metabolic Rate
CMV	Cytomegalovirus
CNS	Central Nervous System
COM	Chronic Otitis Media
COPD	Chronic Obstructive Lung Disease
CPD	Cephalopelvic Disproportion
CPR	Cardiopulmonary Resuscitation
CRBBB	Complete Right Bundle Branch Block
CRF	Chronic Renal Failure
CRH	Corticotropin-releasing Hormone
CRP	C-reactive Protein
CSF	Cerebrospinal Fluid
CSOM	Chronic Suppurative Otitis Media
CSSD	Central Sterile Supply Department
CST	Convulsive Shock Therapy
CT	Cerebral Thrombosis
CVA	Cerebrovascular Accident
CVD	Cardiovascular Disease
CVP	Central Venous Pressure
D&C	Dilatation and Curettage
Dent	Dental
Derm	Dermatology
DI	Diabetes Insipidus
DIC	Disseminated Intravascular Coagulation
Diet	Dietetics
DHEAS	Dehydroepiandrosterone Sulfate
DM	Diabetes Mellitus
DNS	Deviated Nasal Septum
DOA	Date of Admission
DOB	Date of Birth
DOC	Date of Conception
DOD	Date of Discharge or Death

DPT	Diphtheria, Pertussis, and Tetanus (vaccine)
DSA	Digital Subtraction Angiography
DTR	Deep Tendon Reflex
DU	Duodenal Ulcer
DUB	Dysfunctional Uterine Bleeding
D&V	Diarrhea and Vomiting
Dx	Diagnosis
EAM	External Auditory Meatus
EBL	Estimated Blood Loss
EBM	Expressed Breast Milk
EBV	Epstein-Barr Virus
ECCE	Extracapsular Cataract Extraction
ECG or EKG	Electrocardiogram
ECS	Electroconvulsive Shock
ECT	Electroconvulsive Therapy
EDD	Expected Date of Delivery
EEG	Electroencephalogram
EFW	Estimated Fetal Weight
EGA	Estimated Gestational Age
EGD	Esophagogastroduodenoscopy
EH	Essential Hypertension
EHL	Electrohydraulic Lithotripsy
ELISA	Enzyme-linked Immunosorbent Assay
elec	Electra
EMG	Electromyogram
ENA	Extractable Nuclear Antigen
END	Endocrinology
ENT	Ear, Nose and Throat
ER	Emergency Room
ERCP	Endoscopic Retrograde Cholangiopancreatography
ESR	Erythrocyte Sedimentation Rate
EST	Electroshock Therapy
ESWL	Extracorporeal Shock Wave Lithotripsy
EUA	Examination Under Anesthesia
EVD	External Ventricular Drainage
Exp. Lap	Exploratory Laparotomy
Ext. gen	External Genitalia
FB	Foreign Body
FBG	Fasting Blood Glucose
FBS	Fasting Blood Sugar
FD	Forceps Delivery
FDIU	Fetal Death *in Utero*
FDP	Fibrinogen Degradation Product
FFP	Fresh Frozen Plasma
FH	Fetal Heart
FHR	Fetal Heart Rate
FHx	Family History

FiO_2	Fraction of Inspired Oxygen
FIV	Forced Inspired Volume
FM	Fetal Movement
FSH	Follicle-stimulating Hormone
FTA-ABS	Fluorescent Treponemal Antibody Absorption
FT4	Free Thyroxine
FTM	Fractional Test Meal
FTND	Full-term Normal Delivery
FUO	Fever of Unknown Origin
FW	Fetal Weight
Fx	Fracture
G	Gravida
GA	General Anesthesia
GB	Gallbladder
GE	Gastroenterology
G/E	Gastroenteritis
Gen	General
GERD	Gastroesophageal Reflux Disease
Gest.	Gestation
GFR	Glomerular Filtration Rate
GGT	Gamma-glutamyl-transferase
GH	Growth Hormone
GHb	Glycosylated Hemoglobin
GIFT	Glomerular Filtration Rate
GIT	Gastrointestinal Tract
GM	General Medicine
GP	General Practitioner
G6PD	Glucose-6-Phosphate Dehydrogenase
grav.	Pregnancy (Gravida)
GS	General Surgery
G/S	Glucose and Saline
GSH	Glomerular-stimulating Hormone
GTT	Glucose Tolerance Test
GU	Genitourinary
GYN	Gynecology
h	Hour
HASCVD	Hypertensive Arteriosclerotic Cardiovascular Disease
HAV	Hepatitis A Virus
Hb	Hemoglobin
HBc	Hepatitis B Core
HbF	Fetal Hemoglobin
HBs Ab	Hepatitis B Surface Antibody
HBs Ag	Hepatitis B Surface Antigen
HBP	High Blood Pressure
HbS	Sickle-cell Hemoglobin
HBV	Hepatitis B Virus
HBW	High Birth Weight

HC	Head Circumference
hCG	Human Chorionic Gonadotropin
HCO_3	Bicarbonate
Hcrit	Hematocrit
HCV	Hepatitis C Virus
HCVD	Hypertensive Cardiovascular Disease
HD	Heart Disease
HDL	High Density Lipoprotein
HDN	Hemolytic Disease of the Newborn
HDV	Hepatitis D Virus
HEENT	Head, Eyes, Ears, Nose, and Throat
HEM	Hematology
HF	Heart Failure
Hgb	Hemoglobin
HGH	High Growth Hormone
HHA	Hereditary Hemolytic Anemia
HHD	Hypertensive Heart Disease
HIV	Human Immunodeficiency Virus
HLA	Human Lymphocyte Antigen
HMD	Hyaline Membrane Disease
hMG	Human Menopausal Gonadotropin
HPF	High Power Field
HPI	History of Present Illness
HPV	Human Papillomavirus
HR	Heart Rate
HSG	Hysterosalpingography
HSV	Herpes Simplex Virus
HTLV	Human T-cell Lymphotropic Virus
HVD	Hypertensive Vascular Disease
Hx	History
IC	Intensive Care
ICC	Intensive Coronary Care
ICD	International Classification of Disease (WHO)
ICCE	Intracapsular Cataract Extraction
ICCU	Intensive Coronary Care Unit
ICM	Intercostal Margin
ICSI	Intracytoplasmic Sperm Injection
ICU	Intensive Care Unit
I&D	Incision and Drainage
IDDM	Insulin Dependent Diabetes Mellitus
IDK	Internal Derangement of Knee
IDM	Infant of Diabetic Mother
Ig	Immunoglobulin
IGT	Impaired Glucose Tolerance
IH	Infectious Hepatitis
IHD	Ischemic Heart Disease
IM	Internal Medicine

IMB	Intermenstrual Bleeding
Immunol	Immunology
Inj	Injection
INR	International Normalized Ratio
I & O	Intake and Output
IOP	Intraocular Pressure
IP	Inpatient
IPPV	Intermittent Positive Pressure Ventilation
IQ	Intelligent Quotient
ITP	Idiopathic Thrombocytopenic Purpura
IUCD	Intrauterine Contraceptive Device
IUD	Intrauterine Device
IUFB	Intrauterine Foreign Body
IUFD	Intrauterine Fetal Death
IUGR	Intrauterine Growth Retardation
IV	Intravenous
IVF	*In Vitro* Fertilization
IVH	Intraventricular Hemorrhage
IVP	Intravenous Pyelogram
IVSD	Intraventricular Septal Defect
J	Joint
JBE	Japanese B Encephalitis
Jt	Joint
JVP	Jugular Venous Pressure
K	Kilo
Kg	Kilogram
Kj	Knee Jerk
KK	Knee Kick
KUB	Kidney Ureter Bladder
KVO	Keep Vein Open
L1, L2, L3	First, Second and Third Lumbar Vertebrae
LA	Local Anesthesia
lab	Laboratory
LADCA	Left Anterior Descending Coronary Artery
LAG	Lymphangiography
LAO	Left Anterior Oblique
LAP	Leukocyte Alkaline Phosphate
LB	Live Birth
LBB	Left Bundle Branch
LBBB	Left Bundle Branch Block
LBW	Low Birth Weight
LCM	Left Costal Margin
L & D	Labor and Delivery
LDH	Lactate Dehydrogenase
LDL	Low Density Lipoprotein
LFD	Low Forceps Delivery
LFT	Liver Function Test

LGA	Large for Gestational Age
LGV	Lymphogranuloma Venereum
LH	Luteinizing Hormone
LHF	Left Heart Failure
LICS	Left Intercostal Space
LIF	Left Iliac Fossa
lig	Ligament
LIH	Left Inguinal Hernia
LK	Left Kidney
LLE	Left Lower Extremity
LLL	Left Lower Lobe
LLQ	Left Lower Quadrant
LMP	Last Menstrual Period
LOA	Left Occipitoanterior (Fetal Position)
LOP	Left Occipitoposterior (Fetal Position)
LOS	Length of Stay
LOT	Left Occipito Transverse (Fetal Position)
LP	Lumbar Puncture
LPO	Left Posterior Oblique
LSCS	Lower Segment Cesarean Section
LSK	Liver, Spleen, Kidneys
LTCS	Low Transverse Cesarean Section
LTH	Luteotropic Hormone
LUE	Left Upper Extremity
LUL	Left Upper Lobe
LUQ	Left Upper Quadrant
LV	Left Ventricle
LVF	Left Ventricular Failure
LVH	Left Ventricular Hypertrophy
lymphs	Lymphocyes
lytes	Electrolytes
m	Meter
MA	Mental Age
macro	Macrocytic
MAS	Meconium Aspiration Syndrome
maxF	Maxillofacial
MCH	Mean Corpuscular Hemoglobin
MD	Muscular Dystrophy
mEq	Milliequivalent
MetHb	Methemoglobin
mg	Milligram
MFD	Mid Forceps Delivery
MG	Myasthenia Gravis
MH	Marital History
MI	Myocardial Infarction
mL	Milliliter
mm	Millimeter

MPV	Mean Platelet Volume
MR	Mental Retardation
MRI	Magnetic Resonance Imaging
MRSA	Methicillin-resistant *Staphylococcus aureus*
MS	Mitral Stenosis
MSU	Midstream Specimen of Urine
MW	Molecular Weight
n	Nerve
NAD	Nothing Abnormal Detected
NB	Newborn
NBI	No Bone Injury
NBM	Nothing by Mouth
NBW	Normal Birth Weight
N/c	No Complaint
ND	Normal Delivery
NEC	Not Elsewhere Classified
NED	No Evidence of Disease
NEO	Neonatology
NEP	Nephrology
neuro	Neurology
NFTD	Normal Full-term Delivery
NG	Nasogastric
NGf	Nasogastric Feeding
NGT	Nasogastric Tube
NIBP	Non-invasive Blood Pressure
NIC	Neonatal Intensive Care
NICU	Neonatal Intensive Care Unit
NIDDM	Noninsulin Dependent Diabetes Mellitus
NM	Nuclear Medicine
NOS	Not Otherwise Specified
NS	Neurosurgery
NSA	No Significant Abnormality
NSAID	Non-steroidal Anti-inflammatory Drug
N&V	Nausea and Vomiting
NSVD	Normal Spontaneous Vaginal Delivery
NYD	Not Yet Diagnosed
O	Orthopedics
OB-GYN	Obstetrics and Gynecology
OD	Right Eye (Oculus Dexter)
OE	On Examination
O & E	Observation and Examination
OFC	Occipitofrontal Circumference
OG	Orogastric
OGF	Orogastric Feeding
OHSS	Ovarian Hyperstimulation Syndrome
OM	Otitis Media
OMD	Ocular Muscle Dystrophy

OMI	Old Myocardial Infarction
ONC	Oncology
OP	Occipitoposterior
op	Operation
O/P	Outpatient
OPH	Ophthalmology
OPV	Oral Polio Vaccine
OS	Oral Surgery
OS	Left Eye (Oculus Sinister)
OT	Occupation Therapy
P-A	Posteroanterior
P/A	Percussion and Auscultation
Pap	Papanicolaou (pap smear)
PAF	Paroxysmal Atrial Fibrillation
PAS	Pulmonary Artery Systolic Pressure
PAT	Paroxysmal Auricular Tachycardia
Path	Pathology
PA View	Posteroanterior View on X-ray
PCA	Patient Controlled Analgesia
PCB	Postcoital Bleeding
PCOS	Polycystic Ovary Syndrome
PCR	Polymerase Chain Reaction
PCT	Postcoital Test
PCV	Packed Cell Volume
PDA	Patent Ductus Arteriosus
PED	Pediatrics
PED-IC	Pediatric Intensive Care
PEEP	Positive End-expiratory Pressure
PEFR	Peak Expiratory Flow Rate
PERRLA	Pupils, Equal, Round, Reactive to Light and Accommodation
PET	Preeclamptic Toxemia
PFT	Pulmonary Function Test
PGH	Pituitary Growth Hormone
pH	Hydrogen Ion Concentration
Phar	Pharmacy
pH1	Philadelphia Chromosome
PHT	Pulmonary Hypertension
Phys	Physiology
Physio	Physiotherapy
PICC	Peripherally Inserted Central Catheter
PID	Pelvic Inflammatory Disease
PIVD	Protruded Intervertebral Disk
PKU	Phenylketonuria
PL	Plastic
PM	Postmortem
PMA	Progressive Muscular Atrophy
PMB	Postmenopausal Bleeding

PMH	Past Medical History
PMI	Point of Maximal Impulse
PMN	Polymorphonuclear Neutrophil
PMP	Past Menstrual Period
PMR	Physical Medicine and Rehabilitation
PN	Postnatal
PND	Paroxysmal Nocturnal Dyspnea
PNI	Peripheral Nerve Injury
PO_2	Partial Pressure
POC	Products of Conception
POP	Plaster of Paris
PPBS	Postprandial Blood Sugar
PPH	Postpartum Hemorrhage
Ppt	Precipitate
PPU	Perforated Peptic Ulcer
PR	Per Rectum
p.r.n.	As Required (Pro re nata)
PROM	Premature Rupture of Membranes
PSA	Prostate Specific Antigen
PSMA	Progressive Spinal Muscular Atrophy
Psych	Psychiatry
PT	Prothrombin Time
PTC	Percutaneous Transhepatic Cholangiogram
PTCA	Percutaneous Transluminal Coronary Angioplasty
PTH	Parathyroid Hormone
PTT	Partial Thromboplastin Time
PUE	Pyrexia of Unknown Etiology
PUO	Pyrexia of Unknown Origin
PV	Per Vaginum (through the vagina)
P & V	Pyloroplasty and Vagotomy
PVC	Premature Ventricular Contraction
PVP	Portal Venous Pressure
PVR	Pulmonary Vascular Resistance
PVT	Paroxysmal Ventricular Tachycardia
q	Every
q.d.	Every Day (quaque die)
q. 2h	Every 2 hours
q.h	Every hour (quaque hora)
q.i.d.	Four Times Daily (quater in die)
q.m.	Every Morning (quaque mane)
q.n.	Every Night (quaque nocte)
q.n.s.	Quantity Not Sufficient
q.o.d.	Every Other Day
q.o.n.	Every Other Night
q.v.	As much as you please (quantum vis)
q.w.	Every Week
R	Radiology

RA	Rheumatoid Arthritis
RAD	Radiation Absorbed Dose
RAST	Radioallergosorbent Test
RBBB	Right Bundle Branch Block
RBC	Red Blood Cell
RBG	Random Blood Glucose
RCA	Right Coronary Artery
RCM	Right Costal Margin
RCS	Reticulum Cell Sarcoma
RDS	Respiratory Distress Syndrome
RDW	Red Cell Distribution Width
REM	Rapid Eye Movement
Resp	Respiratory
RF	Rheumatic Fever
RFB	Retained Foreign Body
RH	Rheumatology
Rh	Rhesus Blood Factor
Rh+	Rhesus Positive
Rh-	Rhesus Negative
RHD	Rheumatic Heart Disease
RHF	Right Heart Failure
Rhin	Rhinology
RI	Resistance Index
Ri	Rooming in
RIA	Radioimmunoassay
RIF	Right Iliac Fossa
RIH	Right Inguinal Hernia
RLL	Right Lower Lobe
RLQ	Right Lower Quadrant
RM	Radical Mastectomy
RML	Right Mediolateral
RNA	Ribonucleic Acid
R/O	Rule Out
ROA	Right Occipital Anterior
ROIH	Right Oblique Inguinal Hernia
ROM	Rupture of Membranes
ROP	Right Occipital Posterior
ROT	Right Occipital Transverse
RP	Retrograde Pyelogram
RPA	Right Pulmonary Artery
RR	Respiratory Rate
RSV	Respiratory Syncytial Virus
RT	Radiation Therapy (Radiotherapy)
RTA	Road Traffic Accident
RU	Retrograde Urogram
RUE	Right Upper Extremity
RUQ	Right Upper Quadrant

RURTI	Recurrent Upper Respiratory Tract Infection
RVF	Right Ventricular Failure
RVH	Right Ventricular Hypertrophy
Rx	Prescription, therapy
S	Surgery
SAH	Systemic Arterial Hypertension
SAP	Serum Alkaline Phosphatase
SB	Stillbirth
SBE	Subacute Bacterial Endocarditis
SC	Special Care
SCC	Squamous Cell Carcinoma
schiz	Schizophrenia
SGA	Small for Gestational Age
SGPT	Serum Glutamate Pyruvate Transaminase
SBP	Systolic Blood Pressure
SCA	Sickle Cell Anemia
SD	Spontaneous Delivery
Ser	Service
SG	Specific Gravity
SGA	Small for Gestational Age
SGOT	Serum Glutamic Oxaloacetic Transaminase
SHx	Social History
SHBG	Sex Hormone-binding Globulin
SIDS	Sudden Infant Death Syndrome
SLE	Systemic Lupus Erythematous
SMR	Submucous Resection
SOB	Shortness of Breath
s.o.s	If it is Necessary (si opus sit)
SPE	Serum Protein Electrophoresis
SPECT	Single Photon Emission Computerized Tomography
SROM	Spontaneous Rupture of Membrane
SS	Social Service
SSE	Soapsuds Enema
Staph	*Staphylococcus*
Stat.	Immediately (statim)
STD	Sexually Transmitted Disease
SVC	Superior Vena Cava
SVD	Spontaneous Vaginal Delivery
SVT	Supraventricular Tachycardia
SWD	Short Wave Diathermy
Sx.	Symptoms
T3	Triiodothyronine
TA	Tendon Achilles
T&A	Tonsillectomy and Adenoidectomy
tab.	Tablet
TAH	Total Abdominal Hysterectomy
TAL	Tendon Achilles Lengthening
TAO	Thromboangiitis Obliterans

TB	Tuberculosis
TBM	Tuberculous Meningitis
TEV	Talipes Equinovarus
Th	Thoracic
THR	Total Hip Replacement
TIA	Transient Ischemic Attack
TIBC	Total Iron Binding Capacity
t.i.d.	Three Times a Day (ter in die)
TKR	Total Knee Replacement
TL	Tubal Ligation
TM	Tympanic Membrane
TMJ	Temporomandibular Joint
TNS	Transcutaneous Nerve Stimulation
TOP	Termination of Pregnancy
TORCH	Toxoplasmosis, Rubella, Cytomegalovirus and Herpes
TPHA	*Treponema Pallidum* Hemagglutination Assay
TPN	Total Parenteral Nutrition
TPR	Temperature, Pulse and Respiration
TPUR	Transperineal Urethral Resection
TRH	Thyroid Releasing Hormone
TSH	Thyroid-stimulating Hormone
tsp.	Teaspoon
TSS	Toxic Shock Syndrome
TT	Tetanus Toxoid
TTH	Thyrotropic Hormone
TTP	Thrombotic Thrombocytopenic Purpura
TUR	Transurethral Resection
TURB	Transurethral Resection of Bladder (Tumor)
TURP	Transurethral Resection of the Prostate
TVH	Total Vaginal Hysterectomy
TVP	Transvesical Prostatectomy
Tx	Treatment
U/A	Urinalysis
UC	Ulcerative Colitis
UD	Urethral Discharge
UGI	Upper Gastrointestinal
UL	Upper Lobe
Ung.	Ointment
unilat.	Unilateral
UR	Urology
URI	Upper Respiratory Infection
URTI	Upper Respiratory Tract Infection
U/S	Ultrasound
ut.	Uterus
UTI	Urinary Tract Infection
VA	Visual Acuity
Vag	Vagina
VAS	Vascular

VD	Venereal Disease
V&D	Vomiting and Diarrhea
VDRL	Venereal Disease Research Laboratory
VE	Vaginal Examination
vent.	ventilator
VER	Visual Evoked Response
VF	Ventricular Fibrillation
VH	Vaginal Hysterectomy
VHD	Valvular Heart Disease
vit.	Vitamin
VLDL	Very Low Density Lipoprotein
VMR	Vasomotor Rhinitis
vRI	Viral Respiratory Infection
VS	Vital Signs
VSA	Vital Signs Absent
VSD	Ventricular Septal Defect
VT	Ventricular Tachycardia
Vx	Vertex
VZV	Vericella Zoster Virus
WB	Whole Blood
WBC	White Blood Count
WC	Whooping Cough
WCC	White Cell Count
WNL	Within Normal Limits
WPW	Wolff Parkinson White (Syndrome)
wt.	Weight
XDP	Xeroderma Pigmentosum
XM	Cross Match
XR	X-ray
Y	Year
YF	Yellow Fever
YOB	Year of Birth

SYMBOLS

(L)	Left
(R)	Right
(M)	Murmur
.	Start of Operation
x	End of Operation
♂	Male
♀	Female
*	Birth
!	Death
∝	Is Proportional to
Tri	Prism Diopter
Tri t	Time Interval
Tri a	Change in pH

~	Approximately
@	At
⚧	Combined with
>	Greater than
≯	Not greater than
≥	Greater than or Equal to
<	Less than
≮	Not less than
≤	Less than or Equal to
≈	Approximately Equal to
±	Not definite, Plus/Minus
⊠	Decrease
⊠	Increase
⊠	UP
◙	Normal
#	Fracture
Rx	Recipe, Take
°	Degree
1x	Once
2x	Twice
′	Foot
″	Inch
/	Per
:	Ratio (is to)
+	Positive
–	Negative
=	Equals
∞	Infinity
μg	Microgram
μL	Microliter
μ	Micron
M	Murmur
Oz	Ounce
C	With
S	Without
(+)	Significant
(–)	Insignificant
(+)	Possibly Significant
≠	Does not Equal to

Plate 1

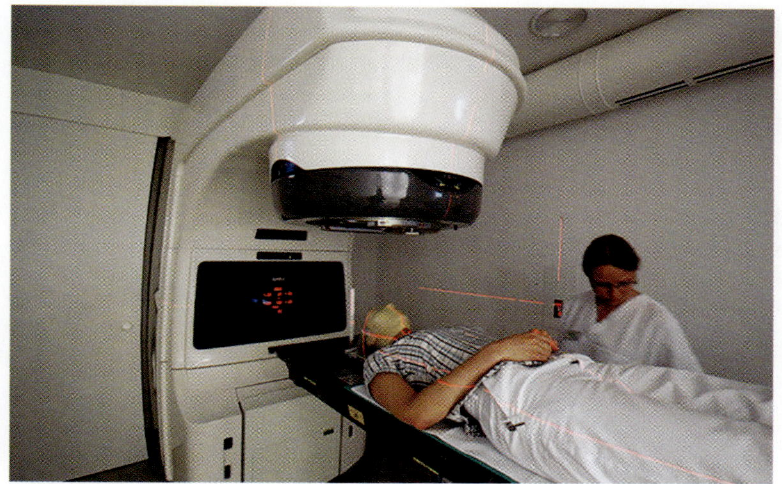

Fig. 6.1 Varian Clinac 2100C Linear Accelerator

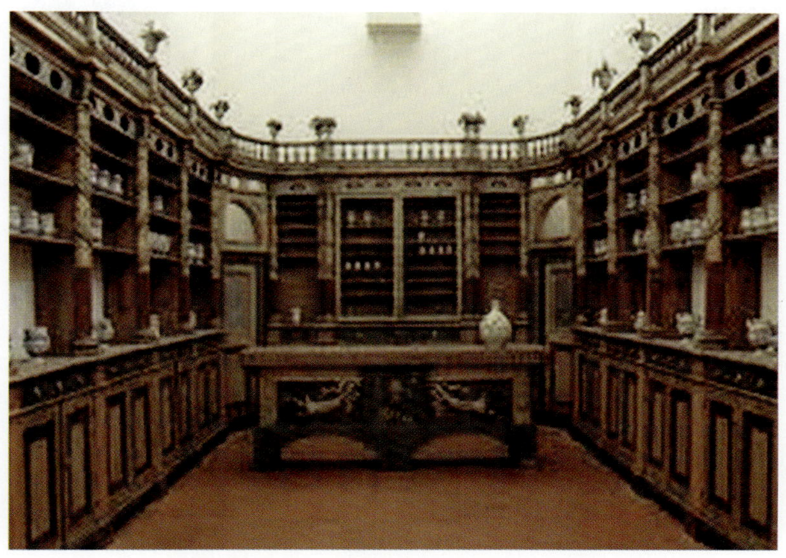

Fig. 9.1 A model of 19th century Italian pharmacy

Plate 2

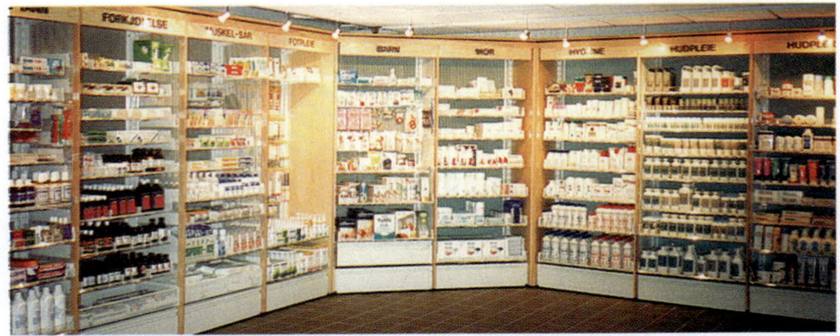

Fig. 9.2 A model of modern pharmacy

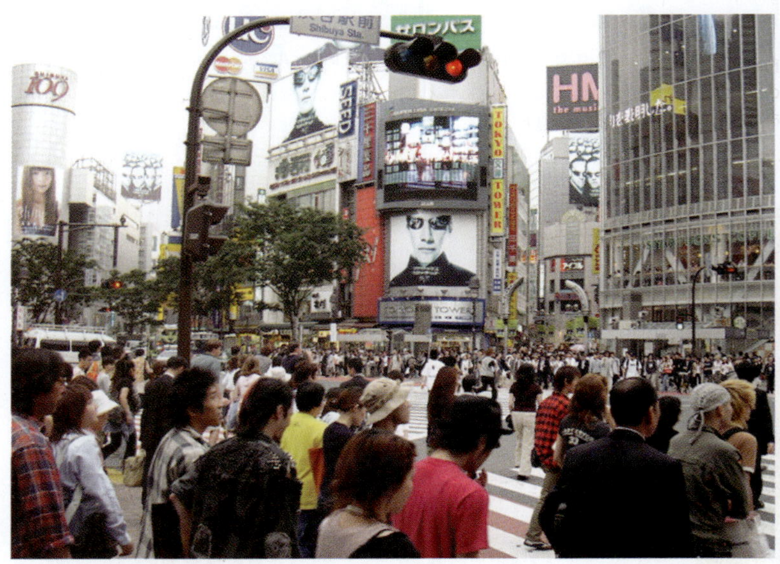

Fig. 12.2 Social psychology studies the nature and causes of social behavior

Plate 3

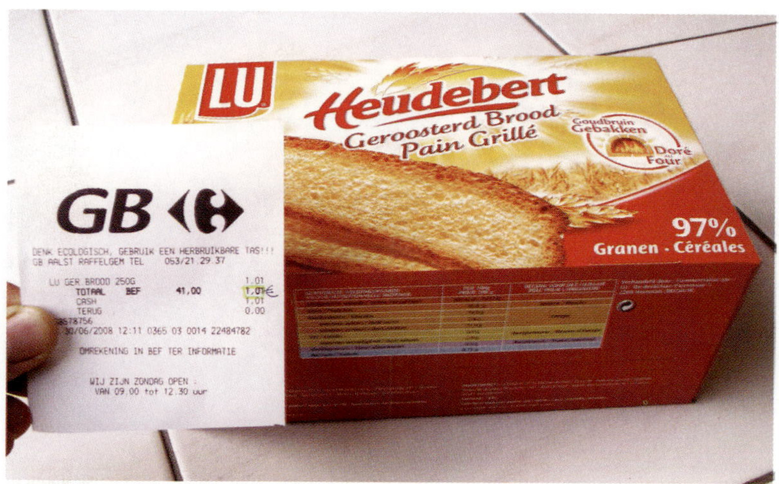

Fig. 16.1 Toasted bread is a cheap, high calorie nutrient usually unbalanced, i.e. deficient in essential minerals and vitamins, largely because of removal of both germ and bran during processing food source

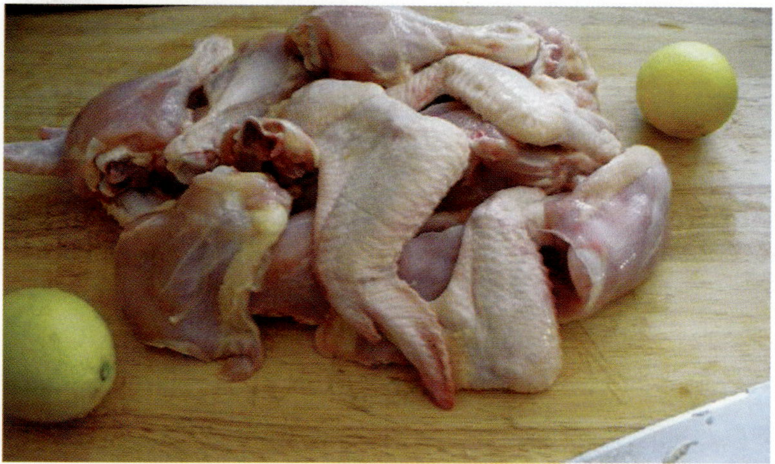

Fig. 16.2 Most meats such as chicken contain all the essential amino acids needed for humans (protein in nutrition)

Plate 4

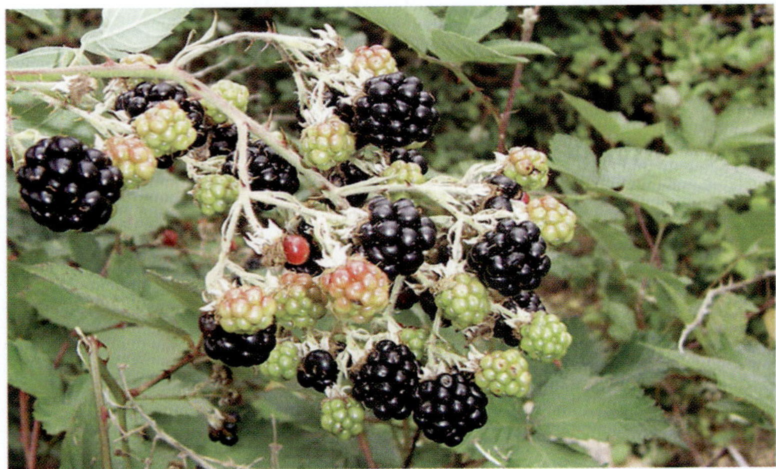

Fig. 16.4 Blackberries are a source of polyphenol antioxidants

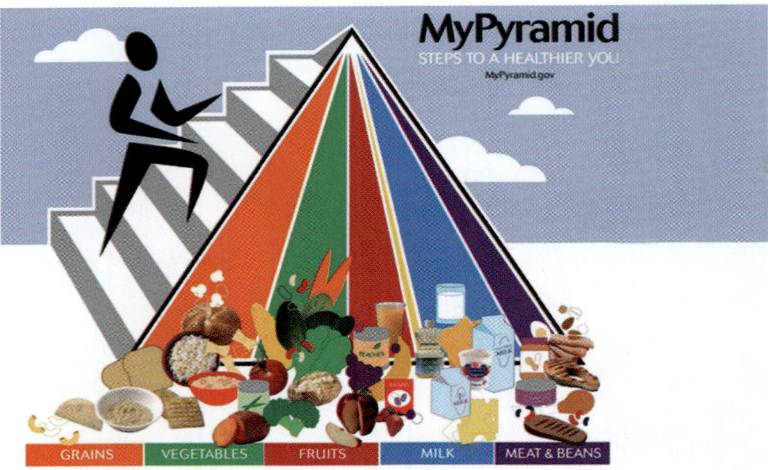

Fig. 16.5 The updated United States Department of Agriculture (USDA) food pyramid, published in 2005, is a general nutrition guide for recommended food consumption for humans

Plate 5

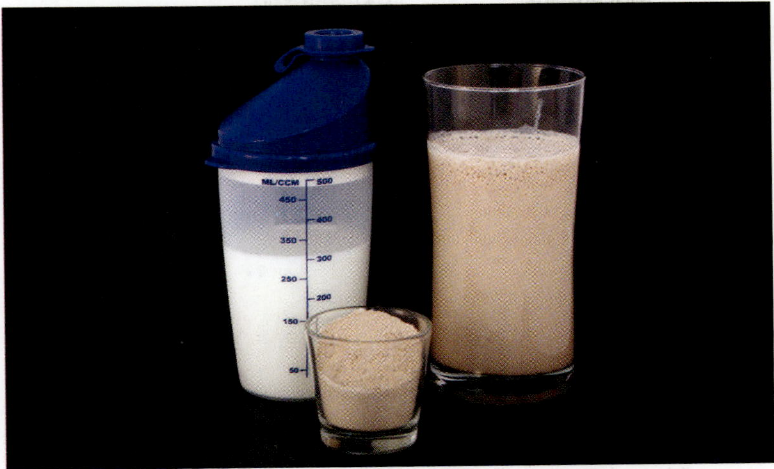

Fig. 16.6 Protein milkshakes, made from protein powder (center) and milk (left), are a common bodybuilding supplement

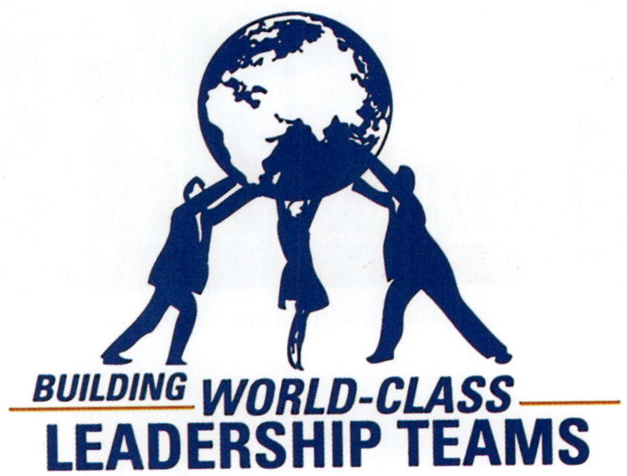

Fig. 24.1 Leadership is to guide and build team to accomplish set goals

Plate 6

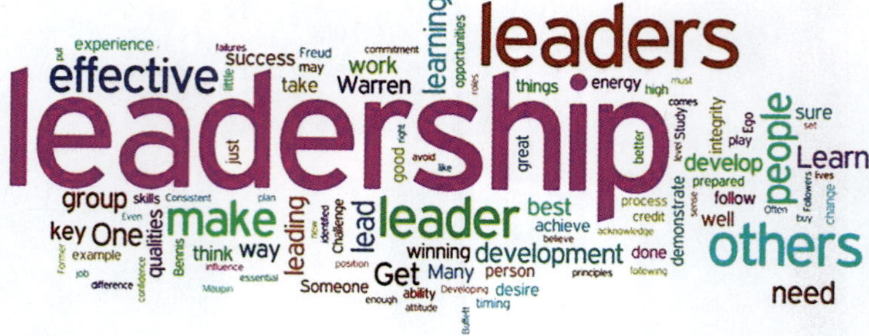

Fig. 24.2 Qualities of a leader

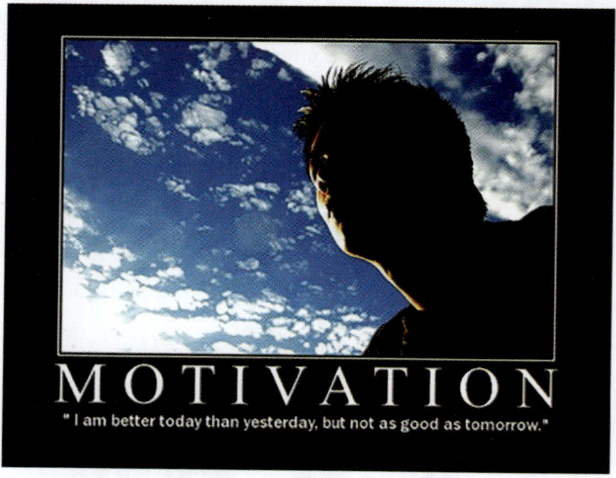

Fig. 25.1 Motivation comes within to heighten your curiosity to achieve set objectives

Plate 7

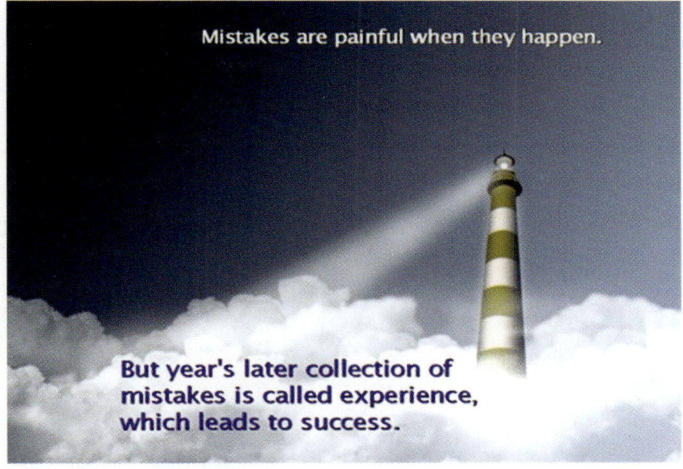

Fig. 25.2 Mistakes and failures of today are learning experience of tomorrow that motivates and leads to success

1 Introduction to Hospital Patient Care Relationship Coordinator

In earlier days of medical practice, the physician alone used to manage the patient care services by recording the patient identification demographic data, taking history and physical examination, dressing the patients for wounds and injuries, taking blood for testing, giving injection and dispensing medicines. And also used to give counseling the patient when to take the medicine, dose, when to see doctor and so on. In simple terms the doctor was doing the services of medical records, nurse, lab technician, pharmacist, social worker and so on. By this method, a physician can see only limited patients, while the number of patients who needed medical services was more. In order to meet the patient care services swiftly and efficiently, the need for some assistants arose. This need has created the allied healthcare professionals, one after one, emanated to assist the busy physician and allow him to deal with medical and complicated cases which need medical background while other allied professionals can contribute greatly to patient care service directly or indirectly with their area of expertise.

ALLIED HEALTH SERVICES

History

The explosion of scientific knowledge that followed World War II brought increasingly sophisticated and complex medical diagnostic and treatment procedures. In addition, increasing medical and healthcare costs provoked a trend away from treating patients in hospitals toward the provision of care in physician's private and group practices, and ambulatory medical and emergency clinics. What followed was an increase in the need for expertly trained healthcare delivery personnel lied professionals have taken the rest?

ALLIED HEALTHCARE WORKERS

Allied healthcare workers are those specialized persons distinct from medicine, dentistry and nursing. They work in an environment of health-care team to make the healthcare system function uninterruptedly and effectively. Evidently, these professionals, who will be associated with medical, nursing and other allied medical professionals in rendering patient care services directly or indirectly, need to have the fundamentals of medical related field's knowledge to enable to contribute effectively. This has become imperative to have a fundamental knowledge and skills of certain subjects, e.g. Anatomy and Physiology, Medical Terminology, Pathology, Laboratory, Radiology, Radiation Therapy, Pharmacology, Pharmacy, Medical Psychology, public Medical Social Work, Medical Records, Public Relations, Medical Secretarial Profession, Communication Skills, Leadership and Motivation, etc.

Allied healthcare professions are clinical healthcare professions distinct from medicine, dentistry, and nursing. They work in an environment of healthcare team to make the healthcare system function effectively and efficiently uninterruptedly.

Professions: Depending on the country and local healthcare system, a limited subset of the following professions may be represented, and may be regulated.

All professionals/professional areas ascribed before belong to the ever growing group of allied health professionals and their subspecialties. The precise titles and roles in the allied health professions may vary considerably from country-to-country.

Since their job descriptions become more specialized, they must adhere to national training and education standards, their professional scope of practice, and often prove their skills through diplomas, certified credentials, and continuing education. Members of the allied health professions must be proficient in the use of many skills. Some of which are medical terminology, acronym and spelling, basics of medical law and ethics, understanding of human relations, interpersonal communication skills, counseling skills, computer literacy, ability to document healthcare information, interviewing skills, and proficiency in word processing, database management and electronic dictation.

As a part of Allied Health Profession which is also known as Paramedical Services. The paramedics generally learn besides their own selected specialty field, also learn subjects like Anatomy, Physiology, Medical Terminology, Medical Records, Fundamentals of Diseases and Diagnostic Procedure. These are Pharmacology, Pharmacy, Physical Therapy, Occupational Therapy, Optometry, Nutrition (Dietetics),

Medical Psychology and many more. Medical Social Work, Public Relations and Medical Secretary have besides condensed combination of the above stipulated subjects such as hospital management program to deal with the day-to-day administrative and patient care issues.

The Allied Health Services have been playing vital role in taking away most of nonprofessional and administrative types of work from the highly qualified professionals, helping them and allowing the professionals to concentrate in their specialized field and not wasting time for nonmedical and for trivial jobs. In fact, in many ways the paramedics service cost much less than the highly paid specialty professionals. This is not only cost effective but also much more than that it contribute in swift and improved patient care resulting great service to general public.

Rapid Growth of Medicine

Medicine being dynamic and with advent of technology, the medical healthcare services are growing much faster and the patients and public expectation from the health institutions have also equally increased. Thus, the need for appropriate allied healthcare services has become essential. These services have been playing a vital role in taking away most of nonprofessional and administrative types of work from the highly qualified medical professionals, helping them and allowing them to contribute in their specialized field not wasting time for nonmedical and for trivial jobs. Yet, in many ways the paramedics service cost much less than the highly paid specialists. This is not only cost effective but much more than that, it contributes in swift, and improved patient care resulting great service to general public.

HOSPITAL PATIENT CARE RELATIONSHIP COORDINATOR

This unique position 'Hospital Patient Care Relationship Coordinator (HPCRC)' is one of allied healthcare professionals with paramedics related educational background, to co-ordinate and liaison between the medical, nursing, other allied healthcare services, administration, finance, transportation, etc. related to the patient care, and the patient, relatives or attendants of patients, referred institution and pubic. To ensure that patient healthcare issues are dealt promptly and judiciously to the utmost satisfaction of all. HPCRC job is to oversee the patient care services from the time of patient's registration or even earlier from the date of booking, and during patient's journey in the hospital as an emergency, outpatient or inpatient till his/her discharge from the hospital. During patient's voyage, the HPCRC has to deal with the medical, nursing, other allied health professionals, lab, radiology, pharmacy, wards, operation theaters, ICCU/CCU, insurance, billing, administration and many, depends on the type of care needed by patient. He has to ensure that patient's medical record including investigation reports are complete in all respects by arranging that related documents are promptly placed in the main patient's record to facilitate the healthcare providers to render their services efficiently. He has to maintain intra, inter-relationship within the hospital, and with the outside healthcare institutions related to continued patient care, insurance, legal and other matters to facilitate the patient or his relatives and institution for smooth functioning of the system. Even after discharge, for some cases, there are many other issues, e.g. death certificates, administrative and legal issues to be settled. Precisely, HPCRC is the envoy of patient as well as the hospital.

Need for a Book for Unique Position

The Author having realized the need for the comprehensive HPCRC book, included fundamentals of Anatomy, Physiology, Medical Terminology, Pathology, Laboratory, Radiology, Radiation Therapy, Pharmacology, Pharmacy, Medical Psychology, Medical Social Work, Medical Records, Public Relations, Medical Secretarial Profession, Communication Skills, Leadership and Motivation. This book would of immense value to the hospitals, hospital patient care coordinators, medical social workers, medical records, medical secretaries, law professionals, medical representatives, insurance companies, and healthcare software developers to serve as textbook in their academic programs, professional career building, besides reference guide throughout. The special features of this position, is when too many people and departments in a healthcare organization playing the role of patient care, it would be hard to locate real setback, while the HPCRC can be handy acting as a single 'window' system concept to clarify and deal with the issue promptly.

SUMMARY

The following are some of the tasks, not limited to, to be performed by HPCRC:

- To create a relationship with patients for cooperation and assistance
- Find out the patient's problems, if any and resolve promptly and judiciously
- Develop good relationship with healthcare providers and other allied health workers

Form No. 1 Paramedical services record

Requesting Physician's Notes	Paramedical Department Notes
Physician:	Name:
Signature: Date:	Signature: Date:
Requesting Physician's Notes	Paramedical Department Notes
Physician:	Name:
Signature: Date:	Signature: Date:

PARAMEDICAL SERVICES RECORD

- Assist the needy patients/relatives or attendants whenever required
- Ensure the patient/relatives are guided and routed appropriately to concerned units
- Explain clearly, the hospital policies and procedures to patients/relatives

- Ensure the patient' record is updated with all relevant information including investigation reports
- Arrange for counseling or any consultation required by patient
- Coordinate and Liaison with the concerned staff/departments regularly
- Follow–up the patient progress during the care as an outpatient, emergency or inpatient
- Alert the hospital departments in advance to provide the services recommended by physician
- Arrange transportation or any other service within the limits of hospital services
- Coordinate with the insurance companies to promptly respond to the institution's requirements and vice versa.
- Deal with outside institutions or public carefully related to patient care services
- Understand and explain the administrative or legal issues relate to patient care
- Maintain intra and inter-relationship within the hospital and with and with the outside healthcare institutions
- Realize that HPCRC is the envoy of patient as well as the hospital
- Understand and clarify any hospital billing issues appropriately
- When patient is in OT, ICU or ICCU or NICU, deal with relatives judiciously
- Represent as an envoy of patient and as well as hospital uniformly
- Maintain cordial relationship with patient/attendant/relatives; before, during and after discharge from the hospital
- Conduct regular orientation programs to enlighten the staff, the patient's difficulties or issues, and how they could be overcome or how to resolve or address amicably
- Obtain the innovative ideas from the staff of different units by brainstorming exercises, how to improve patient care relationship and services
- Act as a 'single window' concept to help the patient promptly by coordinating with concerned
- Harmonize with all the departments with the motto to serve the patient who is a nuclease, around which all the healthcare provider's efforts and services revolve.

2 Anatomy and Physiology: Human Body

CELL

INTRODUCTION

A cell is mass of protoplasm containing a nucleus. It is the unit structure and the fundamental part of life, which carries various functions such as reproduction, respiration, excretion and adaptation to the environment. The human body is made up of a trillion numbers of cells of different types. The size of the cell is about 10–30 mm in diameter.

All cells are similar in that they contain a gelatinous substance composed of water, protein, sugar, acids, fats and various minerals. This substance is called protoplasm. Several parts of a cell are described below and pictured schematically.

STRUCTURE OF CELL (FIG. 2.1)

- *Cell membrane*: Covering or outer layer of the cell which protects the internal environment and determines what passes in and out of the cell.
- *Protoplasm*: A white fluid, like the yolk of an egg, which consists of water, electrolytes, proteins, lipids and carbohydrates. The protoplasm forms the cytoplasm and the nucleus.
- Cytoplasm is the protoplasmic material outside the nucleus. It triggers the work of the cell such as contraction in the muscle cell and transmitting impulses in the nerve cell. The cytoplasm contains mitochondria, endoplasmic reticulum, ribosomes, lysosomes, Golgi bodies, and the centrosome.
- *Mitochondria*: It is responsible for the production of energy in the cell by breaking up the complex food structure into simpler substances. This process is called catabolism. It is also called, kitchen cell (power house).

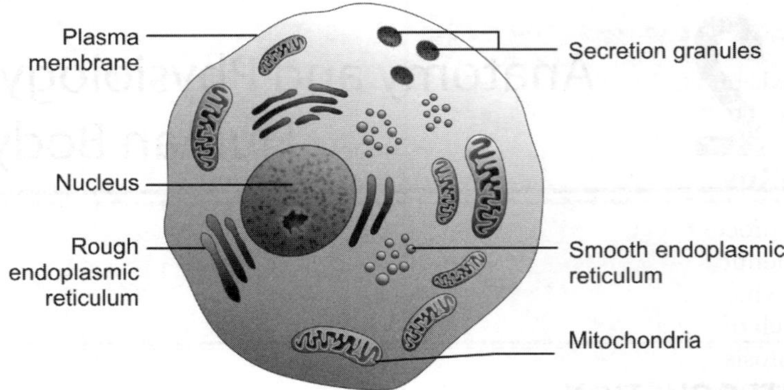

Fig. 2.1 Structure of cell

- *Endoplasmic reticulum*: A tubule like structure. It contains small bodies called ribosomes which help to make substances (proteins) for the cells, this process is called anabolism.
- *Nucleus*: It is the controlling structure of the cell. It controls the cell reproduction, and contains genetic material which determines the functioning and structure of the cell.
- *Chromosomes*: There are 23 pairs of chromosomes, each chromosome consists of a chain of small units called genes made up of deoxyribonucleic acid (DNA) (hereditary information) and ribonucleic acid (RNA). Out of 23 pairs of chromosomes, 22 pairs are autosomes and 1 pair is sex chromosome which decides the sex. A female has 2X (X, X) chromosomes whereas the male has 1X, 1Y chromosomes.

FUNCTIONS OF THE CELL

- *Absorption*: The ability of the cell to absorb or take in oxygen and food substances.
- *Nutrition*: The intake of food substances by the cell.
- *Growth*: It provides the metabolic process to enable the cell to grow to its full size and will be able to function correctly.
- *Reproduction*: On reaching maturity, the cell will divide to form two smaller cells.
- *Removal of waste products*: The removal of waste products produced during metabolism.
- *Movement*: Many cells have the power of movement.

CELL DIVISION

Division of cells are for the growth of the organism and for the replacement of damaged cells. There are two types of cell division:

Mitosis

A process of cell division which produces two new daughter cells (identical to the parent cells), e.g. plants. This involves a series of changes in which there is a rearrangement of centrioles and chromosomes so that each of the two new cells has a nucleus with 23 pairs of chromosomes. Mitosis is the common type of cell division that occurs in the body cells. It consists of four phases—prophase, metaphase, anaphase and telophase.

Prophase: The centrosome divides and the centrioles moves to the opposite poles of the cells with the spindle fibers.

Metaphase: The chromosomes align themselves at the center of the nucleus and become attached to the spindle fibers.

Anaphase: Each chromosome splits into two chromosomes. The separated chromosomes move towards the opposite poles of the cell. The centrioles are divided to form new centrosome.

Telophase: A new nuclear membrane forms around each set of chromosomes, and the spindle fiber disappear. The cytoplasm and cell membrane constrict. Finally, the cell splits into two identical cells.

Meiosis

Cell division occurring in maturation of sex cells, wherein over two successive cell division occur. Each daughter nucleus receives half the number of chromosomes typically to the somatic cells of the species.

The cell division occurring in the human reproductive system is called meiosis. Each person, male or female has 23 pairs of chromosomes comprising of 22 pairs of autosomes and 1 pair of sex chromosomes or somatic chromosomes. In the meiosis cell division, the daughter cell receives equal number of chromosomes from the parent cells, i.e. 22 pairs of autosomes from father and mother, the male has XY sex chromosomes. Whereas the mother has X and X chromosomes. The sex of a child clearly depends on whether it inherits X or Y chromosome from its father.

TISSUE FLUID

Tissue fluids are of two types: intracellular and extracellular. The fluid inside the cell is called intracellular fluid while the fluid outside the cell is called extracellular fluid. Tissue fluid acts as a sort of middle man between the blood and tissues, supplying food and oxygen to the cell and removing waste products from the cell.

TISSUES

A tissue is a group of similar cells working together to do a specific job. A histologist is one who specializes in the study of tissues.

Tissues can be classified into four major types:

1. Epithelium
2. Connective tissue
3. Muscular tissue
4. Nervous tissue.

Epithelium

The various types of epithelial tissues are as follows:

Simple Squamous Epithelium

A single layer of flat cells found in alveoli of lungs, the lining of the interior of the heart and blood vessels and the lymphatic vessels.

Stratified Squamous Epithelium

It is composed of cells which are flat and round. It is found in all parts of the body. The skin is composed of stratified squamous epithelium.

Transitional Epithelium

Cells which provide water tightness. It is found on the lining of urinary tract.

Columnar Epithelium

Cylindrical-shaped cells found in the secretory glands of the body.

Ciliated Epithelium

The free surface of each cell surrounded by fine hair like structures called cilia. It is found in the lining of (nasal cavity, trachea and bronchi) the respiratory system.

Connective Tissue

Connective tissues are fat (also called adipose tissue), cartilage (elastic, fibrous tissues attached to bones), bone, or blood tissues. They are present in different forms in the body. It is a jelly like substance and is hard.

Fibrous Tissue

There are two types of fibrous tissues:

1. White fibrous tissue
2. Yellow elastic tissue.

White fibrous tissue: It consists of bundles of white fibers which cannot stretch. It is found in tendons, ligaments, dura mater and outer layer of the pericardium.

Yellow elastic tissue: It consists of fibers which can stretch. It is found in the walls of arteries, bronchi and alveoli of lungs.

Areolar Tissue

Supporting tissue of the body. Found under the skin, mucous membrane and surrounding blood vessels and nerves.

Adipose Tissue

Found in all parts of the body where fat is deposited or stored, especially under the skin and around the eyes, heart and kidneys.

Cartilage

It is a flexible tissue found mainly in the skeleton. There are three different types of cartilage:

1. Hyaline cartilage
2. Fibrocartilage
3. Yellow elastic cartilage.

Hyaline cartilage: It is bluish white tissue with a smooth glassy surface. It is found covering the ends of the bones, where they form joints (articular cartilage).

Fibrocartilage: It contains white fibrous tissue. It is found in intervertebral disks and semilunar cartilage of the knee joint where great strength combined with certain amount of elasticity is required.

Yellow elastic cartilage: It contains yellow elastic fibers and it is found in the epiglottis and pinna of the ear.

Muscular Tissue

The muscles are structures, which give the power of movements. Muscles are composed of thousands of elongated cells, called muscle fibers. Each contains a small nucleus. Bundles of muscle fibers lie side by side like threads. There are three different types of muscle tissue, they are voluntary, involuntary and cardiac.

Voluntary muscles are found in arms, legs and parts of the body where movement is voluntary. All the muscles attached to the skeleton are of this type and their functions are to move the bones at their respective joints and to help in maintaining the posture of the limbs and body as a whole. The microscopic structure of this muscle is striped in structure, i.e. white and black bands, hence it is also called striated muscle.

Involuntary muscles are found in the internal organs and structures of the body such as stomach, intestine, bladder, bronchi, blood vessels, and is, therefore, sometimes called visceral muscles. It cannot be consciously controlled and its nervous supply comes from the involuntary or autonomic nervous system. It is also called nonstriated or plain muscle.

The cardiac muscle is a special type of muscle found only in the heart. Although, it is an involuntary muscle, it has the form of striated muscle. It has the special property, not observed in other varieties of muscles, of automatic rhythmic contraction which can occur independently of its nervous supply.

Nervous Tissue

Nerve tissues conduct impulses all over the body. The muscles are structures which give the body the power of movements; almost every movement is governed by some portion of the nervous system which acts as a medium between brain and muscle.

ORGANS

Organs are structures composed of several types of tissues. For example, an organ like stomach is composed of muscular tissues, nerve tissues, and glandular epithelial tissues. The medical term for internal organ is viscera (singular: viscus).

Examples:

Eye	Ear	Nose	Tongue
Heart	Lung	Stomach	Intestine
Hand	Leg	Liver	Spleen

SYSTEMS

Systems are groups of organs working together to perform essential fundamental functions of the individual. The different types of systems are skeletal, muscular, nervous, endocrine, circulatory, lymphatic, respiratoy, digestive, urinary, reproductive systems. Although some systems are functioning individually, the functions of various systems are very closely connected and are dependent on each other. For example, mouth, esophagus, stomach, and small and large intestines are organs which compose the digestive system.

The main systems and their organs of the body are as given in **Table 2.1**.

Table 2.1 The main systems and their organs

S. No.	*Name of the system*	*Organs/parts*
1.	Muscular system	*There are three types of muscle tissues:* a. Skeletal, voluntary or striated muscle b. Visceral, involuntary or smooth muscle c. Cardiac muscle
2.	Skeletal system	Bones—there are 206 bones in an adult skeletal system *Joints:* a. Fibrous or fixed joints, b. Cartilaginous or slightly movable joints c. Synovial or freely movable joints
3.	A. Nervous system	A. *The nervous system consist of:* a. Brain b. Spinal cord c. Nerves
	B. Sense organs	B. Sense organs are: a. Eye b. Ear c. Nose d. Tongue e. Skin or integumentary system
4.	Endocrine system (ductless gland)	a. Pituitary gland b. Thyroid gland c. Parathyroid glands d. Thymus gland e. Pancreas (islets of Langerhans) f. Adrenal gland g. Sex glands (ovaries and testes)

Contd...

Contd...

S. No.	*Name of the system*	*Organs/parts*
5.	A. Cardiovascular system or Circulatory system	A. Cardiovascular system consists of: a. Heart b. Aorta, artery, and arteriole c. Vena cava, vein, and venule d. Capillaries
	B. Blood and blood groups	B. Blood and blood groups include: 1. Blood composition a. Plasma b. Blood cells – Leukocytes or white blood cells – Erythrocytes or red blood cells – Thrombocytes or platelets
		2. Blood groups: a. Blood group "A" b. Blood group "B" c. Blood group "AB" d. Blood group "O" e. Rhesus factor (Rh) – Rhesus factor positive (+) – Rhesus factor negative (–)
6.	Lymphatic system	a. Lymph vessels b. Lymph nodes and other lymphatic tissues c. Spleen d. Thymus gland
7.	Respiratory system	a. Nose b. Nasal cavities and paranasal sinuses c. Pharynx d. Larynx e. Trachea f. Bronchi (bronchus—singular) g. Bronchioles h. Alveoli (alveolus—singular) i. Lung capillaries (bloodstream)
8.	Digestive system	A. Gastrointestinal tract a. Oral cavity (mouth) b. Pharynx c. Esophagus d. Stomach e. Enteron (small intestine) – Duodenum – Jejunum – Ileum

Contd...

Contd...

S. No.	*Name of the system*	*Organs/parts*
		f. Colon (large intestine) – Cecum – Ascending colon – Transverse colon – Descending colon – Sigmoid colon – Rectum g. Anus B. Accessory organs a. Salivary glands b. Liver c. Gallbladder d. Pancreas
9.	Urinary system	a. Kidneys b. Ureters c. Urinary bladder d. Urethra
10.	Reproductive system	*Male:* a. Testes b. Scrotum c. Seminiferous tubules d. Epididymis e. Vas deferens f. Seminal vesicles g. Ejaculatory duct h. Prostate gland i. Penis j. Urethra *Female:* a. Ovaries b. Fallopian tubes c. Uterus d. Vagina e. Vulva f. Cervix g. Labia majora h. Labia minora i. Hymen j. Mammary glands (accessory organ)

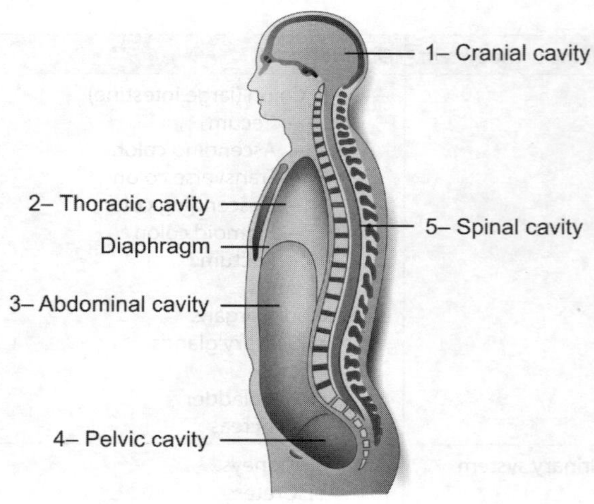

Fig. 2.2 Body cavities

BODY CAVITIES (FIG. 2.2)

A body cavity is a space within the body which contains internal organs (viscera). Some of the important viscera contained within those cavities are listed in **Table 2.2**.

ANATOMICAL DIVISIONS OF THE BODY (FIG. 2.3)

Anatomical divisions of the abdomen are labeled in **Figure 2.3**. These divisions are used in anatomy texts to describe the regions in which organs and structures are found while documenting the patient care. The names of the divisions are:

1. Right hypochondriac regions (upper lateral regions beneath the ribs)
2. Epigastric region (regions of the stomach)
3. Left hypochondriac regions (upper lateral regions beneath the ribs)
4. Right lumbar region
5. Umbilical region (region of the navel or umbilicus)
6. Left lumbar region
7. Right iliac fossa
8. Hypogastric region (lower middle region below the umbilicus)
9. Left iliac fossa.

Table 2.2 Some of the important viscera contained within those cavities

S. No.	*Name of the cavity*	*Organs/parts*
1.	Cranial cavity	Brain
2.	Thoracic cavity	Lungs, heart, esophagus, trachea, thymus gland, aorta The thoracic cavity can be divided into two smaller cavities: a. The pleural cavity—the areas surrounding the lungs. Each pleural cavity is lined with a double-folded membrane called pleura; visceral pleura is closer to the lungs, and parietal pleura is closer to the outer wall of the pleural cavity b. The mediastinum cavity—the area between the lungs. It contains the heart, aorta, trachea, esophagus, and thymus gland
3.	Abdominal cavity	Stomach, small and large intestines, spleen, liver, gallbladder, and pancreas
4.	Pelvic cavity	Ureters, urinary bladder, urethra; uterus and vagina in the female
5.	Spinal cavity	Nerves of the spinal cord runs through vertebrae

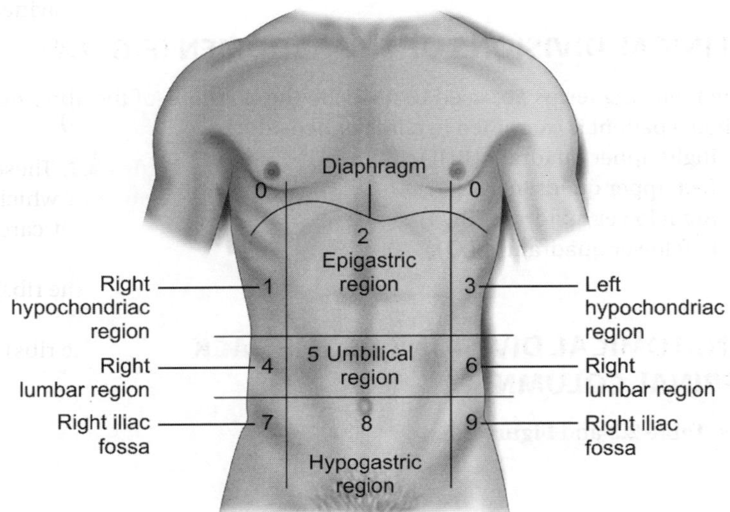

Fig. 2.3 Anatomical divisions of the body

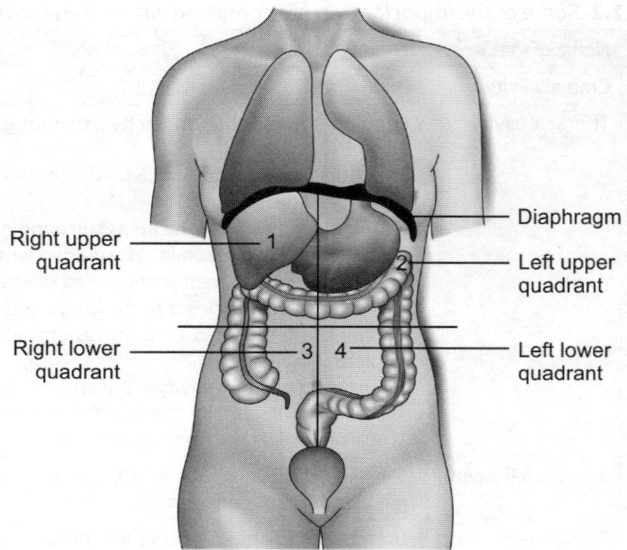

Fig. 2.4 Clinical divisions of the abdomen

CLINICAL DIVISIONS OF THE ABDOMEN (FIG. 2.4)

The following terms are used to describe the divisions of the abdomen when a patient is examined in clinic or bedside:

1. Right upper quadrant (RUQ)
2. Left upper quadrant (LUQ)
3. Right lower quadrant (RLQ)
4. Left lower quadrant (LLQ).

ANATOMICAL DIVISIONS OF THE BACK (SPINAL COLUMN)

See **Table 2.3** and **Figure 2.5**.

Table 2.3 Anatomical divisions of the back

S. No.	*Division of the back*	*Abbreviation*	*Location*
1.	Cervical vertebrae	C	Neck region. There are 7 cervical vertebrae (C1-C7)
2.	Thoracic vertebrae	T or D (Dorsal)	Chest region. There are 12 thoracic vertebrae (T1-T12). Each bone is joined to a rib
3.	Lumbar vertebrae	L	Loin or flank region (between the ribs and the hip bone). There are 5 lumbar vertebrae (L1-L5)
4.	Sacral vertebrae	S	Five bones (S1-S5) are fused to form one bone, the sacrum
5.	Coccygeal	Nil	The coccyx (tailbone) is small bone composed of 4 fused pieces

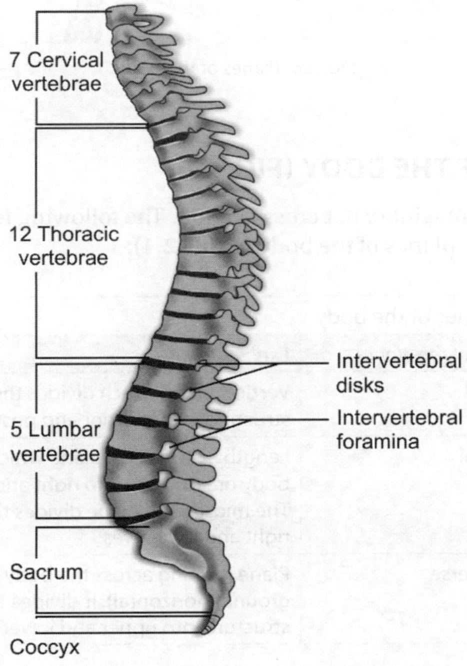

Fig. 2.5 Anatomical divisions of the back (spinal column)

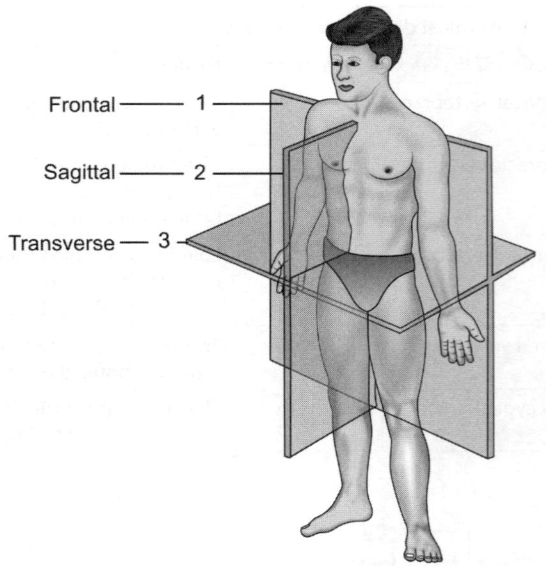

Fig. 2.6 Planes of the body

PLANES OF THE BODY (FIG. 2.6)

A plane is an imaginary flat cross-section. The following terms are used to describe the planes of the body **(Table 2.4)**:

Table 2.4 Planes of the body

S. No.	*Name of the planes*	*Explanation*
1.	Frontal	Vertical plane which divides the body or structure into anterior and posterior portions
2.	Sagittal	Lengthwise vertical plane which divides the body or structure into right and left portions. The midsagittal plane divides the body into right and left halves
3.	Transverse	Plane running across the body parallel to the ground (horizontal). It divides the body or structure into upper and lower portions

POSITIONAL AND DIRECTIONAL TERMS OF THE BODY (TABLE 2.5)

Table 2.5 Positional and directional terms of the body

Position	*Description of the position*
Anterior	In front of the body
Posterior	At the back of the body
Central	Pertaining to the center
Deep	Away from the surface
Superficial	Near the surface
Distal	Away from the beginning of the structure or away from the center
Proximal	Pertaining to the beginning of a structure
Inferior	Below another structure
Superior	Above another structure
Lateral	Pertaining to the sides
Medial	Near to the median of the body (structure)
Supine	Lying on the back
Prone	Lying on the belly
Afferent	Towards the structure
Efferent	Away from the structure

3 Medical Terminology

OBJECTIVES IN STUDYING THE MEDICAL LANGUAGE

- To analyze words structurally.
- To correlate and understand word elements with the basics of anatomy, physiology, and diseases of human body.
- To pronounce and write correct spelling of medical terms.

Basic Word Structure

Studying medical words is similar to learning of a new language. The words at first look strange and complicated although they may stand for commonly known English terms. The words gastralgia, means 'stomach ache,' and ophthalmologist, means 'eye doctor,' are some examples.

The medical language is fascinatingly logical in each term, complex or simple, can be broken into basic components and then understood.

These basic components of medical words are:

Root: Foundation of the word		
Example:	gastr/ic – root (stomach)	
Suffix: Word ending		
Examples:	gastr/itis – suffix (inflammation)	gastric – Suffix (pertaining to)
Prefix: Word beginning		
Examples:	epi/gastr/ic – prefix (above)	Ad/renal – prefix (above)
Combining vowel:	A vowel (usually 'O') links the root with the suffix or to another root	
Examples:	cardi/o/gram root–suffix combining vowel	electr/o/cardi/o/gram root–root–suffix combining vowel

CHIEF SOURCES OF MEDICAL WORDS

ANGLO-SAXON (OLD ENGLISH)

These words are from old English, which are mostly anatomical terms.

Examples:

Arm	Back	Bladder	Blood	Cheek	Chest
Chin	Ear	Eye	Finger	Hair	Nose

Thumb, etc.

GREECO-ROMAN (GREEK AND LATIN)

These words are from Greek and Latin languages.

Examples:

Marrow—the word marrow is derived from the Latin word medulla.

Myelitis (G) originating from the Greek word myelos. The word myelitis is the inflammation of marrow.

Crani (G and L) : Skull
Cerebro (L) : Brain
Illi (L) : Ilium
Rhin (G) : Nose
Pneumo (G) : Lungs, air

ARABIC

Most of these words are used to describe chemical substances.

Examples:

Sharab : Sweet beverage (syrup)
Matter : Mother
Alcohol : Something subtle

MODERN GERMAN

These words are derived from French (Modern German).

Example:

Fahrenheit (German Physicist) for thermometer
Kernicterus : Yellow (Jaundice)

COLORS

S. No.	Color	Medical terms	Examples
1.	White	Albus	Albinism
2.	White	Leukos	Leukocyte
3.	White	Candidus	Candidiasis
4.	Black	Melan	Melanoma
5.	Black	Niger	Nigrometer
6.	Red	Erythros	Erythrocyte
7.	Red	Ruber	Rubricyte
8.	Yellow	Flavus	Flavism
9.	Yellow	Xanthos	Xanthoma
10.	Green	Chloros	Chlorhydria
11.	Green	Glaucos	Glaucoma
12.	Blue	Cynos	Cyanosis
13.	Brown	Cirrhos	Cirrhosis
14.	Violet	Iodes	Iodine
15.	Purple	Porphyros	Porphyrinuria
16.	Ashy	Cinereous	Cinerea
17.	Golden	Aureus	Aureomycin

NUMERALS

S. No.	Numerals	Medical terms	Examples
1.	Half	Semi	Semilunar
2.	Half	Hemi	Hemiplegia
3.	First	Primus	Primigravida
4.	One	Unus	Unilateral
5.	Single	Monos	Monocular
6.	Two	Duo	Duodenum
7.	Second	Secundus	Secundine
8.	Two at a time	Bini	Binocular
9.	Twice	Bi, Dis, Di	Dislocation
10.	Three	Tri	Tricuspid

Contd...

Contd...

S. No.	*Numerals*	*Medical terms*	*Examples*
11.	Four	Quadri, Tetra	Quadriplegia, Tetralogy
12.	Five	Quinique	Quintuplet
13.	Six	Sex, Hex	Sexdigitate, Hexadactylism
14.	Seven	Hepta	Heptagram
15.	Eight	Octa	Octigravida
16.	Nine	Non	Nonipara
17.	Ten	Deca	Decameter
18.	One hundred	Centi	Centimeter
19.	One thousand	Milli	Millimeter
20.	10,000	Myri	
21.	1,00,000	Mega	
22.	1/1,00,000	Micro	

ELEMENTS OF MEDICAL TERMS

SUFFIXES AND COMPOUNDING ELEMENTS

True suffixes refer to a syllable denoting a preposition or adverb attached to the end of a word, root, or stem to modify its meaning. Many endings are adjectives or nouns added to a root to form compound words. They may be combining forms or pseudo-suffixes. To simplify learning, the modifying endings have been classified according to their meanings into diagnostic, operative and symptomatic suffixes and compounding elements.

Diagnostic Suffixes and Compounding Elements

Suffix	*Medical term*	*Definition*
• aemia (G) blood	Hyperglycemia	High blood sugar
• cele (G) hernia, tumor, protrusion	Cystocele Hydrocele Myelocele	Hernia of the bladder Serous tumor as of testis Protrusion of spinal cord through the vertebrae

Contd...

Contd...

Suffix	*Medical term*	*Definition*
• ectasis (G)	Atelectasis	Imperfect expansion of lungs at birth
• neonatorum expansion, dilatation	Bronchiectasis	Abnormal dilatation of a bronchus or bronchi
• graphy (G) act of recording or writing	Electrocardiography Echocardiography	The recording of the electricity flowing through the heart A diagnostic procedure in which pulses of high frequency sound waves (ultrasound) are transmitted into the chest and echoes returning from the surfaces of the heart are electronically plotted and recorded
• iasis (G) condition, formation of, presence of	Lithiasis Cholelithiasis Nephrolithiasis	Formation of stones Presence of calculi in the gallbladder Stones present in the kidney
• itis (G) inflammation	Carditis	Inflammation of the heart
	Gastritis	Inflammation of the stomach
	Poliomyelitis	Inflammation of the gray matter of the spinal cord
• malacia (G) softening	Encephalomalacia Osteomalacia Splenomalacia	Softening of the brain Softening of the bones Softening of the spleen
• megaly (G) enlargement	Cardiomegaly Hepatomegaly Splenomegaly	Enlargement of the heart Enlargement of the liver Enlargement of the spleen
• oma (G) tumor	Adenoma Carcinoma Sarcoma	Glandular tumor Malignant tumor of epithelial tissue Malignant tumor of connective tissue
• osis (G) condition, diseases, increase	Arteriosclerosis Dermatosis Neurosis	Hardening of the arteries Any skin condition Functional disorder of the nervous system

Contd...

Contd...

Suffix	*Medical term*	*Definition*
• pathy (G) disease	Adenopathy Myopathy Myelopathy	Any glandular disease Any diseases of a muscle Any pathologic disorder of the spinal cord
• ptosis (G) falling	Blepharoptosis Gastroptosis Nephroptosis	Drooping or (downward displacement) of the eyelid Downward displacement of the stomach Downward displacement of the kidney
• rhexis (G) rupture	Angiorrhexis Cardiorrhexis	Rupture of a blood vessel or lymphatic Rupture of the heart

Operative Suffixes and Compounding Elements

Suffix	*Medical term*	*Definition*
• centesis (G) puncture	Paracentesis Thoracentesis	Puncture of a cavity Aspiration of the pleural cavity
• ectomy (G) excision	Myomectomy Tonsillectomy	Excision of a tumor of the muscle Removal of tonsils
• desis (G) binding fixation	Arthrodesis Spondylosyndesis	Surgical fixation of a joint Surgical fixation of the vertebrae
• lithotomy (G) incision for removal of stones	Cholelithotomy Nephrolithotomy	Incision into gallbladder for removal of stones Incision into kidney for removal of stones
• pexy (G) suspension or fixation	Hysteropexy Orchiopexy	Abdominal fixation or suspension of the uterus Fixation of an undescended testis
• plasty (G) surgical correction plastic repair of	Arthroplasty Hernioplasty	Reconstructive operation on joint Plastic repair of hernia
• rrhaphy (G) suture	Perineorrhaphy Staphylorrhaphy	Suture of a lacerated perineum Suture of a cleft palate
• scopy (G) inspection or examination	Bronchoscopy Cystoscopy	Examination of the bronchi with an endoscope Inspection of the bladder with a cystoscope

Contd...

Contd...

Suffix	*Medical term*	*Definition*
-ostomy (G) creation of a more or less permanent opening	Colostomy Cystostomy	Creation of an opening into the colon through the abdominal wall Creation of an opening into the urinary bladder through the abdomen
• otomy (G) incision into	Antrotomy Thoracotomy	Incision into the antrum for drainage Opening of the chest
• tripsy (G) crushing or friction	Lithotripsy Phrenicotripsy	Crushing of a calculus in the bladder or urethra Crushing of the phrenic nerve

Symptomatic Suffixes and Compounding Elements

Suffix	*Medical term*	*Definition*
• algia (G) pain	Gastralgia Nephralgia	Stomach pain Renal pain
• genic (G) origin	Bronchogenic Pathogenic	Originating in the bronchi Disease producing
• lysis (G) dissolution or breaking down	Hemolysis Neurolysis	A breaking down of red blood cells Disintegration of nerve tissue
• osis (G) increase or condition	Anisocytosis Lymphocytosis	Inequality of size of cells Excess of lymph cells
• penia (G) deficiency or decrease	Leukopenia Neutropenia	Abnormal decrease of leukocytes in the blood Abnormal decrease of neutrophils in the blood
• rrhage,	Hemorrhage	The escape of blood from the vessels; bleeding
• rrhagia (G) excessive flow bursting forth	Metrorrhagia Otorrhagia	Uterine bleeding Hemorrhage from the ear
• rrhea (G) flowing	Metrorrhea Dysmenorrhea Otorrhea	A free or abnormal uterine discharge Painful menstruation Discharge from the ear

Contd...

Contd...

Suffix	*Medical term*	*Definition*
• spasm (G) involuntary contractions	Chirospasm Dactylospasm	A spasm as contraction of the hand Spasm or cramp in fingers or toes (Writer's cramp)
• stasis (G) stand still	Hemostasis	Interruption of blood flow through any vessel or to any anatomical area
• stenosis (G) narrowing, contraction	Aorticstenosis Mitralstenosis	A narrowing of the aortic orifice of the heart A narrowing of the left atrio-ventricular orifice

ROOTS

The root stem or main body of a word indicates the organ or part of which is modified by a prefix or suffix, or both. Properly, Greek combining forms or roots should be used only with Greek prefixes and suffixes, Latin with Latin. A vowel, usually a, i, or o is often inserted between the combining forms for euphony.

Root	*Medical term*	*Definition*
aden (G) gland	Adenectomy Adenoma	Excision of a gland Glandular tumor
aer (G) air	Aerated Aerobic	Filled with air Pertaining to organism, which lives only in the presence of air
Angio (G) vessel	Angiotomy Angitis	Incision of blood vessels Inflammation of the blood vessels
arth (G) joint	Arthralgia Arthritis	Pain in the joints Inflammation of the joints
blephar (G) eyelid	Blepharitis Blepharoptosis	Inflammation of the eyelid Drooping of the upper eyelid
card (G) heart	Cardiology Electrocardiogram	The science of the heart A graphic record of the heart beat by an electrometer
cerebro (L) brain	Cerebromalacia Cerebrospinal	Softening of the brain Referring to brain and spinal cord

Contd...

Contd...

Root	*Medical term*	*Definition*
cephal (G) head	Cephalalgia Cephalic	Headache Pertaining to the head
cerv (L) neck	Cervicectomy Cervicovesical	Excision of the neck of the uterus Relating to the cervix uteri and bladder
cheil, chil (G) lip	Cheilitis Cheiloplasty	Inflammation of the lip Plastic operation of the lip
chir (G) hand	Chiromegaly Chiroplasty	Abnormal size of the hands, wrists and ankles Plastic repair of the hand
chol (G) bile	Cholangitis Cholecyst	Inflammation of bile duct Gallbladder
chondr (G) cartilage	Chondrectomy Chondroma	Excision of a cartilage A cartilaginous tumor
cost (L) rib	Costochondral Costosternal	Pertaining to a rib and its cartilage Referring to the ribs and breast bone
crani (G,L) skull	Craniotomy Cranial	Surgical opening (incision) of the skull Pertaining to the skull
cysto (G) bladder, sac	Cyst Cystoscope	A bladder; any sac containing a liquid Instrument for interior examination of the bladder
cyt (G) cell	Cytology Erythrocyte	The study of cell life Red blood cell
dacry (G) tear	Dacryocele Dacryocyst	Protrusion of the lacrimal sac The lacrimal sac
dactyl (G) finger, toe	Dactylitis Dactylomegaly	Chronic disease of bone of fingers or toe in young children Abnormal size of fingers and toes
derm (G) skin	Dermatitis Dermopathy	Inflammation of the skin Any skin disease
encephal (G) brain	Encephalitis Encephaloma	Inflammation of the brain Brain tumor
enter (G) intestine (small)	Enteritis Enterocele	Inflammation of the small intestine A hernia of the small intestine
gastr (G) stomach	Gastrectasis Gastroenteritis	Dilatation of the stomach Inflammation of the stomach and the small intestine

Contd...

Contd...

Root	*Medical term*	*Definition*
glyco (G) sweet	Glycemia Glycosuria	Sugar in blood Sugar in urine
hem, haemat (G) blood	Hematemesis Hemophilia	Vomiting of blood Inability of the blood to coagulate
hepat (G) liver	Hepatitis Hepatoma	Inflammation of the liver A liver tumor
hyster (G) metra, uterus	Hysterectomy Hysteropexy	Excision of the uterus Abdominal fixation of the uterus
ile, eile, (L-G) ileum	Ileum Ileostomy	Third part of the small intestine Creation of an opening through abdomen into the ileum
ili (L) ilium	Ilium Iliosacral	The wide, upper part of the hip bone Pertaining to ilium and sacrum
leuk (G) white	Leukocyte Leukopenia	White blood cell Abnormal decrease in number of leukocyte
lip (G) fat	Lipectomy Lipemia	Excision of fatty tissues Fat in the blood
lith (G) stone	Lithiasis Lithoscope	Presence of concretions or stones Instrument for examining stone in bladder
menig (G) membrane	Meningitis Meningioma	Inflammation of the membranes of spinal cord and brain Tumor of the meninges
metra(G) or hyster uterus	Metritis Metrorrhagia	Inflammation of the uterus Bleeding from the uterus
myel (G) marrow	Myelitis Myelosarcoma	Inflammation of spinal cord or bone marrow Malignant tumor of the bone marrow
my (G) muscle	Myitis or myositis Myocardium	Inflammation of a muscle The middle and thickest layer of the heart wall
nephr (G) kidney	Nephropexy Nephrosclerosis	Surgical attachment of a floating kidney Hardening of the kidney
ophthalm (G) eye	Ophthalmology Ophthalmoscope	The study of the eye and its diseases Instrumental examination of the eye

Contd...

Contd...

Root	*Medical term*	*Definition*
osteo (G) bone	Osteoma Osteomalacia	A bony tumor Softening of the bone
pneum (G) and exudation lung, or air	Pneumonia Pneumothorax	Inflammation of the lungs with consolidation Introduction of air into the pleural cavity
proct (G) rectum, anus	Proctoscopy Proctopexy	Instrumental examination of the rectum Suture of the rectum to some other part
psycho (G) soul, mind	Psychiatry Psychopathy	Medical specialty treating mental and neurotic disorders Any mental disease usually related to defective character and personality
pyel (G) pelvis	Pyelitis Pyelogram	Inflammation of the pelvis of the kidney Radiogram of the ureter and renal pelvis
pyloro (G) pylorus, gatekeeper	Pylorus Pylorostenosis	Orifice between stomach and duodenum Constriction of pylorus
pyo (G) pus	Pyogenic Pyometritis	Pus forming Purulent inflammation of the uterus
radi (L) ray	Radiology Radiotherapy	The study of X-rays in the diagnosis and treatment of disease The use of radiation of any type in treating diseases
spondyl (G) vertebra	Spondylitis Spondylolisthesis (olisthesis: slipping)	Inflammation of vertebrae Forward dislocation of lumbar vertebrae with pelvic deformity
trachel (G) orcervi neck	Trachelitis Tracheloplasty	Inflammation of the cervix Plastic operation of the cervix uteri
tubercul (L) tubercle	Tuberculosis Tuberculoma	An infectious disease marked by the formation of tubercles in any tissue A tuberculous abscess or tumor
viser (L) organ	Viscus Viscera	Pertaining to the internal organs Organ

PREFIXES

Prefixes are the most frequently used elements in the formation of medical terms. A prefix consists of one or two syllables placed before a word to modify its meaning. These syllables are often prepositions or adverbs. Some common prefixes are:

Prefix	*Medical term*	*Definition*
ab (L) from, away from	Abductor Abnormal	That which draws away from a common center Away from or not corresponding to rule
a, an (G) without, not	Apnea Anesthesia	Temporary absence of respiration Loss of sensation
ad (L) adherence, increase, near, toward	Adductor Adrenal	That which draws toward a common center A ductless (endocrine) gland above the kidney
ante (L) before	Antenatal Antepartum	Before birth Before the onset of labor
anti (G) against	Antisepsis Antipyretic	The exclusion of putrefactive germs A drug that reduces fever
bi (L) two, both, double	Biconvex Bilateral	Having two convex surfaces as in a lens Affecting both sides
com, con, or sym (L) together, with	Congenital defect Conjunctiva	Born with a defect, hereditary Mucous membrane which lines eyelids
contra (L) against, opposite	Contraception Contraindication	The prevention of conception A condition antagonistic to the line of treatment
dys (G) bad, difficult, painful	Dysentery Dysmenorrhea Dyspepsia Dysphagia Dysphasia Dyspnea Dysuria	Inflammation of intestinal mucous membrane accompanied by pain Painful menstruation Imperfect digestion Difficulty in swallowing Impairment of speech Labored or difficult breathing Pain or difficult urination
ec (G) out	Ectopic pregnancy	Gestation outside the uterine cavity

Contd...

Contd...

Prefix	*Medical term*	*Definition*
ecto (G) outside ex-out	Ectropion of eyelid	Eversion as the edge of the eyelid
em, en (G) in	Empyema Encephalopathy	Pus in a body cavity, especially in the pleural cavity Any disease of the brain
endo (G) within	Endocardium Endocarditis Endocrine gland Endometrium Endometritis Endoscope Endoscopy	Lining membrane of inner surface of the heart Inflammation of the endocardium A ductless gland in which an internal secretion forms The mucous membrane lining the inner surface of the uterus Inflammation of the endometrium Tubular instrument for examining cavities through natural openings Inspection of cavities by use of the endoscope
epi (G) upon, at, in addition to	Epidermis Epigastrium Epiphysis	Cuticle or outer layer of the skin Region over the pit of the stomach A center of ossification at both extremities of long bones
ex (G) out, away from, over	Exacerbation Exophthalmia Expectoration Exudate	Aggrevation of symptoms Abnormal protrusion of the eyeballs Expulsion of mucus from the lungs Accumulation of fluid due to inflammatory condition
hemi (G), or semi (L) half	Hemiplegia Hemiglossectomy	Paralysis of one-half of the body Removal of half a tongue
hyper (G) above, excessive, beyond	Hyperacidity Hypercalcemia Hyperemisis gravidarum Hyperemia Hyperpyrexia Hypertension	An excess of acid in the stomach Excess of calcium in the blood Excessive vomiting during early pregnancy Congestion High fever (above 106 degree Fahrenheit) High blood pressure
hypo (G) beneath, below, deficient	Hypodermic injection Hypoglycemia	Injection under the skin Low blood sugar

Contd...

Contd...

Prefix	*Medical term*	*Definition*
inter (L) between	Intercostal Interfemoral	Between two ribs Between the thighs
meta (G) next, between	Metabolism Metacarpal	The sum of all the physical and chemical processes by which living organized substance is produced and maintained Bone of the metacarpus
para, par (G) beside, around, near, abnormal	Paracentesis Parametritis Paranephritis Parathyroid	Puncture of a cavity with tapping Inflammation of the parametrium Inflammation of suprarenal capsules; of connective tissue above the kidney Ductless gland near the thyroid gland
peri (G) around, about	Pericardium Pericarditis Perimetritis Periostitis	The double membranous sac enclosing the heart Inflammation of the pericardium Inflammation of the serous membrane enveloping the uterus Inflammation of the periosteum
pre (L, G) before, in front of	Precancerous Pericardium Pre-eclampsia Presentation	Before the development of carcinoma Region over the heart Eclampsia before delivery (Eclampsia is major toxemia during pregnancy) Manner of the fetus presenting itself at the cervix
pyo (G) pus	Pyocele Pyocyst Pyonephritis	A collection of pus in the scrotum A cyst containing pus Prulent inflammation of the kidney
post (G)	Postpartum Postnatal	After delivery After birth
retro (L) backward, behind, back of	Retroflexion Retroperitoneal Retroversion	A bending or flexing backward; for example of the uterus Located behind the peritoneum A state of being turned back; for example, of the uterus
semi (L) half	Semicoma Semilunar valves	Mild degree of coma Half-moon shaped valves of the aorta and pulmonary
sub (L) under, beneath, below super,	Subclavicular Subcutaneous Suppuration Supernatant Supraoccipital	Beneath the clavicle Beneath the skin The process of pus formation Floating on surface Situated above the occiput

Contd...

Contd...

Prefix	*Medical term*	*Definition*
supra (L) above, beyond, superior sym,	Suprapubic cystotomy Suprarenal Symphysis of pubis	Surgical opening into the bladder from above the symphysis pubis Adrenal gland above the kidney Fusion of pubic bone on midline anteriorly
sym (G) with, along, together, beside	Synarthrosis Syndactlism	An immovable joint A fusion of two or more fingers or toes; webbing
toxi (G) poison	Toxicology Toxicosis Toxicophobia	The science or study of poisons Any diseased condition due to poisoning Irrational fear of being poisoned
trans (L) across, over	Transection Transfusion Transurethral prostatectomy	Incision across the long axis; cross section Injection of the blood of one person into the blood vessel of another Excision of the prostate gland through the urethra
tri (G) three	Tricuspid Trifacial Trigone	Having three cusps or points; tricuspid valve Fifth cranial nerve A triangular space, especially that of the lower part of the urinary bladder

COMMON ABBREVIATIONS

S.No.	*Abbreviation*	*Term*
1.	ACC	Adenoid cystic carcinoma
2.	AMA	Against medical advice
3.	Ant.	Anterior
4.	b.i.d.	Twice a day (bis in die)
5.	BID	Brought in dead
6.	C	Centrigrade (Centum gradus)
7.	CA(Ca)	Carcinoma
8.	CC	Chief complaint
9.	CSSD	Central sterile supply department

Contd...

Contd...

S.No.	*Abbreviation*	*Term*
10.	DOA	Date of admission
11.	DOD	Date of discharge or death
12.	Dx	Diagnosis
13.	ER	Emergency room
14.	EUA	Examination under anesthesia
15.	FB	Foreign body
16.	F/U	Follow-up
17.	FUO	Fever of unknown origin
18.	GA	General anesthesia
19.	GP	General practitioner
20.	GS	General surgery
21.	GSH	Glomerulus stimulating hormone
22.	HPI	History of present illness
23.	ICD	International classification of disease
24.	IMP	Improved
25.	I and O	Intake and output
26.	IP	Inpatient
27.	IV	Intravenously
28.	LA	Local anesthesia
29.	MH	Marital history
30.	MSW	Medical social worker
31.	NAD	Nothing abnormal detected
32.	NBM	Nothing by mouth
33.	N/C	No complaints
34.	NEC	Not elsewhere classified
35.	NED	No evidence of disease
36.	NOS	Not otherwise specified
37.	NYD	Not yet diagnosed
38.	O/A	On admission
39.	OD	Once a day
40.	OE	On examination

Contd...

Contd...

S.No.	*Abbreviation*	*Term*
41.	O and E	Observation and examination
42.	OP	Outpatient
43.	OPC	Outpatient clinic
44.	OR	Operating room
45.	OT	Operation theater
46.	PH	Past history
47.	PI	Present illness
48.	PM	Postmortem
49.	PO	Postoperative
50.	PP	Postpartum
51.	q.d	Quaque die (everyday)
52.	q.d.h	Quaque duo hora (every two hours)
53.	q.h	Quaque hora (every hour)
54.	q.i.d.	Quarter in die (four times daily)
55.	q.n	Quaquenocte (every night)
56.	q.n.s	Quantum nonstatis (insufficient quantity)
57.	q.q.h	Quaque quarta hora (every four hours)
58.	q.s	Quantum statis (sufficient quantity)
59.	q.t.h	Quaque tri hora (every three hours)
60.	q.v	Quantum vis (as much as desired)
61.	RAD	Radiation absorbed dose
62.	RFB	Retained foreign body
63.	RR	Recovery room
64.	RT	Radiation therapy
65.	Rx	Recipe (take)
66.	Sx	Symptoms
67.	Tx	Therapy
68.	US	Ultrasound
69.	VS	Vital signs
70.	WNL	Within normal limits
71.	XR	X-ray

4 Laboratory Investigation Cookbook

INTRODUCTION

The author has taken care to incorporate this chapter especially for the benefit of users of the *Paramedics 6-in-1 Handbook*. When we talk of general and special investigations that includes test of laboratories such as pathology, microbiology, serology, biochemistry, radiology, diagnostic therapies, electrocardiogram (ECG), electroencephalogram (EEG), ultrasound, CT scan and MRI. Investigations as such are vital part of dynamic medicine. Without these tests detecting, proper diagnoses would not have happened and without established diagnoses, there would not be in any remedial treatment. Precisely, appropriate investigation carried out in patient on time would reveal the health problem of the patient that will help the doctors and medical care providers to plan and treat the disease/injury promptly that remedies the sick and injured not only saves live but also prevents further aggravation and complications. It is hard to measure dimension and role of investigation.

The role of investigations have tremendously increased in curing preventing, promoting and rehabilitating the sick and injured despite of medical education, sophisticated equipment, supersonic technology and extensive global medical research. Hence, investigations find a place in vital part of healthcare delivery system and the professionals especially nursing and paramedical should have a good background picture of names of investigations that are required to establish accurate diagnosis/injuries.

Almost all-important investigations are classified and presented in the following manner to serve as quick 'cookbook' to users:

1. Description of some investigations commonly used to establish diagnoses
2. Selected diagnoses and required investigations
3. Variations of investigations (increase and decrease) with normal values and resulting diagnoses
4. List of normal values of investigations in alphabetical order.

This list will be of great value for all those who are involved in analysis of ambulatory, discharge record analysis, quality assurance, case mix studies, diagnostic related group, cost calculation for investigation and justification of diagnoses, and deviation of investigation studies, etc.

DESCRIPTION OF THE LABORATORY AND RADIOLOGICAL INVESTIGATIONS (SYSTEM WISE)

Blood and Lymphatic System

S. No.	*Name of the test*	*Description*
1.	Hemoglobin	Measurement of the amount of hemoglobin in blood sample
2.	Hematocrit	Percentage of erythrocytes (RBC) in a volume of blood
3.	White blood cell count	Number of white blood cells or leukocytes per cubic millimeter
4.	White blood cell differential count	Numbers of different types of leukocytes (immature and mature forms)
5.	Platelet count	Number of platelets per cubic millimeter of blood
6.	Red blood cell count	Number of erythrocytes per cubic millimeter of blood
7.	Erythrocyte sedimentation	Speed at which erythrocytes settle out of plasma
8.	Prothrombin time	Ability of the blood to clot
9.	Partial thromboplastin time	Determination of the presence of important clotting factors in the blood
10.	Antiglobulin test	This test demonstrates whether the patient's erythrocytes are coated with antibody and is useful in determining the presence of antibodies in infants or 'RH' women

Contd...

Contd...

S. No.	*Name of the test*	*Description*
11.	Bleeding time	A small stab wound is made in the earlobe or forearm and the time required for it to stop bleeding is recorded. This test evaluates the vascular and platelet factors associated with hemostasis. Failure of either of these components leads to a prolonged bleeding time. An increase in noted in thrombocytopenia, ingestion of anti-inflammatory drugs, and infiltration of bone marrow by primary or metastatic tumors
12.	Alpha-fetoprotein (AFP)	A plasma protein found normally in some embryonic tissue. It is also present in the blood of adults with hepatocellular carcinoma and germ cell neoplasms. The AFP levels are used to monitor the effectiveness of cancer therapy in patients with these types of malignancies

Musculoskeletal System

S. No.	*Name of the test*	*Description*
1.	Rheumatoid factor	The serum of a patient with rheumatoid arthritis contains this antibody in elevated levels. The test, however, is not specific since rheumatoid factor is present in aging, scleroderma, acute pulmonary tuberculosis, systemic lupus erythematosus, and other disorders

Skin

S. No.	*Name of the test*	*Description*
1.	Bacterial analysis	Sample of purulent (pus-filled) material or exudates (fluid which accumulates in a space or passes out of tissues) is sent to the laboratory for examination to determine what type of bacteria is present
2.	Fungal tests	Scrapings from skin lesions are placed on a growth medium for several weeks and then examined microscopically for evidence for fungal growth

Endocrine System

S. No.	*Name of the test*	*Description*	
1.	Serum tests	The measurement of the following substances in serum (blood) is important in diagnosing endocrine disorders:	
		Substance	*Endocrine gland function*
		Calcium	Parathyroid gland
		Cortisol	Adrenal cortex
		Electrolytes	Adrenal cortex
		Estradiol (estrogen)	Ovaries
		FSH	Adenohypophysis
		HGH	Adenohypophysis
		Insulin	Pancreas
		LH	Adenohypophysis
		Parathyroid hormone	Parathyroid gland
		Prolactin	Adenohypophysis
		T3	Thyroid gland
		Free thyroxin (not bound to protein)	Thyroid gland
		Testosterone	Testis
		TSH	Adenohypophysis
		The following substances are measured in the urine as indicators of endocrine function:	
		Substance	*Endocrine gland function*
		Calcium	Parathyroid gland
		Catecholamines	Adrenal medulla
		Free cortisol	Adrenal cortex
		Electrolytes	Adrenal cortex
		17-hydroxycorticosteroids	Adrenal cortex
		17-ketosteroids	Adrenal cortex
		Ketones	Pancreas
		Glucose	Pancreas

Contd...

Contd...

S. No.	*Name of the test*	*Description*
2.	Blood sugar	Blood sugar determination helps to estimate the amount of glucose in the blood when the patient is fasting and after the food is consumed. High percent of glucose in the blood indicate the presence of diabetes mellitus and low percent indicates hypoglycemia.
3.	Fasting blood sugar	Used to detect abnormalities of glucose metabolism. The level of glucose in the blood is determined after the patient has fasted for 8 hours
4.	Glucose tolerance test	This test measures the glucose level in a blood sample from a fasting patient (fasting blood sugar) and in specimens taken 50 minutes, 1 hour, 2 hours, and 3 hours after ingestion of 100 g of glucose
5.	Radioimmunoassay	This test measures hormone levels in plasma

Cardiovascular System

S. No.	*Name of the test*	*Description*
1.	Serum enzyme tests	During a myocardial infarction, enzymes released into the bloodstream from the heart muscle can be measured and found as evidence of an infarction
2.	Lipid tests	Lipids are fatty substances found in food and in the bloodstream. Lipid tests measure the amounts of these substances in a blood sample
3.	Lipoprotein electrophoresis	Lipoproteins are fats (lipids) and protein molecules bound together. Protein electrophoresis is the process of physically separating lipoproteins from a blood sample

Respiratory System

S. No.	Name of the test	Description
1.	Pulmonary function tests	This group of tests evaluates ventilation capabilities of the lungs
2.	Tuberculin test	Antigens such as PPD (purified protein derivative) are applied to the skin with multiple punctures (tine tests) or intradermally (mantoux test). A local inflammatory reaction is observed in infected persons after 48–96 hours
3.	Sputum culture and sensitivity (CS)	Bacteriological procedure used to isolate the organism causing disease, especially pneumonia. When the caustic organism is isolated, this test determines which antibiotic will be effective for treatment

Digestive System

S. No.	Name of the test	Description
1.	Liver function tests	Serum glutamic oxyacetic transaminase (SGOT) Serum glutamic pyruvic transaminase (SGPT) These tests reveal the levels of enzymes (SGOT and SGPT) in the blood serum. Enzyme levels are elevated when there is damage to liver cells
2.	Alkaline phosphate (ALP)	This is another enzyme test done on serum. An increased level of alkaline phosphatase is found in liver disease
3.	Serum bilirubin	High level of bilirubin in the blood produces a jaundiced condition in the patient. This test indicates excessive hemolysis, hepatic disorders, or obstructive conditions of the bile ducts. Serum bilirubin is formed from the breakdown of hemoglobin. In the liver, bilirubin is secreted into the bile and then excreted into the intestinal tract through the bile ducts
4.	Stool culture	Feces are placed in a growth medium to test for the presence of microorganisms
5.	Occult blood	Determines bleeding in gastrointestinal disorders. Because this test is so sensitive, the patient is instructed to have a meat-free diet for 3 days before the test. The presence of undigested mean can give a false-positive reading
6.	Stool guaiac	Guaiac is added to a stool sample to reveal the presence of blood in the feces

Urinary System

S. No.	Name of the test	Description
1.	Blood urea nitrogen (BUN)	This test measures the amount of urea in the blood Normally the urea level is low since urea is excreted in the urine continuously. When the kidney is diseased or fails, however, urea accumulates in the blood and this can lead to unconsciousness and death
2.	Urinalysis	One of the most widely used laboratory tests. It provides general information regarding the health of the body as a whole as well as specific information on the conditions of the urinary structures
3.	Creatinine clearance test	This test measures the ability of the kidney to remove creatinine from the blood. A blood sample is drawn and the amount of creatinine concentration is compared with the amount of creatinine excreted in the urine during a 24-hour period. If the kidney is not functioning well in its job of clearing creatinine from the blood, there will be a disproportionate amount of creatinine in the blood, compared with the urine

Female Reproductive System

S. No.	Name of the test	Description
1.	Pap test	Microscopic analysis of the cell smear (spread on a glass slide) can detect the presence of cervical or vaginal carcinoma
2.	Pregnancy test	This test detects the presence or human chorionic gonadotropin (hCG) in the urine or blood
3.	Endometrial biopsy	Used in screening high-risk patients for endometrial cancer. This test is done as an office procedure during the gynecologic examination. Following the administration of a small amount of anesthetic, a thin, hollow curette is used to remove endometrial tissue for laboratory analysis

Male Reproductive System

S. No	*Name of the test*	*Description*
1.	Semen analysis	This test is done for fertility analysis and is also to establish the effectiveness of vasectomy. Sperm cells are counted and examined for motility and shape
2.	Venereal disease research laboratory (VDRL) test	This test is for syphilis. The patient's blood (serum) is placed with the syphilis antigen (spirochete)
3.	Fluorescent treponemal antibody absorption (FTA-ABS) test	This is more specific test for syphilis. The syphilis bacterium is actually searched for under the microscope

Cancer Medicine

S. No	*Name of the test*	*Description*
1.	Carcino-embryonic antigen (CEA) test	Carcinoembryonic antigen can be found in the blood-stream of patients with a variety of tumors of gastrointestinal origin. Measurements of levels in the blood-stream can lead to early identification, resection, and possible cure of some cases
2.	Alpha-fetoprotein test	This test detects the presence of the protein antigen (alpha-fetoprotein) in the serum of patients with liver and testicular cancer
3.	Beta-hCG (human chorionic gonadotropin) Test	This blood test detects the presence of a portion of human chorionic gonadotropin (hCG) in the serum of patients with testicular cancer and is used as a marker for the presence of tumor cells in the body
4.	Estrogen (estradiol) receptor assay	This test measures the concentration of estrogen receptor site on tumor cells of breast cancer patients

SELECTED DIAGNOSIS WITH REQUIRED INVESTIGATIONS

S. No.	*Diagnosis*	*System*	*Investigations*
1.	Achalasia cardia	Gastrointestinal	X-ray, fluoroscopy
2.	Acne vulgaris	Skin	Skin test
3.	Acoustic neuroma	Ear, nose, throat (ENT)	ENT examination, lumbar puncture—CSF culture

Contd...

Contd...

S. No.	*Diagnosis*	*System*	*Investigations*
4.	Acute alcohol intoxication	General	Toxicology test, BP, pupil examination, blood gas analysis, blood examination, blood alcohol level, urine analysis, stool test
5.	Acute bronchitis	Respiratory	Chest X-ray, blood gas analysis, sputum culture
6.	Acute cholecystitis	Gastrointestinal	WBC differential, X-ray
7.	Acute gastritis	Gastrointestinal	Endoscopy
8.	Acute glomerulonephritis	Nephrology	Renal function test, electrolytic examination, erythrocyte sedimentation rate (ESR), BP, 24 hours urine volume, blood culture, hyaline test, specific gravity, urine analysis
9.	Acute leukemia	Hematology	Hematological examination, total WBC, differential WBC, bone marrow test, lymph node examination
10.	Acute mesenteric lymphadenitis	Gastrointestinal	Lymph node aspiration or culture
11.	Acute mesenteric vascular occlusion	Gastrointestinal	WBC differential, hemoglobin
12.	Acute morphine poisoning	General	Toxicology test, BP, pupil examination, blood gas analysis, blood examination, stool test, urine analysis
13.	Acute organic small bowel obstruction	Gastrointestinal	WBC differential, X-ray
14.	Acute otitis media	Ear, nose, throat (ENT	ENT examination, ESR, swap culture, audiometry test
15.	Acute pancreatitis	Gastrointestinal	WBC differential, serum amylase, urine amylase, lipase

Contd...

Contd...

S. No.	*Diagnosis*	*System*	*Investigations*
16.	Acute pyelonephritis	Nephrology	Renal function test, electrolytic examination, ESR, BP, 24 hours urine volume, blood culture, hyaline test, specific gravity, urine analysis and culture
17.	Acute renal failure	Nephrology	Renal function test, electrolytic examination, erythrocyte sedimentation rate (ESR), BP, 24 hours urine volume, blood culture, hyaline test, specific gravity, urine analysis and culture
18.	Acute respiratory failure	Respiratory	BP, chest X-ray, blood gas analysis, ESR, ECG, blood examination, blood and urine culture
19.	Acute retention of urine	Nephrology	Cystoscopy, ultrasound kidney, intravenous pyelogram, X-ray kidney, ureter, bladder
20.	Acute rheumatic fever	Pediatric	Pediatric examination, cardiological consultation, ESR, chest X-ray, differential WBC, ECG, RH factor titer
21.	Addison's disease	Nephrology	BP, total and differential WBC, hematological study, 17-hydroxy-corticoids level
22.	Adult respiratory distress syndrome	Respiratory	WBC total, ESR, X-ray
23.	Agranulocytosis	General	Total WBC, differential WBC, ESR, lymph node examination
24.	Alcoholic hepatitis	Gastrointestinal	Alkaline phosphatase, serum glutamic-oxaloacetic transminase (SGOT), liver biopsy, prothrombin time
25.	Amenorrhea	Gynecological	Irregular menstrual cycle, pregnancy test, tuberculin test, Hb count

Contd...

Contd...

S. No.	*Diagnosis*	*System*	*Investigations*
26.	Amoebiasis	Gastrointestinal	Stool, sigmoidoscopy
27.	Anemia	Pediatric	Pediatric examination, Hb count, ESR, Liver function text (LFT), ultrasound spleen
28.	Anal fissure	Gastrointestinal	Stool, sigmoidoscopy
29.	Anaphylitic shock	General	Toxicology test, BP, pupil examination, blood examination, stool test, urine analysis
30.	Anemia	General	Hemoglobin, RBC, hematocrit
31.	Angina pectoris	Cardiovascular	ECG, angiography, radioisotope
32.	Aortic regurgitation	Pediatric	Pediatric examination, cardiological consultation, chest X-ray, barium X-ray, sputum culture, Rh factor titer, hematological study
33.	Aortic stenosis	Pediatric	Pediatric examination, cardiological consultation, chest X-ray, ECG
34.	Aortic stenosis	Cardiovascular	ECG, X-ray, Doppler echocardiography
35.	Appendicitis	Gastrointestinal	WBC differential, X-ray abdomen, liver function test
36.	Arsenic poisoning	General	Toxicology test, BP, pupil examination, blood gas analysis, blood examination, stool test, urine analysis
37.	Ascites	Gastrointestinal	Diagnostic paracentesis, protein analysis, blood count, blood culture, AFT, amylase, WBC total, WBC differential, LFT
38.	Atelectasis	Respiratory	X-ray, CT scan
39.	Atypical pneumonia	Respiratory	WBC total, sputum culture, X-ray

Contd...

Contd...

S. No.	*Diagnosis*	*System*	*Investigations*
40.	Bacillary dysentery	Gastrointestinal	Stool culture
41.	Barbiturate poisoning	General	Toxicology test, BP, pupil examination, blood examination, stool test, urine analysis
42.	Bee sting	General	Skin test
43.	Bell's palsy	Neurology	Nervous conduction test, EMG, phenatine assay test
44.	Bronchopneumonia	Pediatric	Pediatric examination, chest X-ray, stool test, electrolytic test
45.	Bronchial adenoma	Respiratory	Bronchoscopy
46.	Bronchial asthma	Respiratory	WBC total, WBC differential, ESR, sputum culture, blood gas analysis, PFT, X-ray chest, allergic skin test
47.	Bronchiectasis	Respiratory	WBC total, sputum culture, X-ray, bronchogram
48.	Bronchiolar carcinoma	Respiratory	Sputum, chest X-ray, bronchoscopy, biopsy
49.	Bronchopneumonia	Respiratory	Blood culture, WBC differential, X-ray
50.	Burns	General	Electrolytic analysis, skin test, BP, blood examination
51.	Cancer cervix	Gynecological	Hb count, ESR, differential WBC count, blood culture, lymph biopsy
52.	Cancer colon	Gastrointestinal	Hemoglobin, sigmoidoscopic and X-ray
53.	Cancer esophagus	Gastrointestinal	Hemoglobin, barium swallow
54.	Candidiasis (Thrush)	Gastrointestinal	Skin test
55.	Carcinoma of body of uterus	Gynecological	ESR, urine analysis, Hb count, differential WBC count, pap smear, biopsy cervix, lymph node
56.	Carcinoma of liver	Gastrointestinal	Hemoglobin, liver function test, ultrasound and CT scan, liver scan

Contd...

Contd...

S. No.	*Diagnosis*	*System*	*Investigations*
57.	Carcinoma of stomach	Gastrointestinal	Hemoglobin, stool, gastroscopic and X-ray
58.	Cardiac arrest	Cardiovascular	BP, ECG, chest X-ray, pupil examination, blood gas analysis, blood examination
59.	Cardiogenic shock	Cardiovascular	BP, ECG, chest X-ray, pupil examination, blood gas analysis, blood examination
60.	Cardiogenic shock	Cardiovascular	Urine flow, blood gas analysis, blood pressure, ECG
61.	Cervicitis	Gynecological	Biopsy cervix, histological study, urine analysis, culture
62.	Choledocholithiasis	Gastrointestinal	WBC differential, liver function test, platelet count
63.	Cholera	Gastrointestinal	Stool culture
64.	Cholesteatoma	Ear, nose, throat (ENT)	ENT examination, audiometry test, PNS X-ray
65.	Chronic bronchitis	Respiratory	Sputum, X-ray
66.	Chronic cholecystitis	Gastrointestinal	X-ray
67.	Chronic gastritis	Gastrointestinal	WBC differential, gastroscopy
68.	Chronic lymphatic leukemia	Hematology	Total and differential WBC, HB count, bone marrow test, lymph node examination, hematological study
69.	Chronic obstructive	Respiratory pulmonary disease	Chest X-ray, planogram, CT scan-lungs, WBC total, differential, RBC, spirometry
70.	Chronic simple otitis media	ENT	ENT examination, audiometry test, peripheral nervous system (PNS) X-ray
71.	Chronic myeloid leukemia	Hematology	Total and differential WBC, Hb count, lymph node examination, hematological study, bone marrow test

Contd...

Contd...

S. No.	*Diagnosis*	*System*	*Investigations*
72.	Congenital syphilis	Pediatric	Pediatric examination, Hb count, weight loss, LFT, X-ray of fore and hind bone
73.	Congestive cardiac failure	Cardiovascular	BP, ECG, echocardiogram, chest X-ray, cardiac enzyme test, lipid profile, LFT, serum potassium level
74.	Contact dermatitis	Skin	Skin scrach test
75.	Cushing's syndrome	Endocrine	Plasma cortisol test, ACTH
76.	Deafness	ENT	ENT examination, audiometry test,
77.	Dehydration	General	Electrolytic analysis, skin test, BP
78.	Delaying menstruation	Gynecological	Irregular, menstrual cycle, Hb count
79.	Dermatophytosis	Skin	Scaling skin test
80.	Deviated nasal septum	ENT	ENT examination, PNS X-ray
81.	Datura poisoning	General	Toxicology test, BP, ECG, pupil examination, skin test, blood gas analysis, blood examination, photosensitivity test, urine analysis, stool analysis
82.	Diabetes insipidus	Endocrine	24 urine volume, antidiuretic hormone (ADH) test
83.	Diabetes mellitus	Endocrine	24 urine volume, ADH test, glucose tolerance test (GTT), sugar level, blood sugar level—fasting and postprandial, urine sugar level
84.	Diabetic ketoacidosis	Endocrine	Blood sugar level—fasting and postprandial, electrolytic analysis, ketone test, urine sugar and ketone test, urine analysis
85.	Diphtheria	Pediatric	Pediatric examination, swap culture, ESR

Contd...

Contd...

S. No.	*Diagnosis*	*System*	*Investigations*
86.	Discharge from ear	ENT	ENT examination, swap culture test
87.	Diverticular disease of colon	Gastrointestinal	X-ray, barium enema
88.	Drowning	General	BP, ECG, chest X-ray, pupil examination, blood gas analysis, blood examination
89.	Dumping syndrome	Gastrointestinal	
90.	Duodenal ulcer	Gastrointestinal	Endoscopy
91.	Dysfunctional uterine bleeding		Gynecological Hb count, ESR, differential WBC count, blood culture, lymph biopsy, psychoanalytical test
92.	Dysmenorrhea	Gynecological	Urine analysis, culture, ESR, Hb count
93.	Ectopic pregnancy	Gynecological	Ultrasound uterus, fallopian tube, PV examination
94.	Eczema	Skin	Skin test
95.	Emphysema	Respiratory	Pulmonary function test, X-ray
96.	Empyema	Respiratory	Pus culture
97.	Endocarditis	Cardiovascular	Blood culture, echocardiogram, ECG, ESR, WBC differential, blood culture
98.	Epilepsy	Neurology	Pupil examination, BP, EEG, phentermine assay test, blood gas analysis, blood examination
99.	Epistaxis	ENT	ENT examination, BP test, ECG, differential WBC, ESR, Hb count, prothrombin time
100.	Exfoliative dermatitis	Skin	Skin test
101.	Filaria	General	ESR, blood examination, lymph node test, blood culture, gland biopsy

Contd...

Contd...

S. No.	*Diagnosis*	*System*	*Investigations*
102.	Frostbite	General	Skin test, BP, ECG, blood gas analysis, blood examination, extremity test, ESR
103.	Gastric ulcer	Gastrointestinal	Barium meal and X-ray, gastroscopy
104.	Gonorrhea	Skin	Urine analysis, urine culture
105.	Habitual abortion	Gynecological	Rh-incompatibility test, veneral disease research laboratory (VDRL), thyroid function test, blood sugar
106.	Hemoptysis	Respiratory	Sputum culture, blood culture
107.	Hemorrhoids	Gastrointestinal	Colonoscopy
108.	Hemothorax	Respiratory	Chest X-ray, CT scan, pleural fluid analysis
109.	Heat stroke	General	Skin test, BP, blood gas analysis, blood examination
110.	Hemophilia	Hematology	Partial thromboplastin time (PTT), specific assays factor - VIII and IX
111.	Hepatitis	Gastrointestinal	Blood tests, sonogram imaging, liver biopsy, CAT scan, alpha-fetoprotein (AFT)
112.	Hepatitis	Gastrointestinal	Amino transferase, aspartate aminotransferase-serum glutamic-oxaloacetic transaminase (AST-SGOT), Alanine aminotransferase-serum glutamic pyruvic transaminase (ALT-SGPT), WBC count
113.	Herpes zoster	Skin	
114.	Herpetic stomatitis	Gastrointestinal	WBC differential, blood culture
115.	Hiccup	Gastrointestinal	

Contd...

Contd...

S. No.	*Diagnosis*	*System*	*Investigations*
116.	Hodgkin's disease	Lymphatic system	ESR, blood examination, total and differential WBC, serum copper, serum alkaline phosphate, serum haptoglobin, lymph node biopsy, ultrasound spleen
117.	Hookworm infestation	General	BP, ECG, chest X -ray, blood examination, ESR, skin test, stool test
118.	Hydrothorax	Respiratory	Pleural fluid analysis, total protein, albumin, glucose test, lactate dehydrogenase (LD), carcinoembryonic antigen (CEA), fungal test, acid-fast bacilli (AFB) testing
119.	Hyperemesis gravidarum	Gynecological	Electrolytic analysis
120.	Hyperkalemia	General	BP, ECG, blood examination, skin test, serum potassium level, ADH test
121.	Hypertension	Cardiovascular	BP measurement, ECG, chest X-ray, RBC count, blood urea nitrogen, serum creatinine, potassium level, 17-hydroxycorticosteroids
122.	Hyperthyroidism	Endocrine	Thyroid function test, thyroid scan
123.	Hypoglycemia	Endocrine	Blood sugar level examination, corticosteroids level
124.	Hypothermia	General	Skin test, BP, ECG, blood gas analysis
125.	Hypothyroidism	Endocrine	Thyroid function test, thyroid scan
126.	Incomplete abortion	Gynecological	Ultrasound scanning, Hb count, ESR, differential, total WBC
127.	Indian childhood cirrhosis	Pediatric	Pediatric examination, liver function test, ESR

Contd...

Contd...

S. No.	*Diagnosis*	*System*	*Investigations*
128.	Inevitable abortion	Gynecological	Ultrasound scanning, Hb count, ESR, differential, total WBC
129.	Infantile diarrhea	Pediatric	Pediatric examination, stool examination, ENT examination, oral examination
130.	Infantile eczema	Skin	Skin test, X-ray
131.	Infective arthritis	Musculoskeletal	WBC total, WBC differential, synovial fluid, blood glucose ratio, uric acid, synovial biopsy and culture
132.	Infective polyneuritis	General	ESR, X-ray kidney, ureter and bladder (KUB), blood and urine culture, CSF analysis, adrenocorticotropic hormone (ACTH) test
133.	Injuries to vulva and vagina	Gynecological	Hb count, ESR, blood examination, vaginal examination, urine analysis
134.	Intestinal tuberculosis	Gastrointestinal	Stool culture, X-ray, barium swallow
135.	Intracerebral hemorrhage	Neurology	BP, ESR, coma scale, blood examination, blood gas analysis, pupil examination, X-ray skull, CT scan
136.	Intracranial tumor	Neurology	BP, ESR, coma scale, blood examination, blood gas analysis, pupil examination, X-ray skull, CT scan
137.	Irritable bowel syndrome	Gastrointestinal	Stool analysis
138.	Kwashiorkor	Pediatric	Pediatric examination, skin test, hair examination (pigmentation test), stool examination
139	Lactic acidosis	Digestive	BP, ESR, blood examination, blood gas analysis, plasma level

Contd...

Contd...

S. No.	*Diagnosis*	*System*	*Investigations*
140.	Left ventricular failure	Cardiovascular	BP, ECG, echocardiogram, chest X-ray, cardiac enzyme test, lipid profile, LFT, serum potassium level
141.	Left ventricular failure	Cardiovascular	ECG, chest X-ray, sputum, blood gas analysis
142.	Leukorrhea	Gynecological	Urine analysis, culture pap smear
143.	Leukemias	Hematology	WBC total, WBC differential, bone marrow aspiration, bone biopsy
144.	Lobar pneumonia	Respiratory	WBC differential, sputum culture, chest X-ray
145.	Localized otitis externa	ENT	ENT examination, ESR, swap culture, audiometry test
146.	Lung abscess	Respiratory	Hemoglobin, WBC differential, sputum culture, X-ray
147.	Malaria	General	ESR, blood examination and culture for MP
148.	Marasmus	Pediatric	Pediatric examination, weight loss
149.	Mediastinal tumor	Respiratory	Barium swallow, chest X-ray
150.	Menopause	Gynecological	LDH, FSH test, pap smear, Hb count
151.	Migraine	Neurology	Skull, PNS X-ray, EEG, audiogram, ENT, neurological examination
152.	Mitral regurgitation	Pediatric	Pediatric examination, cardiological consultation, chest X-ray, ECG
153.	Mitral regurgitation	Cardiovascular	ECG, chest X-ray, echocardiogram, BP
154.	Mitral stenosis	Pediatric	Pediatric examination, cardiological consultation, chest X-ray, barium X-ray, sputum culture, Rh factor titer, hematological study

Contd...

Contd...

S. No.	*Diagnosis*	*System*	*Investigations*
155.	Mitral stenosis	Cardiovascular	ECG, chest X-ray, echocardiogram, cardiac catheterization
156.	Mitral value disease	Cardiovascular	ECG, echocardiogram, stress test
157.	Monilial vaginitis	Gynecological	Urine culture, pap smear, ESR, skin scaling test
158.	Multiple myeloma	Neurology	ESR, total and differential WBC, bone morrow test, Bence-Jones protein test, bone scan, BUN, serum creatinine, serum uric acid, serum calcium, X-ray bone
159.	Myasthenia gravis	Nervous	Muscle tone test (EMG), edrophonium and neostigmine test
160.	Myocardial infarction	Cardiovascular	ECG, differential WBC, ESR, CPK-MB, SGOT, LDH, radioisotopes
161.	Nausea and vomiting	Gastrointestinal	Chloride
162.	Nephrotic syndrome	Nephrology	24 hours protein urine, urine albumin, Hb count, lipid profile, LFT
163.	Nodular cirrhosis	Gastrointestinal	Hemoglobin, LDH, SGOT, alkaline phosphates, bilirubin, albumin, liver biopsy
164.	Nonspecific ulcerative colitis	Gastrointestinal	WBC differential, barium enema and X-ray, sigmoidoscopy
165.	Non-Hodgkin's lymphoma	Cancer medicine	ERS, blood examination, lymph node biopsy, total and differential WBC count
166.	Organophosphorus poisoning	General	BP, ECG, pupil examination, blood examination, gastric lavage test, urine analysis, stool analysis

Contd...

Contd...

S. No.	*Diagnosis*	*System*	*Investigations*
167.	Osteoarthritis	Musculoskeletal	ESR, RA factor, radiological study, arthroscopy
168.	Osteomyelitis	Musculoskeletal	Blood culture, X-ray, ESR, WBC, bone marrow test
169.	Pancreatitis	Gastrointestinal	Serum amylase, serum lipase concentration, WBC total, WBC differential, serum calcium concentration, serum albumin, chest X-ray, ultrasonography, CT-pancreas, cholangiography
170.	Paralytic ileus	Gastrointestinal	X-ray
171.	Parkinson's disease	General	Nerve conduction test, ECG, EEG, CT scan and MRI
172.	Pemphigus	Skin	Skin test
173.	Peptic esophagitis	Gastrointestinal	X-ray, biopsy
174.	Peptic ulcer	Gastrointestinal	Endoscopy, fluoroscopy, gastric analysis
175.	Pleural effusion	Respiratory	X-ray, thoracocentesis-definite procedure
176.	Pneumonia	Respiratory	WBC differential, blood gas analysis, sputum culture, X-ray findings, lung scan
177.	Poisoning	General	Toxicology test, BP, pupil examination, blood gas analysis, blood examination, stool test, urine analysis
178.	Premenstrual tension	Gynecological	Breast examination, ECG, BP, psychoanalytical test
179.	Primary biliary cirrhosis	Gastrointestinal	Alkaline phosphatase, liver function test
180.	Profuse vaginal hemorrhage	Gynecological	BP, Hb count, blood examination, ultrasound pelvic, vaginal examination
181.	Psoriasis	Skin	Scaling skin test
182.	Pulmonary edema	Respiratory	X-ray

Contd...

Contd...

S. No.	*Diagnosis*	*System*	*Investigations*
183.	Pulmonary thromboembolism	Respiratory	X-ray, lung scan, ECG, pulmonary angiography
184.	Pulmonary embolism	Respiratory	X-ray, ECG, count blood count (CBC), serum enzyme (AST, LDH), serum bilirubin, lung scan, ultrasound-lungs
185.	Pulmonary tuberculosis	Respiratory	Tuberculin skin test, mantoux test, sputum culture AFB, chest X-ray
186.	Raised intracranial tension	Neurology	BP, ECG, pupil examination, CT scan, skull X-ray
187.	Rectal polyp	Gastrointestinal	High sensitivity focal occult blood tests (FOB)
188.	Regional enteritis (Crohn's disease)	Digestive	Gastrointestinal WBC differential, calcium
189.	Renal colic	Nephrology	ESR, cystoscopy, ultrasound kidney, intravenous pyelogram, X-ray kidney, ureter, bladder, urine examination
190.	Rheumatic fever	Cardiovascular	ESR, rheumatoid factor, antistreptolysin-o' titer
191.	Rheumatoid arthritis	Musculoskeletal	Hb count, U/S spleen, ESR, rheumatoid factors (RFs), WBC total and differential, X-ray joint, arthroscopy
192.	Rickets	Pediatric	Pediatric examination, forelimb X-ray, vitamin D deficiency
193.	Ringworm	Skin	Skin test
194.	Roundworm	General	ESR, blood examination, total and differential WBC count, stool test
195.	Sarcoidosis	Respiratory	Chest X-ray, sputum culture-AFB, limb biopsy
196.	Scabies	Skin	Skin test
197.	Scurvy	Pediatric	Pediatric examination, oral-gum and teeth examination, hindlimb X-ray, vitamin C deficiency
198.	Seborrhoeic dermatitis	Skin	Scaling skin test

Contd...

Contd...

S. No.	*Diagnosis*	*System*	*Investigations*
199.	Secondary biliary cirrhosis	Gastrointestinal	Liver function test
200.	Secondary otitis media	ENT	ENT examination, tuning fork test, audiometry test
201.	Senile vaginitis	Gynecological	Skin test, urine culture, cervical biopsy, cervical cytological test
202.	Sickle cell anemia	Hematology	RBC count, Hb, WBC differential, erythropoietic study
203.	Snake bite	General	Toxicology test, BP, ECG, pupil examination, skin test, blood gas analysis, blood examination, photosensitivity test, urine analysis, stool analysis
204.	Spontaneous pneumothorax	Respiratory	Chest X-ray
205.	Spontaneous pneumothorax	Respiratory	BP, chest X-ray
206.	Sprue syndrome	Gastrointestinal	Stool culture, vitamin deficiency, X-ray
207.	Stroke	General	BP, prothrombin test, EEG, CT scan, blood examination, ECG
208.	Subacute bacterial endocarditis	Cardiovascular	Cardiovascular blood culture, urine analysis, Hb count
209.	Suicidal behavior	Psychiatry	BP, psychoanalytical test, previous history investigation
210.	Syncope	Cardiovascular	ECG, treadmill test, echocardiogram, fasting sugar
211.	Syphilis	Skin	Urine analysis, urine culture, lymph node test
212.	Tapeworm infestation	General	ESR, stool test
213.	Tension pneumothorax	Respiratory	Chest X-ray

Contd...

Contd...

S. No.	Diagnosis	System	Investigations
214.	Thalassemias	Hematology	Hb, hematocrit, RBC count, serum bilirubin, serum ferritin, bone marrow study
215.	Threadworm	General	ESR, stool test
216.	Threatened abortion	Gynecological	Hb count, ESR, urine analysis, culture, beta hCG liter
217.	Tinnitus	ENT	ENT examination, audiometry test
218.	Transfusion reaction	General	BP, skin test, lymph node examination, corticosteroid level
219.	Traumatic pneumothorax	Respiratory	Emergency surgical procedure is required
220.	Trichomonas vaginitis	Gynecological	Urine analysis, erythrocyte sedimentation rate (ESR), skin test, Hb count
221.	Typhoid fever	Gastrointestinal	Widal test, stool
222.	Upper gastrointestinal hemorrhage	Gastrointestinal	WBC differential, stool, liver function test
223.	Uremia	Urology	Urine analysis, skin test, serum creatinine level, chloride level
224.	Vaginitis	Gynecological	Urine analysis, culture, ESR, Hb count, skin test
225.	Vertigo	ENT	ENT examination
226.	Vertigo due to Menier's diseases	ENT	ENT examination, audiometry test
227.	Vincent's stomatitis	Gastrointestinal	Blood test to determine infection
228.	Viral hepatitis	Gastrointestinal	SGOT, SGPT, LDH, liver biopsy
229.	Viral pneumonia	Respiratory	Sputum culture, chest X-ray
230.	Wilson's disease	Gastrointestinal	Liver function test, ceruloplasmin

NORMAL VALUES FOR LABORATORY INVESTIGATIONS

S. No.	Test	Conventional units	SI units
1.	Acid hemolysis test	No hemolysis	No hemolysis
2.	Alkaline phosphatase	Total score 14–100	Total score 14–100

Contd...

Contd...

S. No.	*Test*	*Conventional units*	*SI units*
3.	Cell Counts		
	Erythrocytes		
	Males Females Children Leukocytes, total	4.6–6.2 million/mm^3 4.2–5.4 million/mm^3 4.5–5.1 million/mm^3 4500–11,000/mm^3	4.6–6.2 $\times 10^{12}$/L 4.2–5.2 $\times 10^{12}$/L 4.5–5.1 $\times 10^{12}$/L 4.5–11.0 $\times 10^{9}$/L
4.	Leukocytes, differential		
	Band neutrophils Segmented neutrophils Lymphocytes Monocytes Eosinophils Basophils Platelets Reticulocytes	150–400/mm^3 3000–5800/mm^3 1500–3000/mm^3 300–500/mm^3 50–250/mm^3 15–50/mm^3 150,000–350,000/mm^3 25,000–75,000/mm^3 0.5–1.5% of erythrocytes	150–400 $\times 10^{6}$/L 3000–5800 $\times 10^{6}$/L 1500–3000 $\times 10^{6}$/L 300–500 $\times 10^{6}$/L 50–250 $\times 10^{6}$/L 15–50 $\times 10^{6/}$L 150–350 $\times 10^{9}$/L 25–75 $\times 10^{9}$/L
5.	Coagulation tests		
	Bleeding time (template)	2.75–8.0 min	2.75–8.0 min
	Coagulation time (glass tubes)	5–15 min	5–15 min
	Factor VIII and other coagulation factors	50–150% of normal	0.5–1.5 of normal
	Fibrin split products (Thrombo-Wellcotest)	<10 μg/mL	< 10 mg/L
	Fibrinogen	200–400 mg/dL	2.0–4.0 g/L
	Partial thromboplastic time (PTT)	20–35 sec	20–35 sec
	Prothrombin time (PT)	12.0–14.0 sec	12.0–14.0 sec
6.	Coombs test		
	Direct Indirect	Negative Negative	Negative Negative
7.	Corpuscular Values of erythrocytes		
	Mean corpuscular hemoglobin (MCH)	26–34 pg	0.40 to 0.53 fmol
	Mean corpuscular volume (MCV)	80–96 μm^3	80 to 96 fL
	Mean corpuscular hemoglobin concentration (MCHC)	32–36%	0.32 to 0.36%

Contd...

Contd...

S. No.	*Test*	*Conventional units*	*SI units*
8.	Haptoglobin	26–185 mg/dL	260–1850 mg/L
9.	Hematocrit		
	Males Females Newborns Children	40–54 mL/dL 37–47 mL/dL 49–54 mL/dL 35–49 mL/dL	0.40–0.54 volume fraction 0.37–0.47 volume fraction 0.49–0.54 volume fraction 0.35–0.49 volume fraction
10.	Hemoglobin Males Females Newborns Children (varies with age)	 14.0–18.0 g/dL 12.0–16.0 g/dL 16.5–19.5 g/dL 11.2–16.5 g/dL	 2.17–2.79 mmol/L 1.86–2.48 mmol/L 2.56–3.02 mmol/L 1.74–2.56 mmol/L
11.	Hemoglobin, fetal	<1.0% of total	<0.01% of total
12.	Hemoglobin A_{1c}	3–5% of total	0.03–0.05% of total
13.	Hemoglobin A_2	1.5–3.0% of total	0.015–0.03% of total
14.	Hemoglobin, plasma	0–5.0 mg/dL	0–0.8 μmol/L
15.	Methemoglobin	30–130 mg/dL	4.7–20 μmol/L
16.	Erythrocyte sedimentation rate (ESR) Males Females *Westergren* Males Females	 0–5 mm/hr 0–15 mm/hr 0–15 mm/hr 0–20 mm/hr	 0–5 mm/hr 0–15 mm/hr 0–15 mm/hr 0–20 mm/hr
17.	Acetoacetate plus acetone		
	Qualitative Quantitative	Negative 0.3–2.0 mg/dL	Negative 3–20 mg/L
18.	Acid phosphatase, serum (thymolphthalein monophosphate substrate)	0.11–0.60 U/L	0.11–0.60 U/L
19.	Adrenocorticotropin, plasma (ACTH)		
	6.00 AM 6.00 PM	10–80 pg/mL < 50 pg/mL	10–80 ng/L < 50 ng/L

Contd...

Contd...

S. No.	*Test*	*Conventional units*	*SI units*
20.	Alanine aminotransferase,		
	serum (ALT, SGPT)	7–35 U/L	7–35 U/L
21.	Albumin, serum	3.5–5.5 g/dL	35–55 g/L
22.	Aldolase, serum	1.5–12.0 U/L	1.5–12.0 U/L
23.	Aldosterone, plasma		
	Supine Standing Males Females	3–10 ng/dL 6–22 ng/dL 5–30 ng/dL	0.08–0.30 nmol/L 0.17–0.61 nmol/L 0.14–0.83 nmol/L
24.	Alkaline phosphatase, serum (ALP)	20–90 U/L (30°C)	20–90 U/L/(30°C)
25.	Ammonia nitrogen, plasma	15–49 µg/dL	11–35 µmol/L
26.	Amylase, serum	25–125 U/L	25–125 U/L
27.	Anion gap	8–16 mEq/L	8–16 mmol/L
28.	Ascorbic acid, blood	0.4–1.5 mg/dL	23–85 µmol/L
29.	Aspartate aminotransferase, serum (AST, SGOT)	7–40 U/L	7–40 U/L
30.	Base excess, blood	0 + 2 mEq/L	0 + 2 mmol/L
31.	Bicarbonate		
	Venous plasma Arterial blood	23–29 mEq/L 18–23 mEq/L	23–29 mmol/L 18–23 mmol/L
32.	Bile acids, serum	0.3–3.0 mg/dL	3–30 mg/L
33.	Bilirubin, serum		
	Conjugated Unconjugated Total	0.1–0.4 mg/dL 0.2–0.7 mg/dL 0.3–1.1 mg/dL	1.7–6.8 µmol/L 3.4–12 µmol/L 5.1–19 µmol/L
34.	Calcium, serum	9.0–11.0 mg/dL	2.25–2.75 mmol/L
35.	Calcium, ionized, serum	4.25–5.25 mg/dL	1.05–1.30 mmol/L
36.	Carbon-dioxide, total, serum or plasma	24–30 mEq/L	24–30 mmol/L
37.	Carbon-dioxide tension, blood PCO_2	35–45 mm Hg	35–45 mm Hg
38.	β-Carotene serum	40–200 µg/dL	0.74–3.72 µmol/L
39.	Catecholamines, plasma		
	Epinephrine Norepinephrine	15–55 pg/mL 65–400 pg/mL	82–300 pmol/L 384–2364 pmol/L

Contd...

Contd...

S. No.	*Test*	*Conventional units*	*SI units*
40.	Ceruloplasmin, serum	23–44 mg/dL	230–440 mg/L
41.	Chloride, serum or plasma	96–106 mEq/L	96–106 mmol/L
42.	Cholesterol, serum or EDTA plasma		
	Desirable range LDL Cholesterol HDL Cholesterol	< 200 mg/dL 60–180 mgdL 30–80 mg/dL	< 5.18 mmol/L 600–1800 mg/L 300–800 mg/L
43.	Copper		
	Males Females	70–140 μg/dL 85–155 μg/dL	11–22 μmol/L 13–24 μmol/L
44.	Cortisol, plasma		
	8.00 AM 4.00 PM 10.00 PM	6–23 μg/dL 3–15 μg/dL <50% of 8 AM value	170–635 nmol/L 82–413 nmol/L <0.5% of 8 AM value
45.	Creatine, serum	0.2–0.8 mg/dL	15–61 μmol/L
46.	Creatine kinase, serum (CK, CPK)		
	Males Females	55–170 U/L 30–135 U/L	55–170 U/L 30–135 U/L
47.	Creatine kinase-MB Isoenzyme, serum	0.0–4.7 ng/mL	0.0–4.7 μg/L
48.	Creatinine, serum	0.6–1.2 mg/dL	53–108 μmol/L
49.	Ferritin, serum	20–200 ng/mL	20–200 μg/L
50.	Fibrinogen, plasma	200–400 mg/dL	2.0–4.0 g/L
51.	Folate		
	Serum Erythrocytes	1.8–9.0 ng/mL 150–450 ng/mL	4.1–20.4 nmol/L 340–1020 nmol/L
52.	Follicle-stimulating hormone, plasma (FSH)		
	Males Females Postmenopausal	4–25 mU/mL 4–30 mU/mL 40–250 mU/mL	4–25 U/L 4–30 U/L 40–250 U/L
53.	Y-Glutamyltransferase, serum		
	Males Females	5–38 U/L 5–29 U/L	5–38 U/L 5–29 U/L
54.	Gastrin, serum	0–200 pg/mL	0–200 ng/L
55.	Glucose (fasting), plasma or serum	70–115 mg/dL	3.89–6.38 mmol/L.
56.	Growth hormone also known as human growth hormone (HGH), plasma	0–10 ng/mL	0–10 μg/L

Contd...

Contd...

S. No.	*Test*	*Conventional units*	*SI units*
57.	Haptoglobin, serum	26–185 mg/dL	260–1850 mg/L
58.	Immunoglobulins, serum		
	IgG IgA IgM IgD IgE	550–1900 mg/dL 60–333 mg/dL 45–145 mg/dL 0.5–3.0 mg/dL < 500 ng/mL	5.5–19.0 g/L 0.60–3.3 g/L 0.45–1.5 g/L 5–30 mg/L < 500 μg/L
59.	Insulin (fasting), plasma	5–25 μU/mL	36 to 179 pmol/L
60.	Iron, serum	75–175 ng/dL	13–31 umol/L
61.	Iron-binding capacity, serum		
	Total Saturation	250–410 μg/dL 20%–55%	45–73 μmol/L 0.20–0.55
62.	Lactate		
	Venous blood Arterial blood	4.5–19.8 mg/dL 4.5–14.4 mg/dL	0.50–2.2 mmol/L 0.50–1.6 mmol/L
63.	Lactate dehydrogenase, serum (LD, LDH)	100–190 U/L	100–190 U/L
64.	Lipase, serum	10–140 U/L	10–140 U/L
65.	Lipids, total, serum	450–850 mg/dL	4.5–8.5 g/L
66.	Luteinizing hormone, serum (LH)		
	Males Females Premenopausal Midcycle Postmenopausal	 5–22 mU/mL 3 × baseline >30 mU/mL	 5–22 U/L 3 × baseline >30 U/L
67.	Magnesium, serum	1.8–3.0 mg/dL	0.75–1.25 mmol/L
68.	Osmolality	286–295 mOsm/kg	2.85–2.95 mOsm/kg
69.	Oxygen blood		
	Capacity Content, arterial Saturation, arterial Tension, PO_2	16–24 Vol % 15–23 Vol % 94–100% 75–100 mm Hg	7.14–10.7 mmol/L 6.69–10.3 mmol/L 0.94–1.00 75–100 mm Hg
70.	P_{50}	26–27 mm Hg	26–27 mm Hg
71.	pH, arterial blood	7.35–7.45	7.35–7.45
72.	Phenylalanine, serum	< 3 mg/dL	< 0.18 mmol/L

Contd...

Contd...

S. No.	Test	Conventional units	SI units
73.	Phosphate, inorganic, serum	3.0–4.5 mg/dL	1.0–1.5 mmol/L
74.	Potassium, serum or plasma	3.5–5.0 mEq/L	3.5 to 5.0 mmol/L
75.	Prolactin, serum		
	Males Females	1–20 ng/mL 1–25 ng/mL	1–20 μg/L 1–25 μg/L
76.	Protein, serum		
	Total Albumin α1-Globulin α2-Globulin β-Globulin γ-Globulin	6.0–8.0 g/dL 3.5–5.5 g/dL 0.2–0.4 g/dL 0.5–0.9 g/dL 0.6–1.1 g/dL 0.7–1.7 g/dL	60–80 g/L 35–55 g/L 2–4 g/L 5–9 g/L 6–11 g/L 7–17 g/L
77.	Pyruvate, blood	0.3–0.9 mg/dL	0.03–0.10 mmol/L
78.	Sodium, serum or plasma	136–145 mEq/L	136–145 mmol/L
79.	Testosterone, plasma		
	Males Females Pregnant	275–875 ng/dL 23–75 ng/dL 38–190 ng/dL	9.0–10.0 nmol/L 0.8–2.6 nmol/L 1.3–6.6 nmol/L
80.	Thyroid stimulating hormone,		
	serum (TSH)	0–7 mU/L	0–7 mU/L
81.	Thyroxine, free, serum (FT_4)	1.0–2.1 ng/dL	13–27 pmol/L
82.	Thyroxine, serum (T_4)	4.4–9.9 μg/dL	57–128 nmol/L
83.	Triglycerides, serum	40–150 mg/dL	0.4–1.5 g/L
84.	Triiodothyronine, serum (T_3)	150–250 ng/dL	2.3–3.9 nmol/L
85.	Triiodothyronine resin uptake, (T_3RU)	25–38% uptake	0.25–0.38 uptake
86.	Urate		
	Males Females	2.5–8.0 mg/dL 1.5–7.0 mg/dL	0.15–0.48 mmol/L 0.09–0.42 mmol/L

Contd...

Contd...

S. No.	*Test*	*Conventional units*	*SI units*
87.	Urea, serum or plasma	24–49 mg/dL	4.0–8.2 mmol/L
88.	Urea nitrogen, serum or plasma	11–23 mg/dL	3.9–8.2 mmol/L
89.	Viscosity, serum	1.4–1.8 × water	1.4–1.8 × water
90.	Vitamin A, serum	20–80 µg/dL	0.70–2.80 µmol/L
91.	Vitamin B_{12}, serum	180–900 pg/mL	133–664 pmol/L

URINE INVESTIGATIONS

S. No.	*Test*	*Conventional units*	*SI units*
1.	Acetone and acetoacetate, qualitative	Negative	Negative
2.	Albumin		
	Quantitative	Negative	Negative
	Qualitative	10–100 mg/24 hrs	10–100 mg/24 hrs
3.	Aldosterone	3–20 µg/24 hrs	8.3–55 nmol/24 hrs
4.	δ-Aminolevulinic acid	1.3–7.0 mg/24 hrs	10–53 µmol/24 hrs
5.	Amylase	3–20 U/hr	3–20 U/hr
6.	Amylase/creatinine clearance ratio	1–4%	0.01–0.04%
7.	Bilirubin, qualitative	Negative	Negative
8.	Calcium (usual diet)	<250 mg/24 hrs	<6.3 mmol/24 hrs
9.	Catecholamines		
	Epinephrine	<10 µg/24 hrs	<55 nmol/24 hrs
	Norepinephrine	<100 µg/24 hrs	<590 nmol/24 hrs
	Total free catecholamines	4–126 µg/24 hrs	24–745 nmol/24 hrs
	Total metanephrines	0.1–1.6 µg/24 hrs	0.5–8.1 µmol/24 hrs
10.	Chloride (varies with intake)	110–250 mEq/24 hrs	110–250 nmol/24 hrs
11.	Copper	0–50 µg/24 hrs	0–0.80 µmol/24 hrs
12.	Cortisol, free	10–100 µg/24 hrs	27.6–276 nmol/24 hrs
13.	Creatinine	15–25 mg/kg body weight/24 hrs	0.13–0.22 mmol/kg

Contd...

Contd...

S. No.	*Test*	*Conventional units*	*SI units*
14.	Creatinine clearance (corrected to 1.73 m^2 body surface area)		
	Males Females	110–150 mL/min 105–132 mL/min	110–150 mL/min 105–132 mL/min
15.	Dehydroepiandrosterone		
	Males Females	0.2–2.0 mg/24 hrs 0.2 1.8 mg/24 hrs	0.7–6.9 μmol/24 hrs 0.7–6.2 μmol/24 hrs
16.	Estrogens, total		
	Males Females	4–25 mg/24 hrs 5–100 mg/24 hrs	14–90 nmol/24 hrs 18–360 nmol/24 hrs
17.	Glucose (as reducing substance)	<250 mg/24 hrs	<250 mg/24 hrs
18.	Hemoglobin and myoglobin, qualitative	Negative	Negative
19.	17-Hydroxycorticosteroids		
	Males Females	3–9 mg/24 hrs 2–8 mg/24 hrs	8.3–25 umol/24 hrs 5.5–22 umol/24 hrs
20.	5-Hydroxyindoleacetic acid		
	Qualitative Quantitative	Negative <9 mg/24 hrs	Negative <47 μmol/24 hrs
21.	17-Ketosteroids		
	Males Females	6–18 mg/24 hrs 4–13 mg/24 hrs	21–62 μmol/24 hrs 14–45 μmol/24 hrs
22.	Magnesium	6.0–8.5 mEq/24 hrs	3.0–4.2 μmol/24 hrs
23.	Osmolality	38–1400 mOsm/ kg H_2O	38–1400 mOsm/kg H_2O
24.	pH	4.6–8.0	4.6–8.0
25.	Phenylpyruvic acid, qualitative	Negative	Negative
26.	Phosphate	0.9–1.3 g/24 hrs	29–42 mmol/24 hrs
27.	Porphobilinogen		
	Qualitative Quantitative	Negative <2.0 mg/24 hrs	Negative <9 μmol/24 hrs

Contd...

Contd...

S. No.	*Test*	*Conventional units*	*SI units*
28.	Porphyrins		
	Coproporphyrin Uroporphyrin	50–250 μg/24 hrs 10–30 μg/24 hrs	77–380 nmol/24 hrs 12–36 nmol/24 hrs
29.	Potassium	25–100 mEq/24 hrs	25–100 mmol/24 hrs
30.	Pregnanediol		
	Males Females Proliferative phase Luteal phase Postmenopausal	0.4–1.4 mg/24 hrs 0.5–1.5 mg/24 hrs 2.0–7.0 mg/24 hrs 0.2–1.0 mg/24 hrs	1.2–4.4 μmol/24 hrs 1.6–4.7 μmol/24 hrs 6.2–22 μmol/24 hrs 0.6–3.1 μmol/24 hrs
31.	Pregnanetriol	<2.5 mg/24 hrs	<7.4 mmol/24 hrs
32.	Protein		
	Qualitative Quantitative	Negative 10 to 150 mg/24 hrs	Negative 10–150 mg/24 hrs
33.	Sodium	130–260 mEq/24 hrs	130–260 mmol/24 hrs
34.	Specific gravity	1.003–1.030	1.003–1.030
35.	Urate	200–500 mg/24 hrs	1.2–3.0 mmol/24 hrs
36.	Urobilinogen	<4.0 mg/24 hrs	<6.8 μmol/24 hrs
37.	Vanillylmandelic acid (VMA)		
	(4-hydroxy-3-methoxymandelic acid)	1–8 mg/24 hrs	5–40 μmol/24 hrs

SEMEN ANALYSIS

S. No.	*Test*	*Conventional units*	*SI units*
1.	Volume	2–5 mL	2–5 mL
2.	Liquefaction	Complete in 15 min	Complete in 15 min
3.	Leukocytes	Occasional or absent	Occasional or absent
4.	Count	60–150 million/mL	60–150 × 10^6/mL
5.	Motility	>80% motile	>0.80 motile
6.	Morphology	80–90% normal forms	0.80–0.90 normal forms
7.	Fructose	>150 mg/dL	>8.33 mmol/L

CEREBROSPINAL FLUID

S. No.	*Test*	*Conventional units*	*SI units*
1.	Cells	<5/mm^3, all mononuclear	<5 × 10/L, all mononuclear
2.	Protein electrophoresis	Albumin predominant	Albumin predominant
3.	Glucose	50–75 mg/dL (20 mg/dL. Less than in serum)	2.8–4.2 mmol/L (1.1 mmol less than in serum)
4.	IgG		
5.	Children <14 years	<8% of total protein	<0.08 of total protein
6.	Adults	<14% of total protein	<0.14 of total protein
7.	Ig Index	0.3–0.6	0.3–0.6
8.	CSF/serum IgG ratio		
9.	Oligoclonal banding on electrophoresis	Absent	Absent
10.	Pressure	70–180 mm H_2O	70–180 mm H_2O
11.	Protein, total	15–45 mg/dL	150–450 mg/L

VARIATIONS OF INVESTIGATION VALUES WITH NORMAL VALUES AND RESULTING DIAGNOSES

S. No.	Test name	Normal values	Increasing condition	Decreasing condition
1.	Acetone	Negative	Acetone (Ketone bodies) are found in the urine when the body's fat is metabolized for energy, producing an excess of metabolic end products. This occurs in an uncontrolled diabetes, starvation, severe infection accompanied by vomiting and diarrhea, pregnancy and lactation	
2.	Acid phosphatase	1–3 units/dL	Increased level of acid phosphatase indicates prostatic carcinoma, advanced Paget's disease, and hyperparathyroidism	
3.	Alkaline phosphatase	5–11 units/dL	Alkaline phosphatase is raised when there is an increase in the osteoblastic activity of bone, rickets, Paget's disease, myeloid leukemia, hyperparathyroidism, liver diseases, pregnancy and following ingestion of larger amounts of vitamin D	Hypothyroidism
4.	Amino (nitrogen) acids in blood	3.5–5.5 mg/dL	Liver disease	Severe burns
5.	Ammonia	80–110 µg; 9.5 and 49 µg per deciliter (µg/dL)	Hepatic necrosis	Terminal portal cirrhosis
6.	Aspartate transaminase (AST) (or) Serum glutamic oxaloacetic transaminase (SGOT) Alanine transaminase (ALT) (or) Serum glutamic pyruvic transaminase (SGPT)	Less than 40 IU/l	Both AST and ALT are released from damaged hepatic, cardiac and kidney muscles cells as seen in myocardial infarction and liver diseases	

Contd...

Contd...

S. No.	*Test name*	*Normal values*	*Increasing condition*	*Decreasing condition*
7.	Australia antigen	Negative	Positive results indicates viral hepatitis B	
8.	Bacteria	Nil	Presence of bacteria represents infection within the urinary tract	
9.	Basal metabolic rate (BMR)	Hyperthyroidism	Hypothyroidism	
10.	Basophils	0–1%	Chronic myeloid leukemia, polycythemia, vera, cirrhosis of liver, measles, chickenpox	
11.	Bence-Jones protein in urine	Nil	Bence Jones protein is precipitated between 40°C and 60°C, and it disappears when boiling point is reached. Bence-Jones protein is present in cases of multiple myeloma	
12.	Bicarbonates	23–31 mmol/L		
		23–31 mEq/L	Abnormal increase in the bicarbonates leads to metabolic alkalosis and a decrease in the hydrogen anion concentration of the plasma with a resultant rise in blood pH Increased in respiratory acidosis, emphysema of pneumonia	Abnormal decrease in the bicarbonates result in the decrease of blood pH due to metabolic acidosis. Metabolic acidosis is commonly seen in diabetes mellitus, hyperthyroidism, starvation, severe infections with fever, excessive vomiting which results in the accumulation of ketone bodies Decreased in respiratory alkalosis (Excessive respiration)

Contd...

Contd...

S. No.	*Test name*	*Normal values*	*Increasing condition*	*Decreasing condition*
13.	Bilirubin	0.3–1.1 mg/100 mL	Biliary obstruction (jaundice), chronic hepatitis	
14.	Bleeding time (BT)	1–6 minutes in adults	Prolonged bleeding time occurs in vascular purpuras, thrombocytopenia, chloroform and phosphorus poisoning, and after ingestion of aspirin tablets	
15.	Blood pH (hydrogen iron concentration)	7.35–7.45	Blood pH value is raised in vomiting, hyperpnea, fever, intestinal obstruction, etc.	It is decreased in uremia, acidosis, hemorrhage, nephritis, etc.
16.	Blood picture	Anisocytosis—nil Poikilocytosis—nil Microcytes—nil Macrocytes—nil Hypochromic cells—nil Nucleated—nil Erythrocytes—nil Sickle cells—nil Spherocytes—nil	Anisocytosis—nil anisocytosis—erythrocytes vary in size from normal—is seen in anemias Poikilocytosis tear shaped or club shape RBC seen in severe anemias Microcytes RBC small in size than normal and are seen in microcytic anemia and thalassemia major Macrocytes RBC large in size than normal and are seen in pernicious anemia and folic acid deficiency anemia Hypochromic cells—the RBC with abnormally low Hb content as seen in iron deficiency anemia Nucleated erythrocytes are seen in severe anemia Sickle cells are sickle shaped. RBC are found in sickle cell anemia Spherocytes—erythrocytes are relatively small and round rather than biconcave in shape and are seen in thalassemia major	

Contd...

Contd...

S. No.	*Test name*	*Normal values*	*Increasing condition*	*Decreasing condition*
17.	Blood sugar fasting	55–110 mg/dL postprandial (2 hours) 65–140 mg/dL	Blood sugar level is increased in nephritis, hyperthyroidism, pregnancy, uremia, infections, cerebral lesions, etc.	Blood sugar level is decreased in hyperinsulinism, hypothyroidism. Addison's diseases, extensive hepatic damage
18.	Blood urea	2.5–6.5 mmol/L (or)		
		20–40 mg/dL (or)		
		3.5–5.5 mmol/L	Increase in the blood urea indicates an impairment of renal functions	
19.	Bromsulphthalein test	Less than 5% retention of the dye at 45 minutes	Based on hepatic function	
20.	Casts	Nil	Presence of cast indicates tubular or glomerular diseases	
21.	Ceruloplasmin in serum	23–44 mg/dL	Wilson's disease (hepatocellular degeneration)	
22.	Chlorides	96–106 mEq/L	Acidosis	Vomiting
23.	Chronic gonadotropin (pregnancy test)	Negative	Positive results are seen in pregnancy, chorionepithelioma and hydatidiform mole	

Contd...

Contd...

S. No.	*Test name*	*Normal values*	*Increasing condition*	*Decreasing condition*
24.	Coagulation time (CT)	5–18 minutes in adults	The coagulation time is prolonged whenever there is a defect in the clotting mechanism. The important coagulation disorders are hemophilia, liver diseases, vitamin K deficiency, thrombocytopenia, hypofibrinogenemia, and in patients who receive anticoagulants	Coagulation time is reduced in typhoid, endocarditis
25.	Coomb's test	Direct Coomb's test—negative Indirect Coomb's test negative	Direct Coomb's test is used to test blood from the umbilical cord for the possible presence of erythroblastosis fetalis and to diagnose acquired hemolytic anemia. Indirect Coomb's test is to identify antibodies to erythrocyte antigens in the pregnant mother's serum or in patients developing transfusion reaction against Rh positive blood	
26.	Creatine phosphokinase (CPK)	Male: 5–55 mu/mL Female: 5–35 mu/mL	Myocardial infarction	Muscular dystrophy
27.	Creatinine	18 mmol/24 hrs 0.8–2 g/24 hrs	Increased levels are seen in typhoid fever, *Salmonella* infections, and tetanus degeneration of kidney Renal—diabetes, Cushing's syndrome	Decreased levels are seen in muscular atrophy, anemia, leukemia and advanced in degeneration of kidney

Contd...

Contd...

S. No.	*Test name*	*Normal values*	*Increasing condition*	*Decreasing condition*
28.	Differential WBC count	Polymorphonuclear cells: 50–70% Lymphocytes: 20–40% Monocytes: 4–8% Eosinophils: 0–2% Basophils: 0–1% Band forms: 3–5%	Neutrophilia (increased neutrophils) is found in pyogenic bacterial infections. The severity of the infection and the degree of response of the body are indicated by the degree of increase in neutrophils Lymphocytosis (increased lymphocytes) are seen in children, in certain infections (whooping cough, mumps, measles, influenza, syphilis, TB, typhoid etc.) and in lymphatic leukemia. Monocytosis are found in kala azar, typhpoid, TB, subacute bacterial endocarditis and malaria. Eosinophilia is found in parasitic infestations, allergic conditions and leukemia TB, typhoid, etc) and in lymphatic leukemia. Agranulocytosis (a marked decrease in the number of polymorphonuclear cells) is found in suppression of the bone marrow by drugs and radiation. Asthma, drug allergy, urticaria, bilharziasis, eczema, exfoliative dermatitis, Hodgkins' disease	Neutropenia (decreased neutrophils) are found in certain infections (typhoid, measles, influenza, etc.), anemia, and suppression of the bone marrow by various drugs and radiation. Lymphocytopenia (decreased lymphocytes) are seen in acute stages of infection and excessive radiation. Esonophenia–a plastic anemia. Systemic lupus erythematosus, Cushing's diseases, acromegaly
29.	Erythrocyte sedimentation rate (ESR)	Males: 0–9 mm/1st hour Females: 1–20 mm/1st hour	The ESR is increased in tissue destruction, whether inflammatory, or degenerative and during menstruation, pregnancy and in acute febrile disease	Polycythemia vera, congestive cardiac failure, whooping cough, dehydration

Contd...

Contd...

S. No.	*Test name*	*Normal values*	*Increasing condition*	*Decreasing condition*
30.	Erythrocytes	4.5–5.5 million/cmm	Erythrocyte count is increased in polycythemia vera, in cardiac and pulmonary disorders that are characterized by cyanosis	It is decreased in anemias
31.	Glucose (Fasting)	70–110 mg/100 mL	Diabetes, shock	Hypoglycemia, carcinoma of pancreas
32.	Glucose in CSF	50–75 mg/dL	Encephalitis, syphilis of CNS	Tuberculous, sarcoma, lymphoma
33.	Glucose tolerance test (GTT) oral	Fasting 55–110 mg/dL 1/2 hour—30–60 mg (above fasting) 1 hour—20–50 mg above fasting 2 hours—5–15 mg above fasting 3 hours—fasting level or below	Flat or inverted curve are seen in hyperinsulinism, adrenal cortical insufficiency, hypothyroidism, sprue and celiac diseases, anterior pituitary hypofunctioning	High or prolonged curve suggests diabetes mellitus, hyperthyroidism, adrenal cortical tumor, severe anemia, etc.
34.	Hemoglobin in plasma	Men 13–16 g% Women 12–15 g%	Hb is increased in sickle cell anemia, polycythemias and dehydration	Hb is decreased in hemo-dilution anemias and especially in thalassemia
35.	Icterus index, Protein bound iodine (PBI)	1–6 units 4.0–8.0 ug/dL	Increased in biliary obstruction, hemolytic anemias and hyperthyroidism	Decreased in hypothyroidism
36.	Inorganic phosphate (LDH)		Renal failure, diabetic ketosis	Fanconi syndrome in plasma

Contd...

Contd...

S. No.	*Test name*	*Normal values*	*Increasing condition*	*Decreasing condition*
37.	Iodine	3.5–8 μg/100 mL	Pregnancy, hyperthyroidism	Hypothyroidism
38.	Iron	75–175 mcg/100 mL	Aplastic anemia, hemosiderosis, pernicious anemia	Iron deficiency anemia, nephrosis, chronic renal insufficiency
39.	Lactic acid in blood	<1.2 mmol/L	Anemia	Diabetes
40.	Lactate dehydrogenase	100–140 U/L	Myocardial infarction	Acute hepatitis
41.	Leukocytes	4000–11000/cu mm of blood	Myeloid leukemia, emotional disturbances, bacterial infections, gout, diabetic coma, cirrhosis of liver, intestinal obstructions, uremia, malignant tumors, myocardial infarction	Typhoid fever, paratyphoid fever, brucellosis, miliary tuberculosis, measles, infective hepatitis, malaria, kala-azar, relapsing fever, aplastic anemia, megaloblastic anemia, multiple myeloma
42.	Lipase	0.2–1.5 units/mL	Increased in acute and chronic pancreatitis, biliary obstruction, cirrhosis, hepatitis and peptic ulcer	
43.	Lipids (total)	450–850 mg/dL	Diabetes	
44.	Lithium in serum	Therapeutic: 0.5–1.4 mmol/L Toxic: < 2.0 mmol/L	Psychiatric conditions	

Contd...

Contd...

S. No.	*Test name*	*Normal values*	*Increasing condition*	*Decreasing condition*
45.	Lymphocytes	20–35%	Chronic lymphatic leukemia, tuberculosis, syphilis, infective hepatitis, mumps, measles, chickenpox	Typhoid fever, subacute bacterial endocarditis, malaria, kala-azar, amebiasis, Hodgkin's disease
46.	Malarial parasite (MP)	Negative	Thin and thick smears are used for detecting malarial parasite and microfilaria	Vector control; insecticide, treated, mosquito nets and indoor spraying.
47.	Mean corpuscular hemoglobin (MCH)	27–32 pg	Macrocytic anemia	Hypochromic anemia
48.	Microfilaria (MF)	Negative		
49.	Nonprotein nitrogen (NPN)		Acute and chronic nephritis	
50.	Packed cell volume (PCV) or hematocrit	Men 40–54% Women 36–47%	Hematocrit is increased in polycythemia vera and in hemoconcentration resulting from blood loss, dehydration and shock	It is decreased in severe anemias, anemia of pregnancy, acute massive blood loss
51.	Phosphorus	2.5 to 4.5 mg/dL	Phosphorus is elevated in hypoparathyroidism, chronic nephritis, uremia, and alkalosis. There is an inverse relationship between serum calcium and serum phosphorus	Phosphorus is decreased in hyperparathyroidism, rickets, osteomalacia, steatorrhea

Contd...

Contd...

S. No.	*Test name*	*Normal values*	*Increasing condition*	*Decreasing condition*
52.	Platelet count	1–3.5 lakhs/cmm	Thrombocytosis is usually a symptomatic	Thrombocytopenia is found in acute leukemia, aplastic anemia, in idiopathic thrombocytopenic purpura and during cancer therapy
53.	Protein (urine albumin)	Negative	Albuminuria may be found in nephritis and nephrosis, febrile conditions, poisoning, eclampsia, hypertension, and some forms of cardiovascular diseases	
54.	Protein bound iodine (PBI)		Hyperthyroidism	Hypothyroidism
55.	Prothrombin time (PT)	60–100% of control blood 12–16 seconds	Prothrombin time is increased in liver diseases, vitamin K deficiency, fibrinogen deficiency, other hemorrhagic diseases and in cirrhosis, hepatic, and acute toxic necrosis of the liver. It is also prolonged in decumerol therapy	Blood clot more quickly than normal, disorders such as atrial fibrillation or blood clot in the leg or lung
56.	RBC	Nil	Hematuria often indicates pathology. It is found in glomerulonephritis, tuberculosis of the kidney, renal calculi, sickle cell anemia, tumors of the kidney, systemic lupus erythematosus, anticoagulation therapy, excessive use of analgesics, etc.	Aplastic anemia, cancer

Contd...

Contd...

S. No.	*Test name*	*Normal values*	*Increasing condition*	*Decreasing condition*
57.	Reticulocyte count	Adults—0.2–2% of the total erythrocyte count Infants—2–6% of the total erythrocyte count	Increase with any condition stimulating increase in bone marrow activity, i.e. infection, blood loss, following iron therapy in iron deficiency anemia, erythroblastosis fetalis	Decreased with any condition depressing bone marrow activity, such as leukemia, late stages of anemias
58.	Rheumatoid factor	Negative	The presence of rheumatoid factor may suggests the presence of rheumatoid arthritis, but it is not specific test for rheumatoid arthritis since they are found in other conditions also. A high titer of RF is indicative of a poor prognosis	A negative rheumatoid factor doesn't mean one doesn't have rheumatic arthritis
59.	Serum albumin	3.5–5.5. g/100 mL	Dehydration, hemoconcentration	Glomerulonephritis, leukemia, malnutrition, starvation
60.	Serum amylase	80–200 units/dL	When the serum amylase is elevated over 300 units, it indicates acute pancreatitis. It is also elevated in carcinoma of the head of pancreas, duodenal ulcer, mumps, etc. Elevation is not directly correlated with severity	Decreased in chronic pancreatitis, pancreatic fibrosis and atrophy, cirrhosis of liver, acute alcoholism and toxemia of pregnancy

Contd...

Contd...

S. No.	*Test name*	*Normal values*	*Increasing condition*	*Decreasing condition*
61.	Serum calcium	2.1–2.7 mmol/L 9–11 mg/dL	Calcium excess may be seen in cases of tumor or hyperplasia of parathyroid, hyperparathyroidism, multiple myeloma, hypervitaminosis-D, nephritis with uremia, etc. When the blood calcium levels become high, the serum phosphorus levels become low	Calcium deficit may occur in acute pancreatitis, accidental removal of parathyroid glands following thyroidectomy, diarrhea, celiac diseases, rickets, osteomalacia, malnutrition, nephrosis, renal disorders, pregnancy and lactation hypocalcemia is characterized by tetany
62.	Serum chloride	98–108 mmol/L 98–108 mEq/L	Chloride is elevated in nephritis, cardiac decompensation, urinary obstruction, etc.	Decreased in diarrhea, vomiting, Cushing's syndrome, burns, intestinal obstructions, febrile conditions, etc.
63.	Serum cholesterol	3.5–7.8 mmol/L 100–300 mg/dL	Cholesterol is elevated in cases of myxedema, hypothyroidism, arteriosclerosis and bile duct obstruction, physiological in pregnancy, obesity, nephrotic syndrome	Cholesterol is reduced when severe liver damage reduced the ability of the body to synthesize cholesterol, hyperthyroidism, anemia

Contd...

Contd...

S. No.	*Test name*	*Normal values*	*Increasing condition*	*Decreasing condition*
64.	Serum creatinine	55–125 umol/L 1–2 mg/dL	Increased serum levels of creatinine indicate decreased renal functions. It is more accurate indicator of renal functions tests	Testosterone treatment
65.	Serum fibrinogen	0.2–0.4 g/100 mL	Rheumatic fever, arthritis, glomerulonephritis	Typhoid, anemia, eclampsia of pregnancy, hypofibrinogenemia, liver failure, carcinoma of prostate
66.	Serum globulin	1.5–3 gm/130 mL	Multiple myeloma, infective hepatitis	Lymphatic leukemia
67.	Serum magnesium	108–3.0 mg/dL	Renal failure, liver disease	Chronic alcoholism, chronic hepatitis, hypervitaminosis D
68.	Serum potassium	3.4–5.4 mmol/L 3.4–5.4 mEq/L	Elevated potassium is seen in patients with renal failure, postoperative patients with a poor renal output, those with adrenocortical deficiency and intestinal obstruction with vomiting	Potassium deficit is seen in patients with poor dietary intake, excessive potassium loss due to diuretics, laxatives, gastric and intestinal suction, drainage from colostomies, excessive vomiting and diarrheas, fistulas of small and large intestines
69.	Serum proteins	6.0–8.0 g/dL	Diabetic acidosis, chronic inflammation, or electrophoresis, or tests for celiac disease	Liver disease

Contd...

Contd...

S. No.	*Test name*	*Normal values*	*Increasing condition*	*Decreasing condition*
70.	Serum sodium	135–146 mmol/L 135–146 mEq/L	Elevated serum sodium value (hypernatremia) indicates a state of hyperosmolality. It results from a water deficit or an extracellular solute overload	Lower sodium indicates hypo-osmality. It results from excessive water intake, excessive infusions, inability of the kidneys to excrete water, poor salt intake and excessive use of diuretics
71.	Serum thyroxine (T4)	4.5–11.5 ug/dL 70–160 nmol/L	Increased in hyperthyroidism, thyroiditis administration of oral contraceptives and pregnancy	Decreased in hypo-proteinemia nephrotic syndrome, primary and pituitary hypothyroidism, administration of androgenic and anabolic steroids, and mercurial diuretics
72.	Sodium, chloride, and potassium in sweat	Nil	To confirm cystic fibrosis of pancreas	Can cause cramps and constipation, people can also lose high level of sodium through diarrhea, life threatening paralysis may develop
73.	Thrombocytes	Below 150,000/cu mm	Polycythemia vera, thrombocythemia	Aplastic anemia, multiple myeloma, hypersplenism, megaloblastic anemia

Contd...

Contd...

S. No.	*Test name*	*Normal values*	*Increasing condition*	*Decreasing condition*
74.	Thymol turbidity	1– 4.5 units/mL	Increased in liver diseases, infectious diseases with antibody production	Cephalin flocculation reaction, obstructive or post-hepatic jaundice
75.	Total bilirubin	1.7–15.4 umol (or) 0.1–1.0 mg/dL 0.1–0.2 mg/dL (direct) 0.1–0.8 mg/dL (indirect)	Increased level of bilirubin is seen in case hemolytic anemia, obstructive jaundice, infective hepatitis, pernicious anemia, hemolytic disease of the newborn and eclampsia. In cases of infective hepatitis and obstructive jaundice, the direct bilirubin is high	
76.	Total protein, albumin, globulin A/G ratio	6–8 g/dL 3.5–5.5 g/dL 1.5–3 g/dL 1.5 : 1–2.5 : 1	A change in the A/G ratio indicates chronic hepatitis	Decreased level of plasma proteins indicates malnutrition, hemorrhage, loss of plasma from burns, proteinuria and liver damage
77.	Total WBC count	4500–11,000/mm^3	Leukocytosis (above 10,000/cmm) is found in children, in pregnancy, pyrexia infections, infestations, hemorrhage, and in leukemia	Leukopenia (less than 4,000/cmm) is found in certain infections (such as typhoid, influenza, TB, etc.) anemia, bone marrow depression and in cases of leukemic leukemia

Contd...

Contd...

S. No.	*Test name*	*Normal values*	*Increasing condition*	*Decreasing condition*
78.	Triglycerides	0.3–1.7 mmol/L 25–150 mg/dL	Hypothyroidism, diabetes mellitus, nephrotic syndrome, biliary obstruction	Malabsorption, malnutrition
79.	Tri-iodothyronine (T3)	1.1–2.6 nmol/L (or) 60–150 ng/dL	*Increased condition*: High blood pressure, comparative study of alternatives (T3) and Thyroin- a significant increase in T3 and T4 levels was observed. There have been reports on the clinical association between breast cancer …and T4 circulating in the blood reaches to the ovarian tissue causes Inflammation.	*Decreasing condition*: Several hemostatic abnormalities have been reported in hyper thyroidism levels of FT4, tri-iodothronine (T3) and thyrotropin (TSH).
80.	Urea (blood)	21–43 mg/100 mL	Renal failure	Severe liver disease
81.	Uric acid	0.1–0.4 mmol/L 2.5–8 mg/dL	Increased in gouty arthritis, acute leukemia, lymphomas treated by chemotherapy, and toxemias of pregnancy	Decreased in xanthinuria and defective tubular reabsorption
82.	Urine crystals	Nil	Presence of crystals in the urine is an important predisposing factor in calculus formation	
83.	Urine sugar	Negative	Sugar in the urine (glycosuria) is found in uncontrolled diabetes mellitus, pancreatic disorders and impaired tubular reabsorption. Glycosuria may normally result from eating a heavy meal or from emotional stress	

Contd...

Contd...

S. No.	*Test name*	*Normal values*	*Increasing condition*	*Decreasing condition*
84.	Urobilinogen	Random urine less than 25 mg/dL 24 hours urine in 6.7 umol/24 hrs	Increased level are seen in liver diseases, biliary tract diseases and hemolytic anemias. Reduced excretions are seen in complete or nearly complete biliary obstruction, diarrhea, renal insufficiency	
85.	WBC (urine)	Nil	The presence of WBC in the urine designates an infectious process somewhere in the urinary tract	
86.	Widal test	Typhoid 'O' negative Typhoid 'H' negative Typhoid 'A' negative Typhoid 'B' negative	Typhoid positive titer is 1:160 or more and paratyphoid positive titer is 1:80 or more	Lower titers may be regarded as negative
87.	17-hydroxycorticoids in urine	Male: 3–9 mg/24 hrs Female: 2–8 mg/24 hrs	Cushing's syndrome	

5 Radiology

INTRODUCTION

Radiology is the medical specialty concerned with the study of parts and functions of body by means of X-rays. Nuclear medicine (NM) is a specialty that deals with the characteristics and uses of radioactive substances in the diagnosis and treatment of diseases. Imaging is the latest form of visualizing the part of the body by means of ultrasonography (USG), computerized tomography (CT) and magnetic resonance imaging (MRI). X-rays are a special type of rays which can be absorbed by the body substance (e.g. calcium in bones), they do not reach the photographic plate held behind the patient, and white areas are left in the X-ray film. A substance is said to be radiolucent, if it permits most of the X-rays (lung tissue). Radiopaque substances (bones) are those absorb most of the X-rays.

X-RAYS

In the process of clinical diagnosis X-rays are used to assess the nature of bone fractures, dislocations, vertebral disk prolapse, cardiomegaly, pathological cavities in lungs, by plain X-rays. Radiopaque substances are used to diagnose bowel conditions, and blood vessels (barium enema, angiogram, and intravenous pyelogram).

Special Diagnostic Techniques

Fluoroscopy

This procedure uses a fluorescent screen instead of photographic plate to derive a visual image from the X-rays through the patient. Internal organs like heart, and digestive tracts can be absorbed in motion.

Contrast Technique

Radiopaque fluids of iodine compounds are used in special procedures namely cardioangiogram, arteriogram, venogram, bronchogram and cholecystogram.

Dye Injection

Radiopaque dyes are used in procedures like hysterosalpingogram, intravenous cholangiogram (IVC), intravenous pyelogram (IVP), lymph angiogram, myelogram, retrograde pyelogram and sialogram.

Imaging

Modern developments in biomedical technology have gifted latest diagnosis methods like ultrasonography, computed axial tomography scanning and magnetic resonance imaging.

Tomography

Tomography is a technique for taking series of X-ray pictures, so that X-rays of a desired layer of the body are obtained while at the same time structure in front of and behind that layer are blurred out. Computed tomography is a revolutionary technique in radiological diagnosis. CT scanners attached to computers synthesizes all information in many views in a single composite picture of a specific slide.

Magnetic Resonance Imaging

Sound waves and magnetic field images the parts of the body with high accuracy three dimensionally, the same as CT scan. It is widely used in investigating the disorders of brain and spinal cord.

Mammography

Mammography is used for identifying the malignant and hormonal disorders of breasts.

Ultrasonography

Sound waves are transmitted into specific parts of the human body, and it is imaged into live telecast of the functioning especially, uterus, liver, gallbladder, etc. to examine fetal conditions, abscess of the liver and lithiasis of gallbladder. The ultrasonography is the safe method free from radiation.

Nuclear Medicine

Alpha particles, beta particles, and gamma rays are used in nuclear medicine. Bone scanning Iodine-(^{131}I) uptakes are important nuclear medicine investigations. Nuclear medicines are therapeutically used to destroy tissues and stop the growth of malignant cells. Bone scanning is a specialty of nuclear medicine.

X-RADIATION

This article is about the form of radiation. For the method of imaging, *see* Radiography. For imaging in a medical context, *see* Radiology. For other uses, *see* X-ray (disambiguation) **(Fig. 5.1)**.

Hand mit Ringen (Hand with rings): Print of Roentgen's first 'medical' X-ray, of his wife's hand, taken on 22 December 1895 and presented to Professor Ludwig Zehnder of the Physik Institut, University of Freiburg, on 1 January 1896.

X-radiation (composed of X-rays) is a form of electromagnetic radiation. X-rays have a wavelength in the range of 10–0.01 nanometers, corresponding to frequencies in the range 30 pet hertz to 30 exahertz (3 $\times 10^{16}$ Hz to 3×10^{19} Hz) and energies in the range 120 eV–120 keV. They are shorter in wavelength than UV rays. In many languages, X-radiation is called Roentgen radiation after Wilhelm Conrad Roentgen, who is generally credited as their discoverer, and who had called them X-rays to signify an unknown type of radiation.

X-rays can penetrate solid objects, and their largest use is to take images of the inside of objects in diagnostic radiography and crystallography. As a result, the term X-ray is metonymically used to

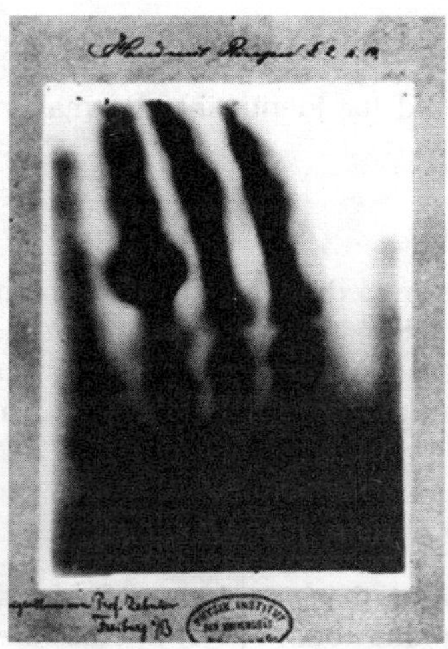

Fig. 5.1 Disambiguation

refer to a radiographic image produced using this method, in addition to the method itself. X-rays are a form of ionizing radiation, and exposure to them can be a health hazard.

X-rays from about 0.12–12 keV (10–0.10 nm wavelength), are classified as soft X-rays, and from about 12 to 120 keV (0.10–0.010 nm wavelength) as hard X-rays, due to their penetrating abilities.

The distinction between X-rays and gamma rays has changed in recent decades. Originally, the electromagnetic radiation emitted by X-ray tubes had a longer wavelength than the radiation emitted by radioactive nuclei (gamma rays). So older literature distinguished between X- and gamma radiation on the basis of wavelength, with radiation shorter than some arbitrary wavelength, such as 10–11 m, defined as gamma rays. However, as shorter wavelength continuous spectrum 'X-ray' sources such as linear accelerators and longer wavelength 'gamma ray' emitters were discovered, the wavelength bands largely overlapped. The two types of radiation are now usually distinguished by their origin: X-rays are emitted by electrons outside the nucleus, while gamma rays are emitted by the nucleus.

Units of Measure and Exposure

The measure of X-rays ionizing ability is called the exposure:

- The coulomb per kilogram (C/kg) is the SI unit of ionizing radiation exposure, and is the amount of radiation required to create 1 coulomb of charge of each polarity in 1 kilogram of matter.
- The Roentgen (R) is an obsolete traditional unit of exposure, which represented the amount of radiation required to create 1 esu of charge of each polarity in 1 cubic centimeter of dry air. 1 Roentgen = 2.58×10^{-4}C/kg.

However, the effect of ionizing radiation on matter (especially living tissue) is more closely related to the amount of energy deposited rather than the charge. This is called the absorbed dose:

- The gray (Gy), which has units of (J/kg), is the SI unit of absorbed dose, and is the amount of radiation required to deposit 1 joule of energy in 1 kilogram of any kind of matter.
- The rad is the (obsolete) corresponding traditional unit, equal to 0.01 J deposited per kg 100 rad = 1 Gy.

The equivalent dose is the measure of the biological effect of radiation on human tissue. For X-rays it is equal to the absorbed dose.

- The sievert (Sv) is the SI unit of equivalent dose, which for X-rays is numerically equal to the gray (Gy).
- The rem is the traditional unit of equivalent dose. For X-rays it is equal to the rad or 0.01 J of energy deposited per kg. 1 Sv = 100 rem.

Medical X-rays are a major source of *manmade* radiation exposure, accounting for 58% in the USA in 1987, but since most radiation exposure is natural (82%) it only accounts for 10% of total USA radiation exposure.

Reported dosage due to dental X-rays seems to vary significantly. Depending on the source, a typical dental X-ray of a human results in an exposure of perhaps, 3, 40, 300, or as many as 900 mrems (30–9,000 Sv).

Medical Physics

X-ray K-series spectral line wavelengths (nm) for some common target materials.

Target	$K\beta$	$K\beta$	$K\alpha$	$K\alpha$
Fe	0.17566	0.17442	0.193604	0.193998
Co	0.162079	0.160891	0.178897	0.179285
Ni	0.15001	0.14886	0.165791	0.166175
Cu	0.139222	0.138109	0.154056	0.154439
Zr	0.070173	0.068993	0.078593	0.079015
Mo	0.063229	0.062099	0.070930	0.071359

X-rays are generated by an X-ray tube, a vacuum tube that uses a high voltage to accelerate electrons released by a hot cathode to a high velocity. The high velocity electrons collide with a metal target, the anode, creating the X-rays. In medical X-ray tubes the target is usually tungsten or a more crack-resistant alloy of rhenium (5%) and tungsten (95%), but sometimes molybdenum for more specialized applications, such as when soft X-rays are needed as in mammography. In crystallography, a copper target is most common, with cobalt often being used when fluorescence from iron content in the sample might otherwise present a problem.

The maximum energy of the produced X-ray photon is limited by the energy of the incident electron, which is equal to the voltage on the tube, so an 80 kV tube cannot create X-rays with energy greater than 80 keV. When the electrons hit the target, X-rays are created by two different atomic processes:

1. *X-ray fluorescence:* If the electron has enough energy it can knock an orbital electron out of the inner shell of a metal atom, and as a result electrons from higher energy levels then fill-up the vacancy and X-ray photons are emitted. This process produces a discrete spectrum of X-ray frequencies, called spectral lines. The spectral lines generated depend on the target (anode) element used and thus are called characteristic lines. Usually these are transitions from upper shells into K shell (called K lines), into L shell (called L lines) and so on.

2. *Bremsstrahlung:* This is radiation given off by the electrons as they are scattered by the strong electric field near the high-Z (proton number) nuclei. These X-rays have a continuous spectrum. The intensity of the X-rays increases linearly with decreasing frequency, from zero at the energy of the incident electrons, the voltage on the X-ray tube.

So the resulting output of a tube consists of a continuous Bremsstrahlung spectrum falling off to zero at the tube voltage, plus several spikes at the characteristic lines. The voltages used in diagnostic X-ray tubes, and thus the highest energies of the X-rays, range from roughly 20–150 kV.

In medical diagnostic applications, the low energy (soft) X-rays are unwanted, since they are totally absorbed by the body, increasing the dose. So a thin metal (often aluminum, but can be one of many X-ray filters) sheet is placed over the window of the X-ray tube, filtering out the low energy end of the spectrum. This is called *hardening* the beam.

Both X-ray production processes are extremely inefficient (~1%) and thus to produce a usable flux of X-rays plenty of energy has to be wasted into heat, which has to be removed from the X-ray tube.

Radiographs obtained using X-rays can be used to identify a wide spectrum of pathologies. Due to their short wavelength, in medical applications, X-rays act more like a particle than a wave. This is in contrast to their application in crystallography, where their wave-like nature is most important.

To take an X-ray of the bones, short X-ray pulses are shot through a body with radiographic film behind. The bones absorb the most photons by the photoelectric process, because they are more electron-dense. The X-rays leave a latent image in the photographic film; when it is subsequently developed, the parts of the image corresponding to higher X-ray exposure are dark, leaving a white shadow of bones on the film.

To generate an image of the cardiovascular system, including the arteries and veins (angiography) an initial image is taken of the anatomical region of interest. A second image is then taken of the same region after iodinated contrast material has been injected into the blood vessels within this area. These two images are then digitally subtracted, leaving an image of only the iodinated contrast outlining the blood vessels. The radiologist or surgeon then compares the image obtained to normal anatomical images to determine if there is any damage or blockage of the vessel.

A specialized source of X-rays which is becoming widely used in research is synchrotron radiation, which is generated by particle accelerators. Its unique features are brightness many orders of magnitude greater than X-ray tubes, wide spectrum, high collimation, and linear polarization.

Detectors

Photographic Plate

The detection of X-rays is based on various methods. The most commonly known methods are a photographic plate, X-ray film in a cassette, and rare earth screens. Regardless of what is 'catching' the image, they are all categorized as 'Image Receptors' (IR).

Before computers and before digital imaging, a photographic plate was used to produce radiographic images. The images were produced right on the glass plates. Film replaced these plates and was used in hospitals to produce images. Now computed and digital radiography has started to replace film in medicine, though film technology remains in use in industrial radiography processes (e.g. to inspect welded seams). Photographic plates are a thing of history, and their replacement (intensifying screens) is now becoming part of that same history. Silver (necessary to the radiographic and photographic industry) is a nonrenewable resource, that has now been replaced by digital (DR) and computed (CR) technology. Where film required wet processing facilities, these new technologies do not. Archiving of these new technologies also saves space.

Since photographic plates are sensitive to X-rays, they provide a means of recording the image, but require a lot of exposure (to the patient), so intensifying screens were devised. They allow a lower dose to the patient, because the screens take the X-ray information and intensify it so that it can be recorded on film positioned next to the intensifying screen.

The part of the patient to be X-rayed is placed between the X-ray source and the image receptor to produce a shadow of the internal structure of that particular part of the body. X-rays are partially blocked ('attenuated') by dense tissues such as bone, and pass more easily through soft tissues. Areas where the X-rays strike darkens when developed, causing bones to appear lighter than the surrounding soft tissue.

Contrast compounds containing barium or iodine, which are radiopaque, can be ingested in the gastrointestinal tract (barium) or injected in the artery or veins to highlight these vessels. The contrast compounds have high atomic numbered elements in them that (like bone) essentially block the X-rays and hence the once hollow organ or vessel can be more readily seen. In the pursuit of a nontoxic contrast material, many types of high atomic number elements were evaluated. For example, the first time the forefathers used contrast it was chalk, and was used on a cadaver's vessels. Unfortunately, some elements chosen proved to be harmful—for example, thorium was once used as a contrast medium (Thorotrast)—which turned out to be toxic in some cases (causing injury and occasionally death from the effects of thorium poisoning). Modern contrast material has improved, and while there is no way to determine who may have sensitivity to the contrast, the incidence of 'allergic-type reactions' is low. The risk is comparable to that associated with penicillin.

PHOTOSTIMULABLE PHOSPHORS

An increasingly common method is the use of photostimulated luminescence (PSL), pioneered by Fuji in the 1980s. In modern hospitals a photostimulable phosphor plate (PSP plate) is used in place of the photographic plate. After the plate is X-rayed, excited electrons in the phosphor material remain 'trapped' in 'color centers' in the crystal lattice until stimulated by a laser beam passed over the plate surface. The light given off during laser stimulation is collected by a photomultiplier tube and the resulting signal is converted into a digital image by computer technology, which gives this process its common name, computed radiography (also referred to as digital radiography). The PSP plate can be reused, and existing X-ray equipment requires no modification to use them.

Geiger Counter

Initially, most common detection methods were based on the ionization of gases, as in the Geiger-Müller counter: a sealed volume, usually a cylinder, with a mica, polymer or thin metal window contains a gas, a cylindrical cathode and a wire anode; a high voltage is applied between the cathode and the anode. When an X-ray photon enters the cylinder, it ionizes the gas and forms ions and electrons. Electrons accelerate toward the anode, in the process causing further ionization along their trajectory. This process, known as a Townsend avalanche, is detected as a sudden current, called a 'count' or 'event'.

In order to gain energy spectrum information, a diffracting crystal may be used to first separate the different photons. The method is called wavelength dispersive X-ray spectroscopy (WDX or WDS). Position-sensitive detectors are often used in conjunction with dispersive elements. Other detection equipment that is inherently energy-resolving may be used, such as the aforementioned proportional counters. In either case, use of suitable pulse-processing (MCA) equipment allows digital spectra to be created for later analysis.

For many applications, counters are not sealed but are constantly fed with purified gas, thus reducing problems of contamination or gas aging. These are called "flow counters".

Scintillators

Some materials such as sodium iodide (NaI) can 'convert' an X-ray photon to a visible photon; an electronic detector can be built by adding a photomultiplier. These detectors are called 'scintillators', film screens or 'scintillation counters'. The main advantage of using these is that an adequate image can be obtained while subjecting the patient to a much lower dose of X-rays.

Image Intensification (Fig. 5.2)

X-rays are also used in 'real-time' procedures such as angiography or contrast studies of the hollow organs (e.g. barium enema of the small or large intestine) using fluoroscopy acquired using an X-ray image intensifier. Angioplasty, medical interventions of the arterial system rely heavily on X-ray-sensitive contrast to identify potentially treatable lesions.

Direct Semiconductor Detectors

Since the 1970s, new semiconductor detectors have been developed (silicon or germanium doped with lithium, Si (Li) or Ge (Li)). X-ray

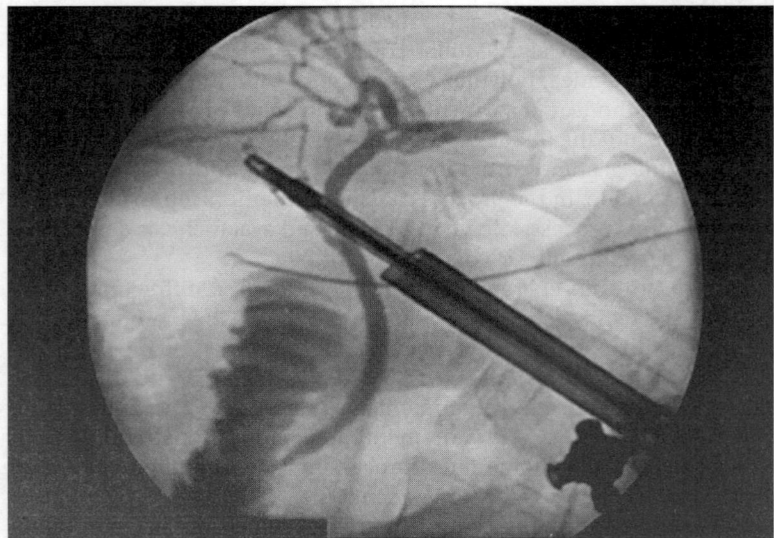

Fig. 5.2 X-ray during angioplasty

photons are converted to electron-hole pairs in the semiconductor and are collected to detect the X-rays. When the temperature is low enough (the detector is cooled by Peltier effect or even cooler liquid nitrogen), it is possible to directly determine the X-ray energy spectrum; this method is called energy dispersive X-ray spectroscopy (EDX or EDS); it is often used in small X-ray fluorescence spectrometers. These detectors are sometimes called 'solid state detectors'. Detectors based on cadmium telluride (CdTe) and its alloy with zinc, cadmium zinc telluride, have an increased sensitivity, which allows lower doses of X-rays to be used.

Practical application in medical imaging started in the 1990s. Currently amorphous selenium is used in commercial large area flat panel X-ray detectors for mammography and chest radiography. Current research and development is focused around pixel detectors, such as CERN's energy resolving Medipix detector.

Note: A standard semiconductor diode, such as a 1N4007, will produce a small amount of current when placed in an X-ray beam. A test device once used by Medical Imaging Service personnel was a small project box that contained several diodes of this type in series, which could be connected to an oscilloscope as a quick diagnostic.

Silicon drift detectors (SDDs)—produced by conventional semiconductor fabrication, now provide a cost-effective and high resolving power radiation measurement. Unlike conventional X-ray detectors, such as Si (Li), they do not need to be cooled with liquid nitrogen.

Scintillators Plus Semiconductor Detectors (Indirect Detection)

With the advent of large semiconductor array detectors it has become possible to design detector systems using a scintillators screen to convert from X-rays to visible light which is then converted to electrical signals in an array detector. Indirect Flat Panel Detectors (FPD) are in widespread use today in medical, dental, veterinary and industrial applications.

The array technology is a variant on the amorphous silicon TFT arrays used in many flat panel displays, like the ones in computer laptops. The array consists of a sheet of glass covered with a thin layer of silicon that is in an amorphous or disordered state. At a microscopic scale, the silicon has been imprinted with millions of transistors arranged in a highly ordered array, like the grid on a sheet of graph paper. Each of these thin film transistors (TFT) is attached to a light-absorbing photodiode making-up an individual pixel (picture element). Photons striking the photodiode are converted into two carriers of electrical charge, called electron-hole pairs. Since the number of charge carriers produced will vary with the intensity of incoming light photons, an electrical pattern is created that can be swiftly converted to a voltage and then a digital signal, which is interpreted by a computer to produce a digital image. Although silicon has outstanding electronic properties, it is not a particularly good absorber of X-ray photons. For this reason, X-rays first impinge upon scintillators made from, e.g. gadolinium oxysulfide or cesium iodide. The scintillators absorbs the X-rays and converts them into visible light photons that then pass onto the photodiode array.

Visibility to the Human Eye

While generally considered invisible to the human eye, in special circumstances X-rays can be visible. Brandes in an experiment a short time after Roentgen's landmark 1895 paper, reported after dark adaptation and placing his eye close to an X-ray tube seeing a faint 'blue-gray' glow which seemed to originate within the eye itself. Upon hearing this, Roentgen reviewed his record books and found he too had seen the effect. When placing an X-ray tube on the opposite side of a wooden door Roentgen had noted the same blue glow, seeming to emanate from the eye itself, but thought his observations to be spurious because he only saw the effect when he used one type of tube. Later he realized that the tube which had created the effect was the only one powerful enough to make the glow plainly visible and the experiment was thereafter readily repeatable. The knowledge that X-rays are actually faintly visible to the dark-adapted naked eye has largely been forgotten today; this is probably due to the desire not to repeat what would now be seen as a recklessly dangerous and potentially harmful experiment with ionizing radiation. It is not known what exact mechanism in the eye produces the visibility: it could be due to conventional detection (excitation of rhodopsin molecules in the retina), direct excitation of retinal nerve cells, or secondary detection via, for instance, X-ray induction of phosphorescence in the eyeball with conventional retinal detection of the secondarily produced visible light.

Though X-rays are otherwise invisible it is possible to see the ionization of the air molecules if the intensity of the X-ray beam is high enough. The beam line from the wiggler at the ID11 at ESRF is one example of such high intensity.

Medical Uses (Figs 5.3 and 5.4)

Since Roentgen's discovery that X-rays can identify bone structures, X-rays have been developed for their use in medical imaging. Radiology is a specialized field of medicine. Radiologists employ radiography

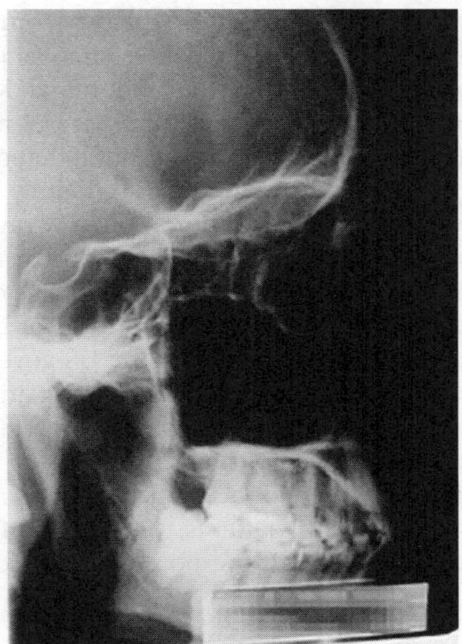

Fig. 5.3 X-ray image of the paranasal sinuses, lateral projection

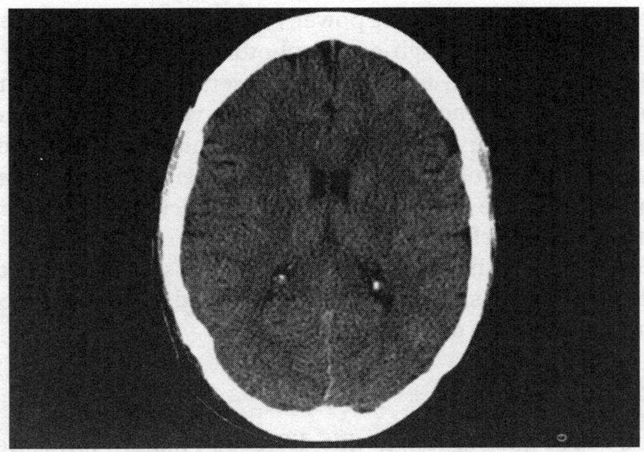

Fig. 5.4 Head CT scan slice—a modern application of X-rays

and other techniques for diagnostic imaging. This is probably the most common use of X-ray technology.

X-rays are especially useful in the detection of pathology of the skeletal system, but are also useful for detecting some disease processes in soft tissue. Some notable examples are the very common chest X-ray, which can be used to identify lung diseases such as pneumonia, lung cancer or pulmonary edema, and the abdominal X-ray, which can detect intestinal obstruction, free air (from visceral perforations) and free fluid (in ascites). X-rays may also be used to detect pathology such as gallstones (which are rarely radiopaque) or kidney stones which are often (but not always) visible. Traditional plain X-rays are less useful in the imaging of soft tissues such as the brain or muscle. Imaging alternatives for soft tissues are computed axial tomography (CAT or CT scanning), magnetic resonance imaging (MRI) or ultrasound. Since 2005, X-rays are listed as a carcinogen by the US government. The use of X-rays as a treatment is known as radiotherapy and is largely used for the management (including palliation) of cancer; it requires higher radiation energies than for imaging alone.

X-rays are a relatively safe method of investigation and the radiation exposure is low. But in pregnant patients, the benefits of the investigation (X-ray) should be balanced with the potential hazards to the unborn fetus.

Shielding Against X-rays

Lead is the most common shield against X-rays because of its high density (11340 kg/m^3), stopping power, ease of installation and low cost. The maximum range of a high-energy photon such as an X-ray in matter is infinite; at every point in the matter traversed by the photon, there is a probability of interaction. Thus there is a very small probability of no interaction over very large distances. The shielding of photon beam is, therefore, exponential (with an attenuation length being close to the radiation length of the material); doubling the thickness of shielding will square the shielding effect.

Table 5.1 shows the recommended thickness of lead shielding in function of X-ray energy, from the recommendations by the Second International Congress of Radiology:

Other Uses (Fig. 5.5)

Each dot, called a reflection, in this diffraction pattern forms from the constructive interference of scattered X-rays passing through a crystal. The data can be used to determine the crystalline structure.

Other Notable Uses of X-rays

- X-ray crystallography in which the pattern produced by the diffraction of X-rays through the closely spaced lattice of atoms in a crystal is

Table 5.1 Function of X-ray energy–recommended thickness of lead shielding

X-rays generated by peak voltages not exceeding	*Minimum thickness of lead*
75 kV	1.0 mm
100 kV	1.5 mm
125 kV	2.0 mm
150 kV	2.5 mm
175 kV	3.0 mm
200 kV	4.0 mm
225 kV	5.0 mm
300 kV	9.0 mm
400 kV	15.0 mm
500 kV	22.0 mm
600 kV	34.0 mm
900 kV	51.0 mm

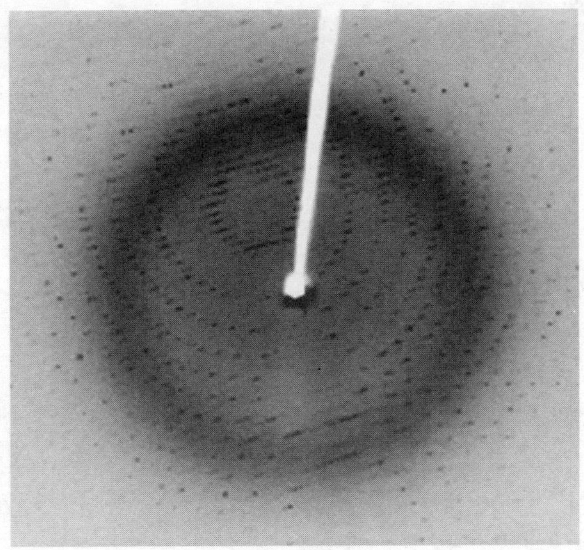

Fig. 5.5 Crystalline structure

recorded and then analyzed to reveal the nature of that lattice. A related technique, fiber diffraction, was used by Rosalind Franklin to discover the double helical structure of DNA.

- X-ray astronomy, which is an observational branch of astronomy, which deals with the study of X-ray emission from celestial objects.
- X-ray microscopic analysis, which uses electromagnetic radiation in the soft X-ray band to produce images of very small objects.
- X-ray fluorescence, a technique in which X-rays are generated within a specimen and detected. The outgoing energy of the X-ray can be used to identify the composition of the sample.
- Industrial radiography uses X-rays for inspection of industrial parts, particularly welds.
- Paintings are often X-rayed to reveal the under drawing and pentimenti or alterations in the course of painting, or by later restorers. Many pigments such as lead white show well in X-ray photographs.
- Airport security luggage scanners use X-rays for inspecting the interior of luggage for security threats before loading on aircraft.
- X-ray fine art photography.
- Roentgen stereophotogrammetry is used to track movement of bones based on the implantation of markers.
- X-ray photoelectron spectroscopy is a chemical analysis technique relying on the photoelectric effect, usually employed in surface science.

Form 1 X-ray request and report

Age Date

Type Of Request: Routine ☐ Emergency ☐ Transport: Wheelchair ☐ Trolley ☐

Allergies: Iodine ☐ Others ______
LNMP__________ Contraceptive Pill: Yes ☐ No ☐ Pregnant: Yes ☐ No ☐

Examination Required:

Brief Clinical Description: Provisional Diagnosis	Date and Time of X-ray Appointment

Previous X-ray

Patients Next Appointment with Clinic

Physician Signature Date

For Use of X-ray Department

Radiographer	Screening Time	X-ray No.
Checked by		

Position	KV	Mas	Total No. of Films

35×43		35×35		35×40		24×30		18×24		FNTAL		OCC

Report

Radiologist Signature Date

X-RAY REQUEST AND REPORT

Form 2 Ultrasound examination form

Age: ______ Nationality: ______ Date and Time Admission: ______

LMP (Arabic)

English ______ Cycle ______ Pill ______ Parity ______

Past History	☐ Twins	☐ Cong Abnor	☐ Type
Family History	☐	☐	☐

Present History ☐ Diabetes ☐ Rh. ☐ Heart Disease ☐ APII ______
☐ Pre-eclampsia ☐ Others
Uterus by Date Presentation
Uterus by Size

Palpation ☐ F M F ☐ F H H
☐ Others ☐ Others

Other Exam Required

Information Requested

Physician ______ Signature ______ Date ______

Serial/Repeat Scan Request		Appointment		
Date	Signature	Date	Time	Signature
		1. ______		
		2. ______		
		3. ______		
		4. ______		

Report

______

______

______

______

______

Physician ______ Signature ______ Date ______

ULTRASOUND EXAM FORM

Form 3 Radiological consultation request/report

RADIOLOGIC CONSULTATION REQUEST/REPORT
(Radiology/Nuclear Medicine/Ultrasound/Computer Tomography Examinations)

<table>
<tr><td rowspan="4">Examination Requested</td><td>Age</td><td>sex</td><td>SSN (Sponsor)</td><td>Ward/Clinic</td><td>Register No.</td></tr>
<tr><td colspan="4">Film No.</td><td>Pregnant
☐ Yes ☐ No</td></tr>
<tr><td colspan="4">Requested by (print)</td><td>Telephone/Page No.</td></tr>
<tr><td colspan="4">Signature of Requestor</td><td>Date Requested</td></tr>
<tr><td colspan="6">Specific Reason for Request (Complaints and findings)</td></tr>
</table>

Date of Examination (Month, day, year)	Date of Report (Month, day, year)	Date of Transaction (Month, day, year)
Radiologic Report		

<table>
<tr><td rowspan="4">Patients Identification (For typed or written entries give Name-last, first, middle, medical facility)</td><td>Location of Medical Records</td></tr>
<tr><td>Location of Radiologic Facility</td></tr>
<tr><td>Signature</td></tr>
<tr><td>Radiological Consultation
Request/Report
2 - Physician</td></tr>
</table>

6 Radiation Therapy

INTRODUCTION

Radiation therapy (in North America), or *radiotherapy* (in the UK and Australia) also called *radiation oncology*, and sometimes abbreviated to external beam radiotherapy (XRT), is the medical use of ionizing radiation as part of cancer treatment to control malignant cells (not to be confused with radiology, the use of radiation in medical imaging and diagnosis). Radiotherapy may be used for curative or adjuvant cancer treatment. It is used as palliative treatment (where cure is not possible and the aim is for local disease control or symptomatic relief) or as therapeutic treatment (where the therapy has survival benefit and it can be curative). Total body irradiation (TBI) is a radiotherapy technique used to prepare the body to receive a bone marrow transplant. Radiotherapy has several applications in non-malignant conditions, such as the treatment of trigeminal neuralgia, severe thyroid eye disease, pterygium, pigmented villonodular synovitis, prevention of keloid scar growth, and prevention of heterotopic ossification. The use of radiotherapy in nonmalignant conditions is limited partly by worries about the risk of radiation-induced cancers.

Radiotherapy is used for the treatment of malignant tumors (cancer), and may be used as the primary therapy. It is also common to combine radiotherapy with surgery, chemotherapy, hormone therapy or some mixture of the three. Most common cancer types can be treated with radiotherapy in some way. The precise treatment intent (curative, adjuvant, neoadjuvant, therapeutic, or palliative) will depend on the tumor type, location, and stage, as well as the general health of the patient.

Radiation therapy is commonly applied to the cancerous tumor. The radiation fields may also include the draining lymph nodes if they are clinically or radiologically involved with tumor, or if there is thought to be a risk of subclinical malignant spread. It is necessary to include a margin of normal tissue around the tumor to allow for uncertainties in daily set-up and internal tumor motion. These uncertainties can be caused by internal movement (for example, respiration and bladder filling) and movement of external skin marks relative to the tumor position.

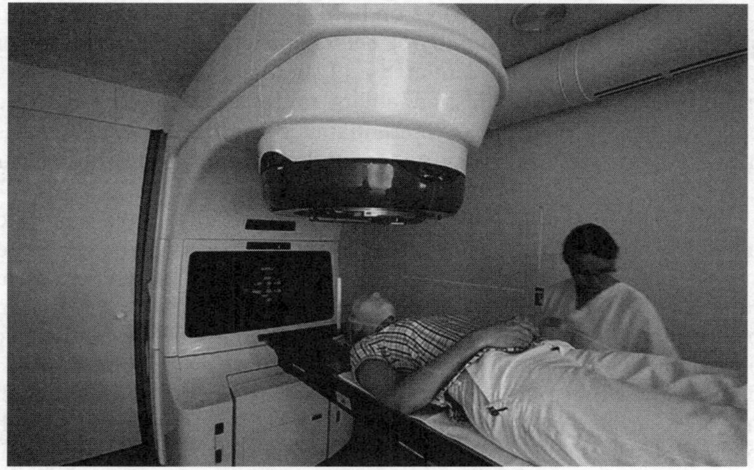

Fig 6.1 Varian Clinac 2100C Linear Accelerator (*For color version, see Plate 1*)

To spare normal tissues (such as skin or organs which radiation must pass through in order to treat the tumor), shaped radiation beams are aimed from several angles of exposure to intersect at the tumor, providing a much larger absorbed dose there than in the surrounding, healthy tissue.

Varian Clinac 2100C Linear Accelerator which is mostly widely selected medical accelerator in the world, treating thousands of patients everyday for treatment of radiology oncology practices. Clinicians around the world depend on Varian system to deliver treatment at the right-time-the instant the tumor is on target. The variant clinac delivers the exact prescribed dose to the patient in the lowest number of monitor units (MUs) possible. Whether it is day-to-day repositioning of the patient or managing motion during treatment. With this machine, clinicians can personalize each patient's care based on their needs and individual clinical protocol **(Fig. 6.1)**.

MECHANISM OF ACTION

Radiation therapy works by damaging the DNA of cells. The damage is caused by a photon, electron, proton, neutron, or ion beam directly or indirectly ionizing the atoms which make up the DNA chain. Indirect ionization happens as a result of the ionization of water, forming free radicals, notably hydroxyl radicals, which then damage the DNA. In the most common forms of radiation therapy, most of the radiation effect is through free radicals. Because cells have mechanisms for repairing

DNA damage, breaking the DNA on both strands proves to be the most significant technique in modifying cell characteristics. Because cancer cells generally are undifferentiated and stem cell-like, they reproduce more, and have a diminished ability to repair sub-lethal damage compared to most healthy differentiated cells. The DNA damage is inherited through cell division, accumulating damage to the cancer cells, causing them to die or reproduce more slowly.

One of the major limitations of radiotherapy is that the cells of solid tumors become deficient in oxygen. Solid tumors can outgrow their blood supply, causing a low-oxygen state known as hypoxia. Oxygen is a potent radiosensitizer, increasing the effectiveness of a given dose of radiation by forming DNA-damaging free radicals. Tumor cells in a hypoxic environment may be as much as 2 to 3 times more resistant to radiation damage than those in a normal oxygen environment. Much research has been devoted to overcoming this problem including the use of high pressure oxygen tanks, blood substitutes that carry increased oxygen, hypoxic cell radiosensitizers such as misonidazole and metronidazole, and hypoxic cytotoxins, such as tirapazamine. There is also interest in the fact that high-LET (linear energy transfer) particles such as carbon or neon ions may have an antitumor effect which is less dependent of tumor oxygen because these particles act mostly via direct damage.

DOSE

The amount of radiation used in radiation therapy is measured in gray (Gy), and varies depending on the type and stage of cancer being treated. For curative cases, the typical dose for a solid epithelial tumor ranges from 60 to 80 Gy, while lymphoma tumors are treated with 20–40 Gy.

Preventive (adjuvant) doses are typically around 45–60 Gy in 1.8–2 Gy fractions (for Breast, Head and Neck cancers respectively). Many other factors are considered by radiation oncologists when selecting a dose, including whether the patient is receiving chemotherapy, whether radiation therapy is being administered before or after surgery, and the degree of success of surgery.

Radiation therapy plans are often evaluated using dose-volume histograms, which allow the clinician to assess the uniformity of the dose to the diseased tissue (tumor) and how well healthy structures are spared.

Fractionation

The total dose is fractionated (spread out over time) for several important reasons. Fractionation allows normal cells time to recover, while tumor cells are generally less efficient in repair between fractions. Fractionation also allows tumor cells that were in a relatively radio-resistant phase of the cell cycle during one treatment to cycle into a sensitive phase of the cycle before the next fraction is given. Similarly, tumor cells that were chronically or acutely hypoxic (and therefore more radioresistant) may reoxygenate between fractions, improving the tumor cell kill. Fractionation regimes are individualized between different radiotherapy centers and even between individual doctors. In North America, Australia, and Europe, the typical fractionation schedule for adults is 1.8–2 Gy per day, five days a week. In the northern United Kingdom, fractions are more commonly 2.67–2.75 Gy per day, which eases the burden on thinly spread resources in the National Health Service. In some cancer types, prolongation of the fraction schedule over too long can allow for the tumor to begin repopulating, and for these tumor types, including head-and-neck and cervical squamous cell cancers, radiation treatment is preferably completed within a certain amount of time. For children, a typical fraction size may be 1.5–1.8 Gy per day, as smaller fraction sizes are associated with reduced incidence and severity of late-onset side effects in normal tissues.

In some cases, two fractions per day are used near the end of a course of treatment. This schedule, known as a concomitant boost regimen or hyper fractionation, is used on tumors that regenerate more quickly when they are smaller. In particular, tumors in the head-and-neck demonstrate this behavior.

One of the best-known alternative fractionation schedules is continuous hyper fractionated accelerated radiotherapy (CHART). CHART, used to treat lung cancer, consists of three smaller fractions per day. Although reasonably successful, CHART can be a strain on radiation therapy departments.

Implants can be fractionated over minutes or hours, or they can be permanent seeds which slowly deliver radiation until they become inactive.

EFFECT ON DIFFERENT TYPES OF CANCER

Different cancers respond differently to radiation therapy. The response of a cancer to radiation is described by its radiosensitivity. Highly radiosensitive cancer cells are rapidly killed by modest doses of radiation. These include leukemia's, most lymphomas and germ cell tumors. The majority of epithelial cancers are only moderately radiosensitive, and require a significantly higher dose of radiation (60–70 Gy) to achieve a radical cure. Some types of cancer are notably radioresistant, that is, much higher doses are required to produce a radical cure than may be safe in clinical practice. Renal cell cancer and melanoma are generally considered to be radioresistant.

It is important to distinguish the radiosensitivity of a particular tumor, which to some extent is a laboratory measure, from the radiation 'curability' of a cancer in actual clinical practice. For example, leukemia's are not generally curable with radiotherapy, because they are disseminated though the body. Lymphoma may be radically curable if it is localized to one area of the body. Similarly, many of the common, moderately radio responsive tumors are routinely treated with curative doses of radiotherapy if they are at an early stage. For example, non-melanoma skin cancer, head and neck cancer, nonsmall cell lung cancer, cervical cancer, anal cancer, prostate cancer. Metastatic cancers are generally incurable with radiotherapy because it is not possible to treat the whole body.

Before treatment, a CT scan is often performed to identify the tumor and surrounding normal structures. The patient is then sent for a simulation so that molds can be created to be used during treatment. The patient receives small skin marks to guide the placement of treatment fields.

The response of a tumor to radiotherapy is also related to its size. For complex reasons, very large tumors respond less well to radiation than smaller tumors or microscopic disease. Various strategies are used to overcome this effect. The most common technique is surgical resection prior to radiotherapy. This is most commonly seen in the treatment of breast cancer with wide local excision or mastectomy followed by adjuvant radiotherapy. Another method is to shrink the tumor with neoadjuvant chemotherapy prior to radical radiotherapy. A third technique is to enhance the radiosensitivity of the cancer by giving certain drugs during a course of radiotherapy. Examples of radiosensitizing drugs include: cisplatin, nimorazole and cetuximab.

TYPES OF RADIATION THERAPY

Historically, the three main divisions of radiotherapy are external beam radiotherapy (EBRT or XBRT) or teletherapy, brachytherapy or sealed source radiotherapy, and systemic radioisotope therapy or unsealed source radiotherapy. The differences relate to the position of the radiation source; external is outside the body, brachytherapy uses sealed radioactive sources placed precisely in the area under treatment, and systemic radioisotopes are given by infusion or oral ingestion. Brachytherapy can use temporary or permanent placement of radioactive sources. The temporary sources are usually placed by a technique called after loading. In after loading a hollow tube or applicator is placed surgically in the organ to be treated, and the sources are loaded into the applicator after the applicator is implanted. This minimizes radiation exposure to healthcare personnel. Particle therapy is a special case of external beam radiotherapy where the particles are protons or heavier ions. Interpretative radiotherapy is a special type of radiotherapy that is delivered immediately after surgical removal of the cancer. This method has been employed in breast cancer (targeted interpretative radiotherapy), brain tumor and rectal cancers.

External Beam Radiotherapy

The following three sections refer to treatment using X-rays:

Conventional External Beam Radiotherapy

Conventional external beam radiotherapy (2DXRT) is delivered via two-dimensional beams using linear accelerator machines. 2DXRT mainly consists of a single beam of radiation delivered to the patient from several directions: often front or back, and both sides. *Conventional* refers to the way the treatment is *planned* or *simulated* on a specially calibrated diagnostic X-ray machine known as a simulator because it recreates the linear accelerator actions (or sometimes by eye), and to the usually well-established arrangements of the radiation beams to achieve a desired *plan.* The aim of simulation is to accurately target or localize the volume which is to be treated. This technique is well-established and is generally quick and reliable. The worry is that some high-dose treatments may be limited by the radiation toxicity capacity of healthy tissues which lay close to the target tumor volume. An example of this problem is seen in radiation of the prostate gland, where the sensitivity of the adjacent rectum limited the A detector system for imaging radiotherapeutic dose distributions in 4D dose which could be safely prescribed using 2DXRT planning to such an extent that tumor control may not be easily achievable. Prior to the invention of the CT, physicians and physicists had limited knowledge about the true radiation dosage delivered to both cancerous and healthy tissue. For this reason, 3-dimensional conformal radiotherapy is becoming the standard treatment for a number of tumor sites.

Stereotactic Radiation

Stereotactic radiation is a specialized type of external beam radiation therapy. It uses focused radiation beams targeting a well-defined tumor using extremely detailed imaging scans. Radiation oncologists perform stereotactic treatments, often with the help of a neurosurgeon for tumors in the brain or spine.

There are two types of stereotactic radiation. Stereotactic radio surgery (SRS) is when doctors use a single or several stereotactic radiation treatments of the brain or spine. *Stereotactic bodyradiation therapy* (SBRT) refers to one or several stereotactic radiation treatments with the body, such as the lungs.

Some doctors say an advantage to stereotactic treatments are they deliver the right amount of radiation to the cancer in a shorter amount of time than traditional treatments, which can often take 6–11 weeks. Plus treatments are given with extreme accuracy, which should limit the effect of the radiation on healthy tissues. One problem with stereotactic treatments is that they are only suitable for certain small tumors.

Stereotactic treatments can be confusing because many hospitals call the treatments by the name of the manufacturer rather than calling it SRS or SBRT. Brand names for these treatments include axesse, cyber knife, Gamma knife, novalis, prim atom, synergy, X-knife, tomotherapy and trilogy. This list changes as equipment manufacturers continue to develop new, specialized technologies to treat cancers.

Virtual Simulation, Three-dimensional Conformal Radiotherapy, and Intensity-modulated Radiotherapy

The planning of radiotherapy treatment has been revolutionized by the ability to delineate tumors and adjacent normal structures in three dimensions using specialized CT and/or MRI scanners and planning software.

Virtual simulation, the most basic form of planning, allows more accurate placement of radiation beams than is possible using conventional X-rays, where soft-tissue structures are often difficult to assess and normal tissues difficult to protect.

An enhancement of virtual simulation is 3-Dimensional Conformal Radiotherapy (3-DCRT), in which the profile of each radiation beam is shaped to fit the profile of the target from a beam's eye view (BEV) using a multileaf collimator (MLC) and a variable number of beams. When the treatment volume conforms to the shape of the tumor, the relative toxicity of radiation to the surrounding normal tissues is reduced, allowing a higher dose of radiation to be delivered to the tumor than conventional techniques would allow.

Intensity-modulated radiation therapy (IMRT) is an advanced type of high-precision radiation that is the next generation of 3-DCRT. IMRT also improves the ability to conform the treatment volume to concave tumor shapes, for example when the tumor is wrapped around a vulnerable structure such as the spinal cord or a major organ or blood vessel. Computer-controlled X-ray accelerators distribute precise radiation doses to malignant tumors or specific areas within the tumor. The pattern of radiation delivery is determined using highly-tailored computing applications to perform optimization and treatment simulation (treatment planning). The radiation dose is consistent with the 3-D shape of the tumor by controlling, or modulating, the radiation beam's intensity. The radiation dose intensity is elevated near the gross tumor volume while radiation among the neighboring normal tissue is decreased or avoided completely. The customized radiation dose is intended to maximize tumor dose while simultaneously protecting the surrounding normal tissue. This may result in better tumor targeting, lessened side effects, and improved treatment outcomes than even 3-DCRT.

3-DCRT is still used extensively for many body sites but the use of IMRT is growing in more complicated body sites such as CNS, head and neck, prostate, breast and lung. Unfortunately, IMRT is limited by its need for additional time from experienced medical personnel. This is because physicians must manually delineate the tumors one CT image at a time through the entire disease site which can take much longer than 3-DCRT preparation. Then, medical physicists and dosimetrists must be engaged to create a viable treatment plan. Also, the IMRT technology has only been used commercially since the late 1990s even at the most advanced cancer centers, so radiation oncologists who did not learn it as part of their residency program must find additional sources of education before implementing IMRT.

Proof of improved survival benefit from either of these two techniques over conventional radiotherapy (2-DXRT) is growing for many tumor sites, but the ability to reduce toxicity is generally accepted. Both techniques enable dose escalation, potentially increasing usefulness. There has been some concern, particularly with 3-DCRT, about increased exposure of normal tissue to radiation and the consequent potential for secondary malignancy. Overconfidence in the accuracy of imaging may increase the chance of missing lesions that are invisible on the planning scans (and therefore not included in the treatment plan) or that move between or during a treatment (for example, due to respiration or inadequate patient immobilization). New techniques are being developed to better control this uncertainty—for example, real-time imaging combined with real-time adjustment of the therapeutic beams. This new technology is called image-guided radiation therapy (IGRT) or four-dimensional radiotherapy.

Particle Therapy

In particle therapy (Proton therapy), energetic ionizing particles (protons or carbon ions) are directed at the target tumor. The dose increases while the particle penetrates the tissue, up to a maximum (the Bragg peak) that occurs near the end of the particle's range, and it then drops to (almost) zero. The advantage of this energy deposition profile is that less energy is deposited into the healthy tissue surrounding the target tissue.

Radioisotope Therapy

Systemic radioisotope therapy (RIT) is a form of targeted therapy. Targeting can be due to the chemical properties of the isotope such as radioiodine which is specifically absorbed by the thyroid gland a thousand fold better than other bodily organs. Targeting can also be achieved by attaching the radioisotope to another molecule or antibody to guide it to the target tissue. The radioisotopes are delivered through infusion (into the bloodstream) or ingestion. Examples are the infusion of metaiodobenzylguanidine (MIBG) to treat neuroblastoma, of oral iodine-131 to treat thyroid cancer or thyrotoxicosis, and of hormone-bound lutetium-177 and yttrium-90 to treat neuroendocrine tumors (peptide receptor radionuclide therapy). Another example is the injection of radioactive glass or resin microspheres into the hepatic artery to radioembolize liver tumors or liver metastases.

A major use of systemic radioisotope therapy is in the treatment of bone metastasis from cancer. The radioisotopes travel selectively to areas of damaged bone, and spare normal undamaged bone. Isotopes commonly used in the treatment of bone metastasis are strontium-89 and samarium (^{153}Sm) lexidronam. In 2002, the United States Food and Drug Administration (FDA) approved ibritumomab tiuxetan (Zevalin), which is an anti-CD20 monoclonal antibody conjugated to yttrium-90. In 2003, the FDA approved the tositumomab/iodine (^{131}I) tositumomab regimen (Bexxar), which is a combination of an iodine-131 labeled and an unlabeled anti-CD20 monoclonal antibody. These medications were the first agents of what is known as radioimmunotherapy, and they were approved for the treatment of refractory non-Hodgkin's lymphoma.

Side Effects

Radiation therapy is in itself painless. Many low-dose palliative treatments (for example, radiotherapy to bony metastases) cause minimal or no side effects, although short-term pain flare up can be experienced in the days following treatment due to edema compressing nerves in the treated area. Treatment to higher doses causes varying side effects during treatment (acute side effects), in the months or years following treatment (long-term side effects), or after retreatment (cumulative side effects). The nature, severity, and longevity of side effects depends on the organs that receive the radiation, the treatment itself (type of radiation, dose, fractionation, concurrent chemotherapy), and the patient.

Most side effects are predictable and expected. Side effects from radiation are usually limited to the area of the patient's body that is under treatment. One of the aims of modern radiotherapy is to reduce side effects to a minimum, and to help the patient to understand and to deal with those side effects which are unavoidable.

The main side effects reported are fatigue and skin irritation, like a mild to moderate sun burn. The fatigue often sets in during the middle of a course of treatment and can last for weeks after treatment ends. The skin irritation will also go away, but it may not be as elastic as it was before. Patients should ask their radiation oncologist or radiation oncology nurse about possible products and medications that can help with side effects.

Acute Side Effects

Damage to the epithelial surfaces: Epithelial surfaces may sustain damage from radiation therapy. Depending on the area being treated, this may include the skin, oral mucosa, pharyngeal, bowel mucosa and ureter. The rates of onset of damage and recovery from it depend upon the turnover rate of epithelial cells. Typically the skin starts to become pink and sore several weeks into treatment. The reaction may become more severe during the treatment and for up to about one week following the end of radiotherapy, and the skin may breakdown. Although this moist desquamation is uncomfortable, recovery is usually quick. Skin reactions tend to be worse in areas where there are natural folds in the skin, such as underneath the female breast, behind the ear and in the groin.

If the head and neck area is treated, temporary soreness and ulceration commonly occur in the mouth and throat. If severe, this can affect swallowing, and the patient may need painkillers and nutritional support/food supplements. The esophagus can also become sore if it is treated directly, or if, as commonly occurs; it receives a dose of collateral radiation during treatment of lung cancer.

The lower bowel may be treated directly with radiation (treatment of rectal or anal cancer) or be exposed by radiotherapy to other pelvic structures (prostate, bladder, female genital tract). Typical symptoms are soreness, diarrhea, and nausea.

Swelling (edema): As part of the general inflammation that occurs, swelling of soft tissues may cause problems during radiotherapy. This is a concern during treatment of brain tumors and brain metastases, especially where there is pre-existing raised intracranial pressure or where the tumor is causing near-total obstruction of a lumen (e.g. trachea or main bronchus). Surgical intervention may be considered prior to treatment with radiation. If surgery is deemed unnecessary or inappropriate, the patient may receive steroids during radiotherapy to reduce swelling.

Infertility: The gonads (ovaries and testicles) are very sensitive to radiation. They may be unable to produce gametes following direct exposure to most normal treatment doses of radiation. Treatment planning for all body sites is designed to minimize, if not completely exclude dose to the gonads if they are not the primary area of treatment.

Medium and long-term side effects: These depend on the tissue that received the treatment; they may be minimal.

Fibrosis: Tissues which have been irradiated tend to become less elastic over time due to a diffuse scarring process.

Hair loss: This may be most pronounced in patients who have received radiotherapy to the brain. Unlike the hair loss seen with chemotherapy, radiation-induced hair loss is more likely to be permanent, but is also more likely to be limited to the area treated by the radiation.

Dryness: The salivary glands and tear glands have a radiation tolerance of about 30 Gy in 2 Gy fractions, a dose which is exceeded by most radical head and neck cancer treatments. Dry mouth (xerostomia) and dry eyes (exophthalmia) can become irritating long-term problems and severely reduce the patient's quality of life. Similarly, sweat glands in treated skin (such as the armpit) tend to stop working, and the naturally moist vaginal mucosa is often dry following pelvic irradiation.

Fatigue: Fatigue is among the most common symptoms of radiation therapy, and can last from a few months to a few years, depending on the quantity of the treatment and cancer type. Lack of energy, reduced activity and overtired feelings are common symptoms.

Cancer: Radiation is a potential cause of cancer, and secondary malignancies are seen in a very small minority of patients, generally many years after they have received a course of radiation treatment. In the vast majority of cases, this risk is greatly outweighed by the reduction in risk conferred by treating the primary cancer.

Death: Radiation has potentially excess risk of death from heart disease seen after some past breast cancer RT regimens.

Cognitive decline: In cases of radiation applied to the head radiation therapy can cause cognitive decline.

Cumulative side effects: Cumulative effects from this process should not be confused with long-term effects—when short-term effects have disappeared and long-term effects are sub clinical, reirradiation can still be problematic.

Form 1 Radiotherapy treatment sheet

Medical Record #:
Hospital Name :
Patient Name :
Date of Birth :
Attending Physician :
Date of Admission :

☐ OPD
☐ IPD

Radiotherapy Treatment Sheet
SR-90 Brachytherapy Application

DIAGNOSIS	

TOTAL PRESCRIBED DOSE (cGy)	
NUMBER OF FRACTIONS	

TOTAL ACTIVITY USED	
DOSE RATE SECOND (cGy/sec)	
TOTAL TIME REQUIRED (sec)	
TIME PER FRACTIONS (sec)	
DOSE PER FRACTION (cGy)	

DATE	FR NO	TIME (sec)	DOSE (cGy)	CUM DOSE (cGy)

Comments

Medical physicist Date

Radiotherapist Date

HOS-08-0002-01 Oncology/Radiotherapy Treatment Sheet SR-90 Brachytherapy Application

Form 2 Radiation therapy (thoracic) form

RADIATION THERAPY (THORACIC) FORM

Name Age Sex Service Ward Bed		Mar. Status Hos. No Occ. Religion Income
DIAGNOSIS: Location:		PALLATIVE/CURATIVE Biopsy Report No. Date, etc.

S1. N0.	Date	Dose given	Total Dose	Diagnostic Radiology Comment	Radiotherapists Comment	Clinicians Comments (including counts) symptomatology, etc.)

MR : 143

RADIATION THERAPY (THORACIC) FORM

7 Optometry

INTRODUCTION

Optometry is a healthcare profession concerned with eyes and related structures, as well as vision, visual systems, and vision information processing in humans.

Like most professions, optometry education, certification, and practice is regulated in most countries. Optometrists and optometry-related organizations interact with governmental agencies, other healthcare professionals, and the community to deliver eye and vision care. Optometry is one of three eye care professions, the others being ophthalmology (which is a branch of surgery) and orthoptics (a sub-specialty of ophthalmology primarily dealing with strabismus).

BACKGROUND

The term 'optometry' comes from the Greek word *optos*, meaning *eye* or *vision*, and *metria*, meaning *measurement*.

The eye, including its structure and mechanism, has fascinated scientists and the public in general since ancient times. Many of the expressions in the English Language that mean to understand are equivalent vision terms. 'I see', to mean I understand.

Many patients when told that they may have an eye problem will be more concerned about diseases that affect vision than other, more lethal diseases. Being deprived of sight can have a devastating effect on the psyche, as well as economic and social effects, as many blind individuals require significant assistance with activities of daily living and are often unable to continue gainful employment previously held while seeing.

The maintenance of ocular health and correction of eye problems that decrease vision contribute greatly to the ability to appreciate the longer lifespan that all of medicine continues to allow. Given the importance of vision to quality of life, many optometrists consider their job to be rewarding, as they are often able to restore or improve a patient's sight.

Behavioral optometry is a related area of nonstrabismus vision therapy that some optometrists practice. Generally, ophthalmologists and orthoptists do not practice this.

In the United States, optometrists have obtained from state legislatures the right to treat more eye conditions and to perform certain laser surgeries. Optometrists have been successful in getting the right to use some types of medication, depending on if the medication is given as pills, eyedrops, or injections. In the United States, all states except for Oklahoma do not allow the optometrists to perform any type of surgeries. However, in Oklahoma, optometrists are allowed by the state legislature to perform laser surgery.

HISTORY

Optometric history is tied to the development of:
- Vision science (related areas of medicine, microbiology, neurology, physiology, psychology, etc.)
- Optics, optical aids
- Optical instruments, imaging techniques **(Fig. 7.1)**
- Other eye care professions.

The word optometry comes from two Greek words—*opto* which means sight, and *metron* which means measure. The history of optometry can be traced back to the early studies on optics and image formation by the eye.

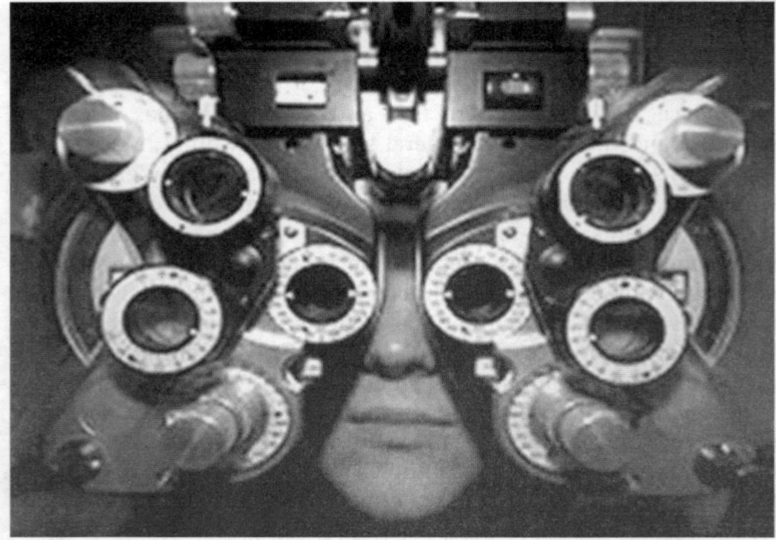

Fig. 7.1 An optical refractor (phoropter) in use

8 Pharmacology

INTRODUCTION

Pharmacology is the science that deals with the origin, nature, chemistry, effects and use of drugs. Pharmacist is the one who is licensed to prepare, and sell or dispense drugs, and compounds and makeup prescriptions. Pharmacopeia is an authoritative treatise on drugs and their preparations; a book containing a list of the products, used in medicines with descriptions, chemical tests for determining identity, purity and formulae for certain mixtures of these substances with statement of average dosage. Pharmacy is the place where the drugs are stored, and dispensed by the pharmacists.

Chemotherapy is the study of those drugs that destroy micro-organisms, parasites or malignant cells within the body.

Toxicology is the study of the harmful chemicals and their effects on the body.

Antidotes are the substances, which are given to neutralize the unwanted effects of drugs.

DRUGS

Drugs are chemical substances used in medicine, in the treatment of disease. A drug can have three different names: (1) Chemical name—name(s) of the main chemicals used; (2) Generic name or official name—unique name universally known through the pharmacopeia; (3) Brand name or trade name—manufacturer's special identity name.

ADMINISTRATION OF DRUGS

The administration of drugs is of different types:

- Oral administration—given by mouth and absorbed into the blood-stream through the intestinal wall
- Sublingual administration—drugs placed under the tongue and allowed to dissolve in the saliva so as to be absorbed into the blood

stream to start acting rapidly, e.g. nitroglycerine (sorbitrate) drug used for angina pectoris.

- Rectal administration—some drugs are administered through the rectum when the patient is constantly nauseated and vomiting. Enema is also given through the rectum.
- Parenteral administration (injection)—there are several types of injections, they are:
  - Subcutaneous/hypodermic injection—given just under the skin
  - Intradermal injection—made into upper layers of the skin mainly used in skin testing for allergic reactions.
  - Intramuscular injection (IM)—this injection is usually given in the buttock or in the deltoid muscle of the hand.
  - Intravenous injection (II)—this injection is given directly into the veins. Most intravenous fluids like dextrose, saline, etc. are administered through this method.
  - Intrathecal injections—this injection is made into sheath of membranes (meninges) which surround the spinal cord and brain.
  - Dermal application—it is locally applied on skin like antiseptics pain relievers, antifungal, etc. It is also called topical application.
  - Inhalation—some vapors and gasses are taken through the nose or mouth by inhalation, e.g. bronchodilators, etc.

CLASSIFICATIONS OF DRUGS

The drugs are classified into various types:

Drugs	*Action*	*Examples*
Vaccines	A suspension of killed microorganisms administered for prevention and treatment of infectious diseases	Tetanus, polio, hepatitis, measles vaccines
Analgesic	Pain relievers	Paracetamol, ibuprofen
Stimulants	Drugs that acts on the brain to speed up the vital process of heart and respiration	
Depressants	An agent that reduces functional activity and vital energies	Diazepam, barbiturates
Sedatives	Drugs that relax and calm nervousness	Hypnotics, alcohol, morphine, codeine, acetylsalicylic acid

Contd...

Contd...

Drugs	*Action*	*Examples*
Cardiovascular drugs	Drugs acting on heart and blood vessels namely antiarrhythmics, calcium channel blocker, antianginal, vasodialators, diuretics, ACE inhibitors and vasoconstrictors	
Autonomic drugs	Drugs those influence the body in the manner similar to the normal action of autonomic nerves	Epinephrine, reserpine, acetylcholine
Gastrointestinal drugs	Used mainly to relieve gastrointestinal discomforts	Antacids, blockers
Antibiotics	Chemical substance produced by a microorganism to stop the growth or kill the bacteria, fungi or parasites	Penicillin, streptomycin, tetracycline, sulfonamides
Antihistamines	These drugs block the action of histamine, which is normally released when foreign antigens enter causing allergic symptoms	Diphenhydramine, chlorpheniramine
Antifungal	Chemical substance produced by a fungi to stop the growth or kill the fungi	
Antiemetics	The drugs relieve nausea and vomiting and overcome vertigo, dizziness, and motion sickness	
Laxatives	Drugs which promotes the motility of the intestine, to excrete the fecal matters	
Blockers	Drug that induces adrenergic blockage at receptors	
Vitamins and minerals	Micronutrients substances essential for proper health and growth	Vitamin A, B_1, B_2, B_6, B_{12}, Niacin, Vitamin C, D, E, K and folic acid
Anesthetics	Agent that reduces or eliminates sensation, local, spinal or general	xylocaine is used for local anesthesia, pethidine is administered for general anesthesia

Contd...

Contd...

Drugs	*Action*	*Examples*
Anticoagulant	Drug that prevents the clotting of blood	Heparin
Anticonvulsants	Reduces the severity of convulsions in various types of epilepsy	
Antidepressant	Drugs that treats the symptoms of depression	
Antidiabetic	Drugs used to treat diabetes mellitus such as oral hypoglycemic and injections of insulin	
Endocrine drugs	Direct hormonal substitutes	Androgens, estrogens, progestines, and glucocorticoids
Gastrointestinal drugs	Drugs act on gastrointestinal tracts	Antacids, antidiarrheal, laxatives
Respiratory drugs	Acts on respiratory tract	Bronchodilators and inhalers
Tranquilizers	Drugs that control anxiety	Valium (diazepam)

9 Pharmacy

INTRODUCTION

Pharmacy is the health profession that links the health sciences with the chemical sciences, and it is charged with ensuring the safe and effective use of pharmaceutical drugs.

The scope of pharmacy practice includes more traditional roles such as compounding and dispensing medications, and it also includes more modern services related to healthcare, including clinical services, reviewing medications for safety and efficacy, and providing drug information. Pharmacy is the term for an establishment where pharmacy in the first sense is practiced in drugstore. Pharmacists are the primary health professionals who optimize medication use to provide patients with positive health outcomes.

The word pharmacy is derived from its root word pharma which was a term used since the 1400–1600s. Apart from the pharma responsibilities, it offered general medical advice and a range of services that are now performed solely by other specialist practitioners, such as surgery and midwifery. The pharma generally operated through a retail shop which, in addition to ingredients for medicines, sold tobacco and patent medicines. The pharmas also used many other herbs in their practice.

In its examination of herbal and chemical ingredients, the work of the pharma may be regarded as a forerunner of the modern sciences of chemistry and pharmacology, prior to the formulation of the scientific method.

The field of pharmacy can generally be divided into three primary disciplines:

1. Pharmaceutics
2. Medicinal chemistry and pharmacognosy
3. Pharmacy practice

The limits between these disciplines and with other sciences, such as biochemistry, are not always clear-cut; and often, collaborative teams from various disciplines research together.

Pharmacology is occasionally considered a fourth discipline of pharmacy. Pharmacology is essential to the study of pharmacy, but it is not just specific to pharmacy, it is usually considered to be of the broader sciences.

PHARMACISTS

Pharmacists are highly-trained and skilled healthcare professionals who perform various roles to ensure optimal health outcomes for their patients. Many pharmacists besides practicing do have their own pharmacy business.

Types of Pharmacy Practice Areas (Figs 9.1 and 9.2)

Pharmacists practice in a variety of areas including retail shops, hospitals, clinics, nursing homes, drug industry, insurance companies, and accreditation agencies. Pharmacists can specialize in various areas of practice including many fields such as hematology/oncology, infectious diseases, ambulatory care, nutrition support, drug information, critical care, pediatrics, etc.

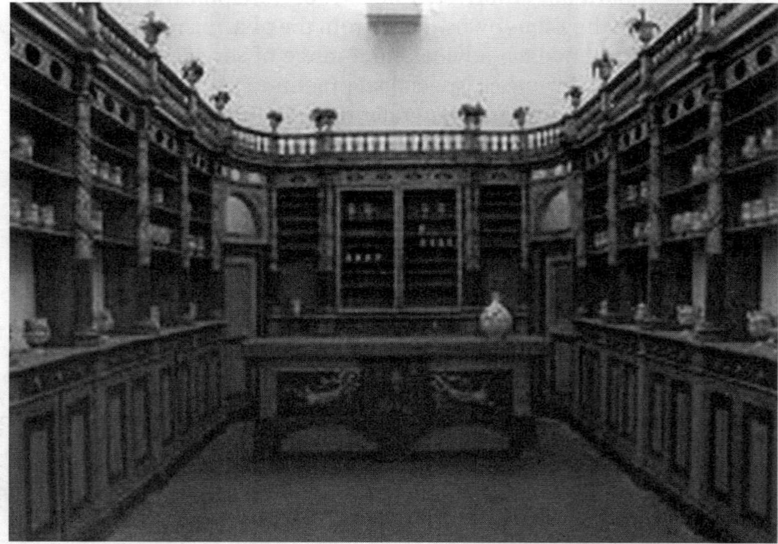

Fig. 9.1 A model of 19th century Italian pharmacy (*For color version, see Plate 1*)

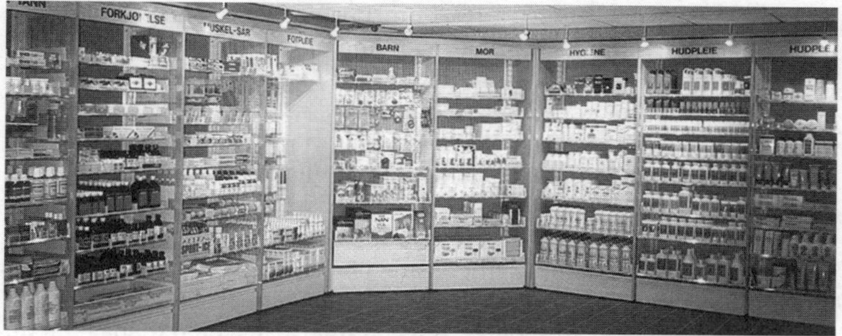

Fig. 9.2 A model of modern pharmacy (*For color version, see Plate 2*)

Community Pharmacy

A *pharmacy* is the place where most licensed pharmacists practice the profession of pharmacy. It initiated as the community pharmacy to deal with community needs and as profession grown and expanded to variety of pharmacy services.

Community pharmacies in early years usually consist of a retail storefront with a dispensary where medications are stored and dispensed. The dispensary is subject to pharmacy legislation; with requirements for storage conditions, compulsory texts, equipment, etc. specified in legislation. Normally, the pharmacists most of their time spent in the dispensary compounding/dispensing medications; and also communicating with patients related the way the drugs are to be used.

All pharmacies are required to have a registered pharmacist on-duty at all times when operational. Apart from having independent pharmacy stores, there are many pharmacies are located in departmental stores and grocery shops. In addition to medicines and prescriptions, many now sell a diverse arrangement of additional household items such as cosmetics, shampoo, office supplies, confectionary, and snack foods. Invariably, most of large pharmacies are located nearby hospitals and nursing home vicinity with 24/7 service.

Hospital Pharmacy

Pharmacies within hospitals differ considerably from general pharmacy stores or pharmacy in departmental stores. The hospital pharmacies may have more complex clinical medication management issues whereas pharmacists in pharmacy stores often have more multifaceted business and customer related issues. The hospital pharmacies size, locations and method of operation varies from hospital-to-hospital. There are main pharmacy, emergency pharmacy and outpatient pharmacy, etc.

In view of the complexity of medications, effectiveness of treatment regimens, safety of medications (i.e. drug interactions) and patient compliance issues in the hospital, many pharmacists working in hospitals have to be well-experienced with appropriate professional qualification. Persons who are specialized in clinical pharmacy are referred to as clinical pharmacists and they often specialize in various disciplines of pharmacy. For example, there are pharmacists who specialize in hematology/oncology, HIV/AIDS, infectious disease, critical care, emergency medicine, toxicology, nuclear pharmacy, pain management, psychiatry, anticoagulation clinics, herbal medicine, neurology/epilepsy management, pediatrics, neonatal pharmacists and more.

Hospital pharmacies can usually be found within the premises of the hospital. Hospital pharmacies usually stock a larger range of medications, including more specialized medications. Most hospital medications are unit-dose, or a single dose of medicine. Hospital pharmacists and trained pharmacy technicians compound sterile products for patients including total parenteral nutrition (TPN), and other medications given intravenously. This is a complex process that requires adequate training of personnel, quality assurance of products, and adequate facilities. The large hospitals with huge patient turnout in ambulatory and inpatient services do prefer outsource high-risk preparations and some other compounding functions to companies who specialize in compounding as a cost contained mechanism or due to shortage of well-qualified pharmacists.

Clinical Pharmacy

Clinical pharmacists care for patients in all healthcare settings especially inside hospitals and clinics and they often collaborate with physicians and other healthcare professionals to improve pharmaceutical care. Clinical pharmacists are now an integral part of the interdisciplinary approach to patient care. They work collaboratively with physicians, nurses and other healthcare personnel in various medical and surgical areas and participate in patient care rounds and drug product selection. In most hospitals in the United States, potentially dangerous drugs that require close monitoring are dosed and managed by clinical pharmacists.

Compounding Pharmacy

Another important function of pharmacist is compounding that is practice of preparing drugs in new forms. For example, if a drug manufacturer only provides a drug as a tablet, a compounding pharmacist might make a medicated lollipop that contains the drug. Patients who have difficulty swallowing the tablet may prefer to suck the medicated lollipop instead. Another form of compounding is by mixing different strengths, (g, mg, mcg) of capsules or tables to yield the desire therapy indicated by the doctor. The pharmacists who specialize in compounding, also dispense the noncompounded drugs to that patients.

Consultant Pharmacy

The field of pharmacy as old as medicine, in the course of its practice, the profession has reached to provide consultancy services and those senior professionals with vast experience are called consultant pharmacists. This practice focuses more on medication regimen review (i.e. 'cognitive services') than on actual dispensing of drugs. Consultant pharmacists most typically work in nursing homes, but are increasingly branching into other institutions and noninstitutional settings. Traditionally consultant pharmacists were usually independent business owners, though in the United States many now work for several large pharmacy management companies. This trend may be gradually reversing as consultant pharmacists begin to work directly with patients, primarily because many elderly people are now taking numerous medications but continue to live outside of institutional settings. Some community pharmacies employ consultant pharmacists and/or provide consulting services. The need for general pharmacists and consultant pharmacist is growing to prevent adverse medication reactions and deaths.

Internet Pharmacy

Since about the year 2000, a growing number of internet pharmacies have been established worldwide. Many of these pharmacies are similar to hospital or community pharmacies, and in fact, many of them are actually operated by pharmacies that serve consumers online without going to pharmacist or drug store. The primary difference is the method by which the medications are requested and received. Some customers consider this to be more convenient and private method rather than traveling to a drugstore where another customer might overhear about the drugs that they take. Internet pharmacies (also known as Online Pharmacies) are also recommended to some patients by their physicians if they are homebound. Many refills are prescribed over internets and patient instead of going to physician's office or clinic can have repeated same drugs or new drug prescribed and collected directly from drug or pharmacy stores.

The most internet pharmacies sell prescription drugs on a valid prescription; some internet pharmacies sell prescription drugs without requiring a prescription in certain drugs. Many customers order drugs from such pharmacies to avoid the 'inconvenience' of visiting a doctor or to obtain medications which their doctors were unwilling to prescribe. However, this practice has been criticized as potentially dangerous, especially by those who feel that only doctors can reliably assess contraindications, risk/benefit ratios, and an individual's overall suitability for use of a medication.

What is most important concern is with internet pharmacies is the ease with which people, especially youth, can obtain controlled substances via the internet without a prescription issued by a doctor/practitioner who has an established doctor-patient relationship. There are many instances where a practitioner issues a prescription, brokered by an internet server, for a controlled substance to a 'patient' s/he has never met. In the United States, in order for a prescription for a controlled substance to be valid, it must be issued for a legitimate medical purpose by a licensed practitioner acting in the course of legitimate doctor-patient relationship. The filling pharmacy has a corresponding responsibility to ensure that the prescription is valid. Often, individual state laws outline what defines a valid patient-doctor relationship.

Canada is home to dozens of licensed internet pharmacies, many of which sell their lower-cost prescription drugs to US consumers, who pay one of the world's highest drug prices. In recent years, many consumers in the US and in other countries with high drug costs have turned to licensed internet pharmacies in India, Israel and the UK, which often have even lower prices than in Canada.

In the United States, there has been a push to legalize importation of medications from Canada and other countries, in order to reduce consumer costs. In most cases importation of prescription medications violates Food and Drug Administration (FDA) regulations and federal laws, therefore, enforcement is generally targeted at international drug suppliers, rather than consumers.

Recently-developed online services like Australia's *Medicine Name Finder* and the Walgreens' *Drug Info Search* provide information about pharmaceutical products but do not offer prescriptions or drug dispensations. These services often promote generic drug alternatives by offering comparative information on price and effectiveness.

Veterinary Pharmacy

Veterinary pharmacies, sometimes called *animal pharmacies* may fall in the category of hospital pharmacy, retail pharmacy or mail-order pharmacy. Veterinary pharmacies stock different varieties and different strengths of medications to fulfill the pharmaceutical needs of animals. Because the needs of animals as well as the regulations on veterinary medicine are often very different from those related to people, veterinary pharmacy is often kept separate from regular pharmacies.

Nuclear Pharmacy

Nuclear pharmacy focuses on preparing radioactive materials for diagnostic tests and for treating certain diseases. Nuclear pharmacists undergo additional training specific to handling radioactive materials, and unlike in community and hospital pharmacies, nuclear pharmacists typically do not interact directly with patients.

Military Pharmacy

Military pharmacy is an entirely different working environment due to the fact that technicians perform most duties that in a civilian sector would be illegal. State laws of technician patient counseling and medication checking by a pharmacist do not apply.

PHARMACY INFORMATICS

The importance of pharmacy informatics has grown due to development of pharmacy software to be used in healthcare institutions. Pharmacy informatics is the combination of pharmacy practice science and applied information science. Pharmacy informaticist's work in many practice areas of pharmacy, however, they may also work in information technology departments or for healthcare information technology vendor companies. As a practice area and specialist domain, pharmacy informatics is growing quickly to meet the needs of major national and international patient information projects and health system interoperability goals. Pharmacists are well trained to participate in medication management system development, deployment and optimization.

ISSUES IN PHARMACY

Separation of Prescribing from Dispensing

In most jurisdictions (such as the United States), pharmacists are regulated separately from physicians. These jurisdictions also usually specify that only pharmacists may supply scheduled pharmaceuticals to the public and that pharmacists cannot form business partnerships with physicians or give them 'kickback' payments. However, the American Medical Association (AMA) Code of Ethics provides that physicians may dispense drugs within their office practices as long as there is no patient exploitation and patients have the right to a written prescription that can be filled elsewhere. Seven to ten percent of American physician's practices reportedly dispense drugs on their own.

In other jurisdictions, doctors are allowed to dispense drugs themselves and the practice of pharmacy is sometimes integrated with that of the physician, particularly in traditional Chinese medicine.

In Canada it is common for a medical clinic and a pharmacy to be located together and for the ownership in both enterprises to be common, but licensed separately.

The reason for the majority rule is the high-risk of a conflict of interest and/or the avoidance of absolute powers. Otherwise, the physician has a financial self-interest in 'diagnosing' as many conditions as possible, and in exaggerating their seriousness, because he or she can then sell more medications to the patient. Such self-interest directly conflicts with the patient's interest in obtaining cost-effective medication and avoiding the unnecessary use of medication that may have side effects. This system reflects much similarity to the checks and balances system of the US and many other governments.

A campaign for separation has begun in many countries and has already been successful. As many of the remaining nations move towards separation, resistance and lobbying from dispensing doctors who have pecuniary interests may prove a major stumbling block.

FUTURE OF PHARMACY

It is expected that the pharmacists to become more integral within the healthcare system in the future, rather than simply dispensing medication, pharmacists will be paid for their patient care services.

This transformation has already commenced in some countries; for instance, pharmacists in Australia receive remuneration from the Australian Government for conducting comprehensive Home Medicines Reviews. In Canada, pharmacists in certain provinces have limited prescribing rights (as in Alberta and British Columbia) or are remunerated by their provincial government for expanded services such as medications reviews (MedsChecks in Ontario). In the United Kingdom, pharmacists who undertake additional training are obtaining prescribing rights. They are also being paid for by the government for medicine use reviews. In the United States, pharmaceutical care or clinical pharmacy has had an evolving influence on the practice of pharmacy. Moreover, the Doctor of Pharmacy (Pharm D) degree is now required before entering practice and some pharmacists now complete one or two years of residency or fellowship training following graduation. In addition, consultant pharmacists who traditionally operated primarily in nursing homes are now expanding into direct consultation with patients, under the banner of 'senior care pharmacy'.

10 Oncology

INTRODUCTION

Oncology is the study of tumors. Unrestrained and excessive multiplication of body cells producing lump or swelling, known as tumor or neoplasm. The neoplasm may be either benign or malignant. Malignant tumors or neoplasm accumulate as growth, which penetrate, compress and ultimately destroy the surrounding normal tissue. The malignant cells from the primary tumor site find their way into lymph channels or blood vessels and are carried to remote body structures by which secondary malignant neoplasm develop. This is called metastasis. Benign neoplasms are new growths that develop in body tissues. They are composed of the same type of cells as the tissue in which they are growing. When they grow bigger in size, then they harm the place by exerting pressure on surrounding structures. In general, benign tumors are not life-threatening; once they are removed they usually do not reoccur.

DIFFERENCES BETWEEN THE MALIGNANT AND BENIGN NEOPLASM

See **Table 10.1**.

Carcinomas

Carcinomas, the largest group, are solid tumors, which are derived from epithelial tissue. Epithelial tissue is found on external and internal body surfaces, including skin, glands, digestive, urinary and reproductive organs. Almost all-malignant neoplasm are carcinomas.

Sarcomas

Sarcomas are a rare type of cancer when compared to carcinomas and are derived from supportive and connective tissue, such as bone, fat,

Table 10.1 Differences between the malignant and benign neoplasm

S. No.	Malignant	Benign
1.	Rapid growth could be seen	Grows slowly
2.	Invasive and infiltrative	Encapsulated
3.	Composed of tissue that does not resemble the tissue in which the neoplasm arises	Composed of highly organized and specialized tissue, that closely resembles the tissue in which the neoplasm arises
4.	If left untreated, establish a new tumor site by infiltrating through blood and lymphatic vessels in the remote regions of the body	Does not spread to remote areas to form a secondary tumor
5.	If left untreated, poses a risk to the patient	Generally poses little risk, if any, to the patient

muscle, cartilage, bone marrow, and lymphatic tissue, or from blood cells. Sarcomas account approximately 10% of all malignant neoplasm.

MIXED TISSUE TUMORS

Mixed tissue tumors are derived from tissue, which is capable of differentiating into epithelial as well as connective tissue. The tumors are thus composed of several different types of cells. Examples are: mixed tissue tumors can be found in kidney, ovaries and testes.

STAGING

Staging is an attempt to define the extent of cancer by classifying it into three categories: T, N, and M. T represents the primary tumor site or place of origin; N represents local or regional node involvement; and M indicates whether metastasis is there or not. When the primary site contains classifications of T_1, T_2, T_3 or T_4, the higher number indicate progressive increases in tumor size and involvement. Similarly N_0, N_1, N_2, or N_3, represent progressively advancing nodular involvement. Finally, M_0, or M+ defines absence or presence of metastasis, respectively **(Table 10.2)**.

GRADING

Grading is concerned with the microscopic appearance of the tumor cells, in other words, the degree of anaplasia. Generally, four grades are

Table 10.2 Staging		
	T	Primary tumor
	N	Regional lymph nodes
	M	Distant metastasis
Tumor		
	T_0	No evidence of primary tumor
	TIS	Carcinoma in situ
	T_1, T_2, T_3, T_4	Progressive increase in tumor size and involvement
	T_X	Tumor cannot be assessed
Nodes		
	N_0	Regional lymph nodes not demonstrably abnormal
	N_1, N_2, N_3, etc.	Increasing degrees of demonstrable abnormality of regional
		lymph nodes
	N_X	Regional lymph nodes cannot be assessed clinically
Metastasis		
	M_0	No evidence of distant metastasis
	M_1, M_2, M_3	Ascending degrees of distant metastasis, including metastasis to distant lymph nodes TNM assignments may be grouped into small number of stages

employed, which are numbered from 1 through 4. Neoplasms that are composed of cells that closely resemble the tissue from which they arise are given a grade 1 rating. The tissue demonstrates a minimum amount of anaplasia. Patients with grade 1 tumors have high survival rate, while patients with grades 2, 3, and 4 tumors, have a poorer survival rate. At the other extreme is grade 4, in which there is a great deal of anaplasia within the tumor. Such tumors are more serious and the prognosis is very poor. Grades 2 and 3 are intermediate grades between these two extremes.

CANCER TREATMENT

Cancer is treated by three major approaches namely, surgery, radiation therapy and chemotherapy.

Surgery

The surgery is performed when the tumor is localized, and gets the effective means of cure. Some common cancers in which surgery may be curative are, those of the stomach, large bowel, breasts and endometrium, especially the accessory organs of the system.

Radiation Therapy

The goal of the radiation therapy is to deliver a maximal dose of ionizing radiation to the tumor tissue and a minimal dose to the surrounding normal tissue. In reality, this goal is difficult to obtain and usually one accepts a degree of residual normal cell damage as a sequel to the destruction of the tumor. The effect of high-dose radiation to cells is to produce damage to DNA and thus inhibit cell replication and growth.

Chemotherapy

Chemotherapy is the treatment of cancer using drugs. It is probably the most important factor responsible for long-term survival in several types of cancer. Chemotherapy may be used alone or in combination with surgery and radiation.

11 Psychiatry

INTRODUCTION

The branch of medicine, which deals with study, treatment and prevention of mental illness. Madness is different from psychiatry. A psychiatric condition, if untreated, may develop into insane condition, which may become madness.

Psychotherapy is the treatment of emotional problems by psychological techniques. There are different techniques involved in psychotherapy **(Table 11.1)**:

Table 11.1 Different types of technique in psychotherapy

S. No.	*Types*	*Explanation*
1.	Behavior therapy	Conditioning the primary feelings of the patients
2.	Group therapy	Patients are educated through group discussions in front of invited audience
3.	Sex therapy	Mainly deals with solving psychosexual disorders such as frigidity, impotence, and premature ejaculation
4.	Family therapy	This deals with the common problems of a family
5.	Psychoanalysis	This is a long-term form of psychotherapy, to resolve internal conflicts, by allowing the patients, to bring their unconscious emotions, such as free association, and transference (recollecting the early past incidence)
6.	Hypnosis	Therapy by recovery of deeply repressed memories
7.	Play therapy	Therapy given to children through toys, and plays to express conflicts, and feelings, which he or she is unable to communicate directly
8.	Electroshock therapy	Treatment applied to the brain by producing convulsions, through electric current, chiefly for severe depressions
9.	Drug therapy	Treatment by drugs such as antianxiety agents (diazepam), antipsychotic tranquilizers (chlorpromazine), lithium, antidepressants, etc.

PSYCHIATRY DISORDERS

Affective Disorders

Disorder of mood, e.g. manic depressive illness, major depressions, etc. Manic depressive illness is characterized by alternating moods of mania such as excitement, activity, exalted feelings and decreased in need for sleep. Major depression, involves, severe, dysphoric mood like sadness, hopelessness, irritability and worry, etc.

Anxiety Disorders

These disorders are characterized by the experience of unpleasant tension, distress, and troubled feelings, like phobias and anxiety states.

Somatoform Disorders

These disorders in which the patient's mental conflicts, are expressed as physical symptoms, like abdominal pain, nausea, vomiting, chest pain, loss of functions in parts of body (difficulty in swallowing), loss of voice, deafness, etc. In conversion disorders (hysterical neurosis), the patient usually has a feared but unconscious conflict, which threatens to escape from repression. Hypochondriosis, is a somatoform disorders, in which the patient has preoccupation, with body pains, and discomforts.

Disassociate Disorders (Hysterical Neurosis)

The symptoms of this disorder are psychogenic amnesia and multiple personality. This disorder is characterized by inability to remember important personal information, unexpected travel away from home or work (with amnesia).

Psychosexual Disorders

These disorders includes sexual perversion, in which the patient's psychological sexual identity from his or her gender identity.

Transvestism

Dressing in the clothes of opposite sex.

Exhibitionism

Compulsive need to expose one's genitals.

Sexual Masochism

Achievement of sexual pleasure from suffering.

Trans-sexualism

Desire to change anatomic sexual characteristics, stemming from the fixed conviction that one is a member of the opposite sex. Such a person often seeks medical and surgical treatment to bring their anatomy into conformity with their belief.

Fetishism

Achieving sexual gratification by substituting an inanimate object for a human love object.

Voyeurism

An abnormal desire, to look at sexual organs or acts.

Sexual Sadism

Achievement of sexual pleasure, by inflicting physical or psychological pain.

Personality Disorders

These are behavioral disorders acceptable to the individuals, but produce, conflict with others who interact with the same individuals.

Antisocial

No loyalty or concern for others and without moral standards.

Passive Aggression

Showing aggressive feelings in passive ways, such as stubbornness, helplessness, etc.

Histrionic

Emotional immaturity, and dependent having general dissatisfaction with themselves and angry feelings about the world.

Narcissistic

Pompous sense of self-importance, and preoccupation, with the fantasy of success and power.

Paranoid

Pervasive, suspiciousness, and mistrust of people, jealous and quick to take offence.

Delirium

Mental disturbances associated with illness characterized by mental cloudiness, and visual hallucinations.

Dementia

Characterized by loss of memory and intelligence. The most common is Senile Dementia.

Schizophrenic Disorders

This is a major psychotic disorder characterized by withdrawal from reality into inner world of disorganized thinking and feeling. Symptoms are bizarre delusions, auditory hallucinations, hearing imaginary voices, and incoherent speech.

Paranoic Disorders

In this disorder, patient will have persistent delusions or persecution and jealousy.

Chronic Alcoholism

Addition to alcohol consumption, may present psychological symptoms such as hallucinations, amnesia, with physical ailments, such as cirrhosis of liver, and brain damage. Patient will be unable to remember and resorts to confabulation (lying).

Drug Dependence (Substance Induced Disorders)

Diseases due to addiction to drugs like opioids (heroin, morphine, etc.), sedatives (barbiturates, diazepam, etc.), cocaine and hallucinogen-type drugs.

12 Medical Psychology

INTRODUCTION

Psychology (literally means 'study of the soul' or 'study of the mind') is an academic and applied discipline which involves the scientific study of human or animal mental functions and behaviors. In the field of psychology, a professional researcher or practitioner is called a psychologist. In addition or opposition to employing scientific methods, psychologists often rely upon symbolic interpretation and critical analysis, although less frequently than other social sciences such as sociology.

Psychologists generally study such observable fact such as perception, cognition, attention, emotion, motivation, personality, behavior and interpersonal relationships, and also consider the mind. A neuropsychologists attempt to understand the role of mental functions in individual and social behavior, in order to explore the underlying physiological and neurological processes.

Psychological knowledge is applied to various areas of human activity including the family, education, employment, and the treatment of mental health problems. Psychology includes many subfields as diverse as human development, sports, health, industry, media and law and integrate research from the social sciences, natural sciences, and humanities.

Psychology encompasses a vast domain, and includes many different approaches to the study of mental processes and behavior. Below are the major areas of inquiry that comprise psychology. A comprehensive list of the subfields and areas within psychology can be found at the list of psychology topics and list of psychology disciplines.

ABNORMAL

Abnormal psychology is the study of abnormal behavior in order to describe, predict, explain, and change abnormal patterns of functioning. Abnormal psychology studies the nature of psychopathology and its causes, and this knowledge is applied in clinical psychology to treat patients with psychological disorders.

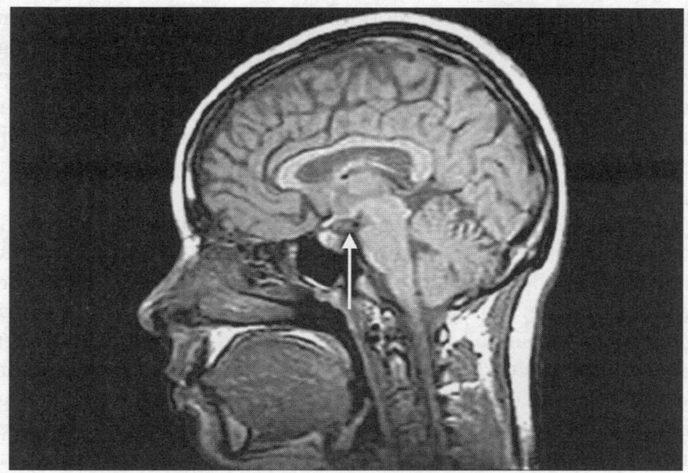

Fig. 12.1 The magnetic resonance imaging depicting the human brain. The arrow indicates the position of the hypothalamus

It is normally difficult to draw the line between normal and abnormal behaviors. In general, abnormal behaviors must be maladaptive and cause an individual significant discomfort in order to be of clinical and research importance. According to the DSM-IV-TR, behaviors may be considered abnormal if they are associated with disability, personal distress, the violation of social norms, or dysfunction **(Fig. 12.1)**.

Biological psychology is the scientific study of the biological, status of behavior and mental states. Bearing in mind all behavior as entangled with the nervous system, biological psychologists feel it is sensible to study how the brain functions in order to understand behavior. This is the approach taken in behavioral neuroscience, cognitive neuroscience, and neuropsychology. Neuropsychology is the branch of psychology that aims to understand how the structure and function of the brain relate to specific behavioral and psychological processes. Neuropsychology is particularly concerned with the understanding of brain injury in an attempt to work out normal psychological function. Cognitive neuroscientists often use neuroimaging tools, which can help them to observe which areas of the brain are active during a particular task.

CLINICAL

Clinical psychology includes the study and application of psychology for the purpose of understanding, preventing, and relieving psychologically related distress or dysfunction and to promote subjective well-being and personal development. The psychological assessment and psychotherapy are part of general study, and clinical psychologists may also engage in research, teaching, consultation, and program development and administration. Some clinical psychologists may focus on the clinical management of patients with brain injury which is known as clinical neuropsychology. In many countries clinical psychology is a profession that deals with mental health.

The clinical psychologist perform the work that be likely to be influenced by various therapeutic approaches, all of which involve a formal relationship between professional and client that could be an individual, couple, family, or small group of community. The various therapeutic approaches and practices are associated with different theoretical perspectives and employ different procedures anticipated to form a therapeutic alliance, explore the nature of psychological problems, and persuade new ways of thinking, feeling, or behaving. There are four major theoretical perspectives that are psychodynamic, cognitive behavioral, existential-humanistic, and systems or family therapy. There has been a growing movement to integrate the various therapeutic approaches, especially with an increased understanding of issues regarding culture, gender, spirituality, and sexual-orientation. With the advent of more vigorous research findings regarding psychotherapy, there is evidence that most of the major therapies are about of equal effectiveness, with the key common element being a strong therapeutic association. In view of new findings and conducting various training programs, psychologists are now adopting an eclectic therapeutic orientation that has been found very useful and significant outcome.

COGNITIVE

Cognitive psychology studies cognition, the mental processes underlying mental activity. The research that made interesting to explore more on learning, perception, problem solving, reasoning, thinking, memory, attention, language and emotion and other related areas. Classical cognitive psychology is associated with a school of thought known as cognitivism, whose adherents argue for an information processing model of mental function, that consist of functionalism and experimental psychology.

As far as the cognitive science is concerned is an interdisciplinary enterprise of cognitive psychologists, cognitive neuroscientists, researchers in artificial intelligence, linguists, human-computer interaction, computational neuroscience, logicians and social scientists. In order to stimulate phenomena of interest computational models are occasionally used. Computational models provide a tool for studying the functional organization of the mind and neuroscience provides measures of brain activity. To understand the activities of both models play an important role.

COMMUNITY

In a social welfare state, community is one of fundamental ingredient in the society and in that community psychology plays a vital role and deals with the relationships of the individual to communities and the wider humanity. Community psychologists seek to understand the quality of life of individuals, families, communities, and society. Their aim is to enhance improve quality of life through collaborative research and efficient practice.

Community psychology as a routine makes use of various perspectives within and outside of psychology to address issues of communities, the relationships within them, and people's attitudes and behaviors about them. Through collaborative research and practice, community psychologists hunt for to understand and to enhance to improve quality of life for individuals, families, communities, and society as whole. Community psychology besides curative, takes a public health approach and focuses on prevention and early intervention as a means to solve problems in addition to treatment. The psychologist had in-depth deliberations and discussions found that the perspective of community psychology as an ecological perspective with the person-environment fit being the focus of study and action instead of attempting to change the person or the environment when an individual or family is seen as having a problem. Timely understand the problem and providing appropriate solution would improve greatly.

COMPARATIVE

Comparative psychology refers to the study of the behavior and mental life of human being as well as animals. It is extended disciplines outside of psychology that study animal behavior such as etiology. Although the field of psychology is primarily concerned with humans, their behavior and mental processes of animals is also an important part of psychological research. This being either as a subject in with strong emphasis about evolutionary links, and somewhat more controversially, as a way of gaining an insight into human psychology.

COUNSELING

Counseling psychology seeks to facilitate personal and interpersonal functioning across the lifespan with a focus on emotional, social, vocational, educational, health-related, developmental, and organizational concerns. Counselors are primarily clinicians, using psychotherapy and other interventions in order to treat patients and potential patients. As conventionally, counseling psychology has been focusing more on normal developmental issues and on a daily basis stress rather than psychopathology, but this distinction has softened over time. Counseling psychologists are employed in a variety of settings, including hospitals, schools, universities, governmental organizations, businesses, private practice, and community mental health centers and also nonprofit religious healthcare organizations.

CRITICAL

Critical psychology its name indicates the seriousness that applies the methodology of critical theory to psychology. Accordingly, it seeks the supportive roles that psychology and psychologists play, often inadvertently, in oppressive ideologies, and it tries to replace these roles with ones that can transform oppressive social structures. Critical psychology operates on the belief 'that mainstream psychology has institutionalized a narrow view of the field's ethical mandate to promote human welfare,' and critical psychology endeavors to broaden the view of that mandate. The critical psychology is under transformation to find new ways and methods to deal cases in an effective ways.

A critical psychologist might ask whether a case with work stress necessitate efforts to change the macrolevel systems that control the work, rather than to treat in isolation those individuals who experience the anxiety and pressure. One might also ask why peoples efforts fail to incorporate a focus on human rights and social justice in complex societies. In short, critical psychology seeks, where it considers appropriate, to raise psychology's level of analysis from the individual to family and society, and to render psychology more transformative than superficially ameliorative. Critical psychology has been applied to a wide range of psychologies other subfields and many of its practitioners are employed in conventional psychological professions. As the lifestyle of people all over the globe is changing in a rapid manner, the critical psychology's role would become inevitable.

DEVELOPMENTAL

The growth of the human mind through the course of life time, the developmental psychology seeks to understand how people come to understand, perceive, and act within their lifespan and how these processes transform as the child grow older. This change focuses mainly on intellectual, cognitive, neural, social, or moral development. Researchers who study children use a number of different types of research methods and techniques to make observations in natural settings or to employ them in experimental situation to find the results. Such methods and techniques often applied in especially designed games and activities that are both enjoyable for the child and scientifically useful to the executors and researchers to study the mental processes of small infants and children of less IQ. In addition to studying children, developmental psychologists also study aging and processes throughout the lifespan, from the infant stage to child growth, youth, adolescent and old age. Developmental psychologists has become a regular and continuous field to conduct research to evolve news techniques and methods to deal with newly emanating problems in the individual, families and community as a whole.

EDUCATIONAL

The work of child psychologists such as Lev Vygotsky, Jean Piaget and Jerome Bruner has been influential in creating teaching methods and educational practices. Educational psychology is often included in the syllabus of teacher education programs, at least in North America, Australia, and New Zealand. Educational psychology is the study of how humans learn in educational settings, the effectiveness of educational interference within the set educational program, add value to the effective teaching psychology, and the social psychology. The institutions where the child psychology and social psychology are imparted have to bear the practical needs of modern medicine and psychological issues that are in vogue.

EVOLUTIONARY

Evolutionary psychology explores the genetic roots of mental and behavioral patterns, and that common patterns may have emerged because they were highly adaptive for humans in the environments of their evolutionary past. Fields closely related to evolutionary psychology are animal behavioral ecology, human behavioral ecology, dual inheritance theory, and sociobiology. Memetics, founded by Richard Dawkins, is a related but competing field that proposes that cultural evolution can occur in a Darwinian sense but independently of Mendelian mechanisms; it is therefore, examines the ways in which thoughts, or memes, may evolve independently of genes in an evolutionary span of period.

FORENSIC

The legal especially medical legal are closely related with forensic psychology. The subject encompasses a broad range of practices including the clinical evaluations of defendants, reports to judges and attorneys, and courtroom testimony on given issues. Forensic psychologists are appointed by the court or hired by attorneys to evaluate defendants' competency to stand trial, competency to be executed, sanity, and need for involuntary commitment. Forensic psychologists are involved in variety of psychological cases related to evaluate sex offenders and treatments, and provide recommendations to the court through written reports and testimony. Many of the questions the court asks the forensic psychologist are generally concerned to legal issues. As a psychologist in some instance cannot answer all legal questions. For example, there is no definition of sanity in psychology. Rather, sanity is a legal definition that varies from place-to-place throughout the world. Therefore, a prime qualification of a forensic psychologist is an intimate understanding of the law, especially criminal law and now this has become a practicing profession, many lawyers have adopted as their specialized profession.

GLOBAL

The global psychology expands the aim of psychology to macrolevel trends; it examines the overwhelming consequences of global warming, economic destabilization and other large-scale phenomena, while recognizing that global sustainability can best be achieved by psychologically marinating sound individuals and cultures that could be useful to society. Global psychologists advocate a comprehensive, psychology, whose strength is its focus on the long-term well-being of all of humanity. Global psychology is matter of fact is a subfield of psychology that addresses the issues raised in the global sustainability debate for solutions to various psychological issues that emanate time-to-time.

HEALTH

Health psychology is mainly related to health illness and healthcare of needy clients. As we have seen the clinical psychology focuses on mental health and neurological illness. The health psychology is mainly concerned with the psychology of a much wider range of health-related behavior including healthy eating and living. The health psychology closely create working link between the doctor-patient relationship, a patient's understanding of health information, and viewpoint about illness. Health psychologists generally involved in public health campaigns, examining the impact of illness or health policy on quality of life as a preventive promotive of psychological impact of health and social care that would build up healthy society.

INDUSTRIAL/ORGANIZATIONAL

Industrial and organizational psychology (I/O) applies psychological concepts and methods to optimize human potential in the industrial and organizational workplaces. Personnel psychology, a subfield of industrial and organizational psychology that applies the principles and methods of psychology in selecting and evaluating workers. The I/O psychology's and organizational psychology, surveys the effects of work environments and its conditions, management involvement on worker motivation, job satisfaction, and welfare of workers in addition to maximize the productivity.

Legal

In the modern days with competitive society, along with the advancements in all the fields, there also parallel growing of criminality, unethical methods and sexual abuses and accidental, suicidal and homogenous issues are creeping heavily all over the globe. The need for legal settlements has become of part of judiciary and prevent the growth, need for legal psychologist is inevitable. Legal psychology is a specialized field to study various issues prevalent in the society, public areas to explore the possibility of assisting the judiciary and society in minimizing the crime and other prevailing legal issues related to human elements that could be addressed. This profession has been engaged as an advisory body in policy makers for the security and well-being of people.

OCCUPATIONAL HEALTH PSYCHOLOGY

Occupational health psychology (OHP) is a discipline that emerged out of health psychology, industrial/organizational psychology, and occupational health. The OHP is concerned with identifying psycho-social characteristics of workplaces that give rise to problems in physical and mental health, e.g. depression. The OHP is concerned with psychosocial characteristics of workplaces as workers' way of working and employers decision and attitudes of supervisors in getting the work done. The OHP also concerns itself with interference that can prevent or improve work-related health problems. Such interventions have definite beneficial implications for the employees and employers and economic success of organizations. The OHP spends more on research areas of concern include workplace violence, unemployment, and workplace safety.

PERSONALITY

Personality psychology studies enduring patterns of behavior, thought, and emotion in individuals, commonly referred to as personality. Theories of personality vary across different psychological schools of thought. According to Freud, personality is based on the dynamic interactions of the ego, superego. Trait theorists, in contrast, attempt to analyze personality in terms of a discrete number of key traits by the statistical method of factor analysis. The number of proposed traits has varied widely. An early model proposed by Hans Eysenck suggested that there are three traits that comprise human personality: extraversion-introversion, neuroticism, and psychoticism. Raymond Cattell proposed a theory of 16 personality factors. The 'Big Five', or Five Factor Model, proposed by Lewis Goldberg, currently has strong support among trait theorists. The personality theory carry different assumptions about such issues as the role of the childhood experience, behavior, forgetness, strong and weak personality.

QUANTITATIVE

The term 'Quantitative psychology' is relatively new and gradually gaining the ground as specialize branch of psychology. This covers the longer standing subfields psychometrics and mathematical psychology. Quantitative psychology involves the application of mathematical and statistical modeling in psychological research, and the development of statistical methods for analyzing and explaining behavioral data. Psychometrics is the field of psychology concerned with the theory and technique of psychological measurement, which includes the measurement of knowledge, abilities, attitudes, and personality traits. Measurement of these phenomena is difficult, and much research has been developed to define and analyze such phenomena. Psychometric research typically involves two major research tasks, namely: (i) the construction of instruments and procedures for measurement; and (ii) the development and refinement of theoretical approaches to measurement.

MATHEMATICAL PSYCHOLOGY

Mathematical psychology is the subdiscipline that is concerned with the development of psychological theory in relation with mathematics and statistics. Basic topics in mathematical psychology include measurement theory and mathematical learning theory as well as the modeling and analysis of mental and motor processes. Psychometrics is more associated with educational psychology, personality, and clinical psychology. Mathematical psychology is more closely related to psychonomics/experimental and cognitive, and physiological psychology and (cognitive) neuroscience.

SOCIAL PSYCHOLOGY (FIG. 12.2)

The social psychology is playing very important role in hospital and patient care environment. These professionals have become indispensable in the care of patients social psychology is the study of social behavior and mental processes, with an emphasis on how humans think about each other and how they relate to each other. Social psychologists are especially interested in how people react to social situations. They study such topics as the influence of others on an individual's behavior, and the formation of beliefs, attitudes, and stereotypes about other people. Social cognition fuses elements of social and cognitive psychology. In

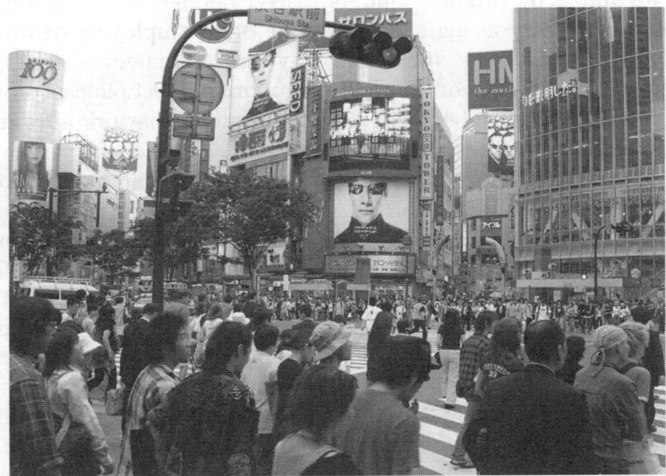

Fig. 12.2 Social psychology studies the nature and causes of social behavior *(For color version, see Plate 2)*

order to understand how people process, remembers, and distort social information. The study of group dynamics reveals information about the nature and potential optimization of leadership, communication, and other phenomena that emerge at least at the microsocial level. In recent years, many social psychologists have become increasingly interested in implicit measures, mediational models, and the interaction of both person and social variables in accounting for behavior.

SCHOOL PSYCHOLOGY

School psychology is also an integral part of educational psychology and clinical psychology to understand and treat students with learning disabilities, to promote the intellectual growth of students in general and weak and below average students in particular. The main object is also promoting safe, supportive, and effective learning environments. School psychologists are trained in educational and behavioral assessment, intervention, and prevention and these psychologist are called professional 'psychologist'.

RESEARCH METHODS (FIG. 12.3)

Psychology leans to be drawing on knowledge from other fields to help explain and understand psychological phenomena. Additionally, psychologists make extensive use of the three modes of inference that were identified by Charles Sanders Peirce: deduction, induction and abduction (hypothesis generation). While often employing deductive-nomological reasoning, they also rely on inductive reasoning to generate explanations. For example, evolutionary psychologists propose explanations of human behavior in terms of such behaviors' advantages for hunter-gatherers.

Academic psychologists may focus purely on research and psychological theory, aiming to further psychological understanding in a specific area, while other psychologists may work in applied psychology to deploy such knowledge for immediate and practical benefit. These approaches are not mutually exclusive, and many psychologists will be involved in both researching and applying psychology at some point during their career. Many clinical psychology programs aim to develop in practicing psychologists both knowledge of and experience with research and experimental methods, which they may interpret and employ as they treat individuals with psychological issues.

When an area of interest requires specific training and specialist knowledge, especially in applied areas, psychological associations are formed and the association in collaboration with educational

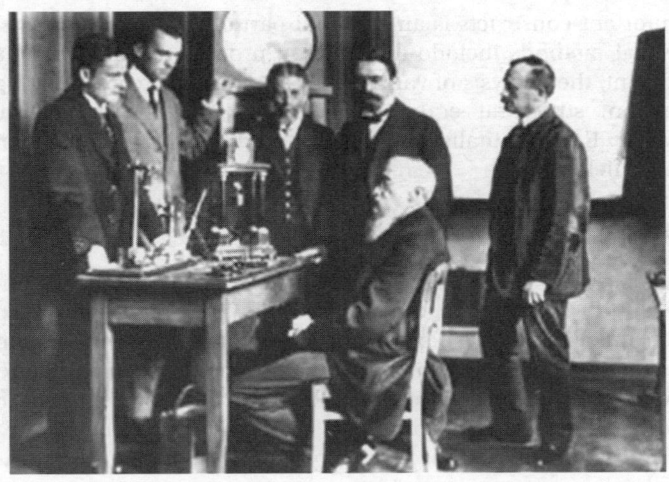

Fig. 12.3 Wilhelm Maximilian Wundt (seated) was a German psychologist, generally acknowledged as a founder of experimental psychology

institutions establish educational and training requirements. These requirements may be laid down for institutional diplomas or university degrees in psychology, so that students acquire an adequate knowledge in a number of areas in order to provide manpower in this specialty where psychologists are required to offer treatment.

QUALITATIVE AND QUANTITATIVE RESEARCH

Qualitative psychological research methods include interviews, first-hand observation, and participant observation. Qualitative researchers aim to enrich interpretations or critiques of symbols, subjective experiences, or social structures. Research in most areas of psychology is conducted in accordance with the standards of the scientific method. Psychological researchers seek theoretically interesting categories and hypotheses from data, using qualitative or quantitative methods or both to explore the unknown to known knowledge. Similar hermeneutic and critical aims have also been served by 'quantitative methods', as in Erich Fromm's study of Nazi voting or Mailgram's studies of obedience to authority.

Quantitative psychological research renders itself to the statistical testing of hypotheses. Quantitatively oriented research designs include the experiment, quasi-experiment, cross-sectional study, case-control study, and longitudinal study. The measurement and operationalization of important constructs is an essential part of these research designs. Statistical methods include the Pearson product-moment correlation coefficient, the analysis of variance, multiple linear regression, logistic regression, structural equation modeling, and hierarchical linear modeling. The quantitative and qualitative research is gaining foothold in all the fields.

PRACTICE

Some observers distinguish a gap between scientific theory and its application—in particular, the application of unsupported or unsound clinical practices. Critics say there has been an increase in the number of mental health training programs that are mainly remain theoretical knowledge and do not inspire scientific competence that help in practice. One disbeliever asserts that practices, such as 'facilitated communication for infantile autism'; memory-recovery techniques including body work; and other therapies, such as rebirthing and reparenting, may be doubtful or even dangerous, despite their qualification to practice. In 1984, Allen Neuringer had made a similar point regarding the experimental analysis of behavior. The institutions impart more practical knowledge and required skills to practice efficiently.

13 Nursing Services

INTRODUCTION

Nursing is a *discipline,* profession, and an area of practice. As a discipline, nursing is centered-around knowledge development. As a profession, nursing has a social mandate to be responsible and accountable to the public it serves.

Nursing is *the integral part of the healthcare system,* and as such encompasses the promotion of health, prevention of illness, and care physically ill, mentally ill, and disabled people of all ages, in all healthcare and other community settings. Within this broadspectrum of healthcare, the particular concern to nurses is individual, family and group responses to actual or potential health problems". The human responses range broadly from health-restoring reactions to an individual episode of illness to the development of policy in promoting the long-term health of a population.

Nursing is *both an art and science* involving the total patients, as promoting spiritual, mental and physical health; stressing health education and health preservation, ministering to the sick, caring for the patient environment and giving health service to the family, the community and the individual (Mother Olivia Gowan, 1943).

Nursing is a *profession in transition.* The trends and issues that underline this phenomenon hold important implications for the management of hospitals and other healthcare institutions and agencies. Nursing service is a critical component in fulfilling hospital, long-term care, and other health service organization objectives for patient care. The nursing profession exists in response to a need of a society and holds ideals related to man's health throughout his lifespan **(Table. 13.1)**.

DEFINITIONS

Nursing Diagnosis

Nursing diagnosis is the process of assessing potential or actual health problems, including those pertaining to a family or community, that fall within the scope of nursing practice; also, a judgment or conclusion reached as a result of such assessment or derived from assessment data.

Nursing Audit

Nursing audit is a method of evaluating nursing practice by reviewing records that document the care provided to patients.

OBJECTIVES

- To provide professional care for patients' recovery and physical and mental health.
- To provide nonprofessional care for patients' comfort and safety such as bed making.

Table 13.1 Job responsibilities, qualification and training and experience of nursing staff

Job	*Responsibilities*	*Education, training and experience*
Director of Nursing	• Directs and supervises all nursing staff and activities • Determines and implements nursing policies and procedures • Plans and directs nurses' introduction and in-service training • Evaluates quality of care	PhD/MSc in nursing with 5 years nursing administration
Assistant Director of Nursing	• Assists Director of nursing and assumes most of the duties and authority during absence • Analyses and evaluates nursing care quality and corrective measures	PhD/MSc degree in nursing with 3 years nursing administration
Nursing Supervisor	• Oversees administration and nursing care for a group of Wards or a Special Care Unit and coordinates them with other departments	BSc degree in nursing with 5 years experience as a head nurse
Night Supervisor	• Represents the Administrator at nights • Visits nursing areas, some patients and other departments • Admits and transfers patients when postponement to day time would be inadvisable	Senior staff-nurse with previous experience as a head nurse

Contd...

Contd...

Job	*Responsibilities*	*Education, training and experience*
Ward Sister	• Supervises and manages ward independently in teaching hospitals. Teaches nursing students in GNM and BSc level	BSc degree in nursing with 3 years experience
Senior Staff-nurse	• Functions as ward in charge, supervises junior staff nurses, auxiliary nurses/midwives and nursing aides	General Nursing and Midwifery trained with 5 years experience as staff nurse in a reputed hospital
Staff Nurses	• Provide nursing services in wards, OPD, A&E, operation theaters, labor room CSSD, radiology, etc. under the supervision of senior staff nurse/ ward sister/nursing supervisor	General nursing and midwifery trained
Auxiliary Nurses	• Assist staff nurses in wards, OPD, A&E, CSSD, labor room, radiology, etc. Auxiliary Nurse Midwife (ANM) under the supervision of senior staff trained nurse/ward sister	Auxiliary Nursing and Midwifery (ANM)
Ward Aides/ Medical Orderlies	• Assist nurses, provides patient transportation/messenger services	Secondary school certificate with formal training in a reputed hospital
Ward Clerks	• Inventory control, collection of patient records, laboratory results, responding admitting office queries, laundry, CSSD affairs, etc.	Secondary school certificate with good handwriting

- To perform administrative duties such as safe-custody of drugs and maintenance of equipment and materials in satisfactory condition.
- To provide continuing education for professional nurses and nursing assistants.
- To undertake understanding, or assist with, research for improved nursing care.
- To provide, where necessary, clinical experience for student nurses.

POLICIES

- To restore patients to the highest level of health individually possible.

- To get patients' families to participate where appropriate, in tasks such as patients' feeding, washing, and dressing.
- To group patients in large wards by degree of illness with groups needing most care located nearest the Nurses' Station.
- To change locations in ward periodically for long stay patients' psychological benefit.

PROCEDURES

Patient Care

- Receiving admitted patients
- Administration of medication
- Assisting physicians
- Performing simple diagnostic procedures
- Collecting and sending specimens to laboratory
- Recording and maintaining medical records
- Recording of vital signs
- Performing gastric lavage and giving enema
- Preoperative preparations
- Delivering bedside nursing
- Coordinating patient care with other team members
- Maintaining clean and safe environment
- Bed making and providing privacy to patients.

Ward Management

- Supervising, directing and controlling staff
- Diet ordering
- Maintaining poisonous and narcotic drug controls and registers
- Communicating
- Maintaining records pertaining to patient care, investigation reports, inventory, medicolegal cases, etc.
- Nursing education
- Safe custody of patients' valuables
- Visitors control
- Discharge and bill settlement.

Operation Theater Management

- Aseptic environment maintenance
- Autoclaving
- Receiving patients from wards
- Coordinating trolley traffic
- Assisting surgeon and anesthetist

- Indenting and procuring surgical instruments and surgical sundries
- Maintaining records and reports
- Safe maintenance of theater equipment and apparatus.

Labor Room Management

- Preparation of expectant mother for aseptic safe delivery
- Conducting normal deliveries
- Assisting doctors in obstetrical emergencies
- Assisting difficult and abnormal deliveries
- Taking care of newborn and premature babies
- Indenting and procuring drugs, linen, etc.
- Maintaining records and reports pertaining to labor room.

Psychiatry Unit Management

- Assisting doctors in admission and discharges
- Preparing patients for electroconvulsive therapy (ECT), therapies and other procedures
- Assisting management of aggressive patients and that with suicidal motives
- Maintaining records, reports and registers.

Postoperative/ICU/Burns Unit Management

- Indenting and procuring drugs, equipment and oxygen cylinders
- Operating ECG, EEG, cardiac resuscitation
- Assisting physicians in operating other high-tech equipment and apparatus.

Educational

- Orientation of new staff and students
- Teaching and guiding staff
- Teaching individual or group of patients
- Clinical teaching
- Demonstrating methods and procedures
- In-service education programs
- Assisting in research programs.

FUNCTIONS

Independent Functions

- The supervision of a patient involving the whole management of care, requiring the application of principles based upon the biological, physical and social sciences.

- The observations of symptoms and reactions, including symptoms of physical and conditions and needs, requiring evaluation or application of principles based upon the biological, the physical and social sciences.
- The accurate recording and reporting of facts, including evaluation of the whole care of the patient.
- The supervision of others, except physicians, contributing to the care of the patient.
- The application and the execution of nursing procedures and techniques.
- The direction and education to secure physical and mental care.

Dependent Function

The application and the execution of legal orders of physicians concerning treatments and medications with an understanding of cause thereof.

PROFESSIONAL NURSING PRACTICE

Professional nursing practice includes:
- Assessment, planning, intervention and evaluation of human responses to health and illness.
- Provision of nursing care to individuals to restore optimum health.
- Procurement, coordination and management of essential patient resources.
- Provision of health counseling and education.
- Establishment of standards of practice for nursing care.
- Development of policies, procedures and protocols.
- Supervision of those assist in the practice of nursing.
- Administration of medications and treatment as prescribed by qualified medical professionals.

ORGANIZATION (FLOW CHART 13.1)

Specialized Nursing Fields

- Medical surgical
- Obstetrics and gynecology
- Pediatric
- Psychiatry
- Community
- Operation theater technique
- Intensive care unit
- Trauma care
- Coronary care.

Flow chart 13.1 Hospital including nursing organization

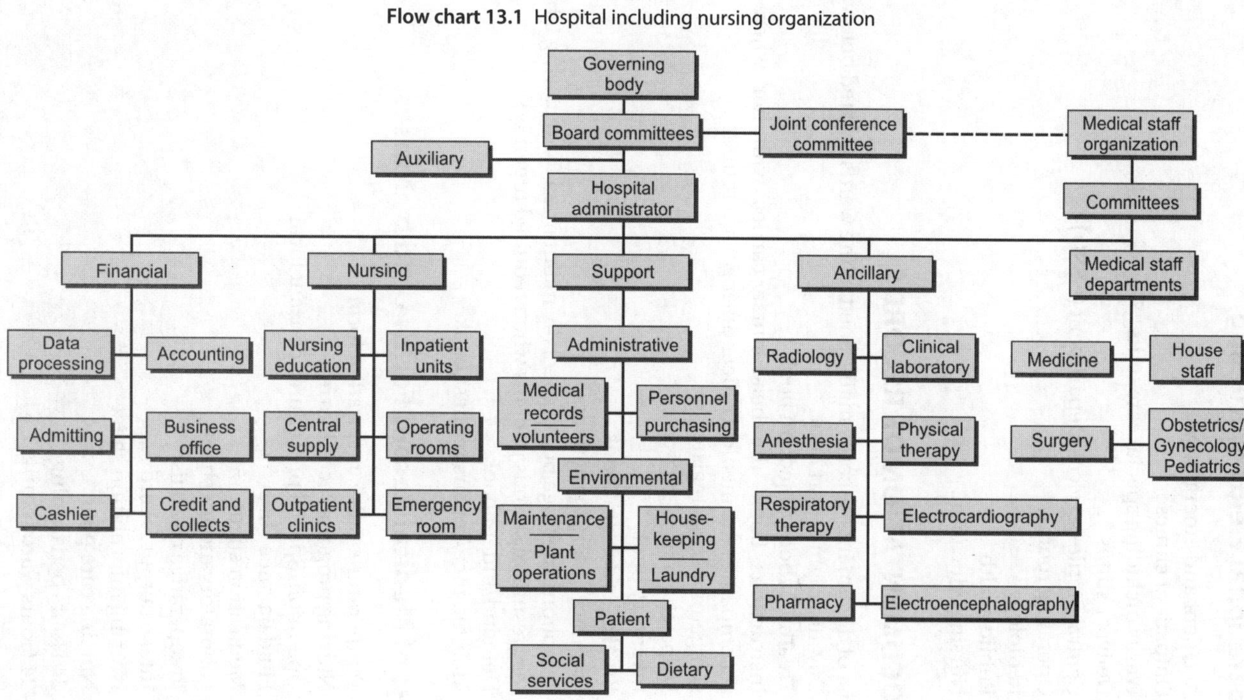

Operational Fields of Nursing

- Accident and emergency
- Outpatient clinics
- Wards including special care units
- Delivery suites
- Central Sterile Services Department (CSSD)
- Operating rooms
- Radiology
- Public health
- Nursing education.

DOCUMENTATION OF RECORDS

A list of documents/records maintained in the wards is listed below:

- Day and night report book
- Treatment book/injection book
- Instructions book—the head nurse carries with her when she accompanies the medical officer during ward rounds
- Dangerous drugs register
- Dispatch book
- Inventory book
- Breakages account book
- Standing orders for patients
- Telephone message book (specially maintained for receiving laboratory results of serious patients when required urgently)
- Demand/indent book
- Maintenance/repairs request book.

List of Medical Record Forms Used by Nurses

- Temperature, pulse, respiration form
- Nursing progress record form
- Operation/Special procedures consent form
- Fluid balance sheet
- Medication sheet
- Laboratory mount sheet
- Preoperative checklist
- Intake output record
- Nursing information sheet
- Nursing care plan
- 24 Hours bed turning
- 24 Hours ward returns

- Diet orders
- Report form—absconded patient
- Incident report form.

Approaches to Staff Development Programs

- Providing information about the current developments in nursing (by magazines, video program, inviting experts for lectures/demonstrations, continuing medical education programs)
- Formal programs
- Unit programs
- Workshops and conferences.

Quality of Nursing Care

The Head Nurse of each ward or special care unit controls the quality of nursing care, primarily, and in detail. Nursing Department Office staff make routine and may be unannounced, overall observations, of 'rounds' of ward activities. Remedial action is implemented through the Head Nurse. Such control may relate to the patients' condition (for controlled pain and anxiety), nurses' professional attitude (for example, attention to patients and families), nursing practices (for example, outdated medications returned to Pharmacy department and materials stored properly), and Medical Records (for example, Nurses' notes recorded up-to-date and without erasures). Other matters controlled by the Nursing Department Office include staff meetings (for example, discussions documented adequately and decisions implemented), and nursing environment (for example, corridors clean, equipment working satisfactorily and materials labeled properly.

Communications

Oral communication includes meetings with nursing staff groups for better use of resources and for better patient care. The public address system, using a coded message summons physicians and especially trained nurses to cardiac arrest patients.

Written communication includes the daily patients' census. The administration manual should include guidance for the Night Supervisor to deal with situations such as power failures and with workers unfit to remain on duty.

Visual communication includes style and color of nurses' uniforms, caps, and belt to signify rank, and lapel pins to signify training school and own name.

Coordination

Coordination is needed:

- Between Nursing Department Office and wards for efficient use of nurses for effective care
- With Medical Staff, while accompanying physicians to patients' bedside
- With Admissions Department to provide accommodation to patients
- Patients selected for clinical lectures and bedside clinics must be available readily for Medical Staff.

Methods of Assigning Nursing Personnel

- *Case method:* It is the set of activities undertaken by a single nurse to mobilize, monitor and evaluate all resources used by a patient during the episode of an illness.
- *Functional nursing*: The responsibilities of the unit are assigned to selected people (Head Nurse) according to their expertise.
- *Team nursing:* In team nursing, ancillary personnel collaborate in providing care to a group of patients under the direction of a professional nurse.
- *Progressive patient care:* A method in which patient care areas provide various levels of care such as Intensive care unit, postintensive care unit, regular care units, convalescent unit and self-care unit
- *Primary nursing:* The primary nurse assumes responsibility for planning the care of one or more patients from admittance to discharge.
- *Modular nursing:* It is a method of nursing assignment in which each nurse is given total responsibility for planning, executing and evaluating nursing care for 4–6 patients.

Public Health Nursing: Functions

- To promote Maternal and Child Health Program (MCH)
- To promote health and nutrition education activities
- To coordinate the activities of health visitors in MCH, Family Planning and Health and Nutrition Education
- To coordinate and conduct Immunization programs
- To help in school health program in the district
- To ensure regular supply of equipment, records, registers, drugs, vaccines and other sundries for MCH program
- To ensure the maintenance of prescribed records and submission of periodical progress of MCH/Family Planning/Nutrition programs

- To help the Statistical Officer in compiling periodical progress reports of programs
- To review the progress of public health programs
- To supervise and give technical guidance and support to ANMs and Health Visitors
- To investigate complaints against public health workers
- To provide continuing education for public health workers
- To work with other functionaries of Social Welfare, Rural Development and voluntary organizations.

Utilization of Nursing Resources

- Nurses' time should be spent on nursing, example, providing direct patient care; adequate staffing levels of clinical and nonclinical support services are required.
- Staffing patterns should utilize levels of education, competence, and experience among nurses. Automated information systems and other labor saving devices should be developed and utilized.
- Costing, budgeting, reporting, and tracking nursing resource utilization should be developed and implemented.

Quality Control

Quality control refers to activities that evaluate, monitor, or regulate services rendered to patients, which can be achieved through the following steps:

- Determination of minimum standards
- Collection of information to determine whether standards are met
- Comparing collected information with established criteria
- Making judgment on quality
- Adopting corrective measures if the standards are not met.

Staff Development

Staff development activities include the following:

- *Induction training:* Briefing philosophy, purpose policies and procedures during first two or three days of employment.
- *Job orientation:* Intended to acquaint a new employee with job responsibilities, work place and routines.
- *In-service education and training:* Ongoing on-the-job education given to enhance performance with advanced techniques.
- *Continuing education:* Educational activity primarily designed to keep the nurses abreast of their field of interest/specialty by updating skills and knowledge.

Nurse Decision-making

- Policy-making and regulatory bodies that have an impact on healthcare should foster greater representation and active participation of the nursing profession
- Employers should ensure active nurse participation in governance, administration and management
- Employers of nurses and physicians should recognize the appropriate clinical decision-making authority of nurses in relationship to other healthcare professionals foster communication and collaboration among the healthcare team, and ensure that the appropriate provider delivers the necessary care; close cooperation and mutual respect between nursing and medicine is essential.

Standards

- *Standard* is a practice that enjoys general recognition and conformity among professionals or an authoritative statement by which the quality of practice, service or education can be judged
- *Standard* are an established rules or basis of comparison in measuring or judging capacity, quantity and value of other products in the same category
- *Standard* is a broad statement of quality
- *Standard* is an acknowledged measure of comparison for quantitative and qualitative values, criterion and norm
- *Standard* is a means of determining what something should be.

Nursing Care Standards

Planning a nursing care standard can be setting a target or a gauge. The following statements visualize the relationship of nursing care standards relating to planning and control devices:

An *objective* is a concrete statement of intention or goal. A *criterion* is the description of variable believed to be an indicator of patient care quality. A *norm* is the current level of performance of a specific criterion, determined by the description of the target population.

By means of objectives, criterion, and norms, the nursing policies and procedures shall be drawn and followed in letter and spirit to establish and maintain required nursing care standards.

Professional Issues

The environment within which every organization function is more stressful than it was in the past. Nursing, traditionally an occupation for women faces additional pressures from the changing opportunities and expectations for women. Nursing, as the largest health profession, has probably received the brunt of the rapid changes in healthcare services.

On the other hand, physicians delegate more responsibility to nurses. Nurses' responsibilities must be coordinated with many other professions. Organization management is much more aggressive in monitoring and controlling patient care practices.

One of the most persistent problems faced by nursing is that of defining what nursing is and what is distinctive about it. Although nurses understand nursing and perhaps most physicians understand nursing, the difficulty in translating nursing to hospital managers remains an enigma, and both nursing and patient care can suffer. This of course stems from the close historical relationship between medicine and nursing and their joint involvement in the clinical care of the patient. In trying to define the nurse's role in relation to the physician's role, some have suggested *nurse's primary emphasis is concerned with care while medicine is concerned with cure.*

Nursing care is not a series of tasks provided to, at, or for someone, but represents *holistic care* individually rendered and *based on needs* of the patient and family. Such nursing output is not easily measured. This lack of quantification can be a source of frustration for some managers. Long-term patient/family outcomes may be the ultimate evaluation of nursing care. But institutions are not directed to improved patient outcome; indeed the converse may be true; for example, under fee-for service reimbursement systems, there are additional financial rewards for complications, such as infection.

Another model suggested by nursing groups emphasizes a decision-making role for nurses. Although it designates a separate domain of expertise and practice, this approach views nursing interacting with the physicians and other health workers. It sees nursing separated into professional decision-making and leadership and technical (cure and care services) activities. This approach stems from increased emphasis on the behavioral sciences. It also represents a determined effort by the profession to develop a science of nursing that will permit accurate prediction and control of the outcomes of nursing intervention.

Negligence

Negligence is the failure to exercise that a prudent (shrewd in the management of practical affairs) person usually exercises marked by a carelessly easy manner.

A nurse may be held liable under negligence in the following incidents:

- Failure to use aseptic technique where required
- Leaving a foreign body inside a patient's body during surgery (mistakes in sponge, instrument or needle count in surgical cases
- Failing to respond promptly on patient symptoms, in critically ill conditions
- Failing to protect an unstable patient from falling or sustaining injuries by any other means
- Disclosure of patient's information to unauthorized persons/agency
- Administering wrong medicine or over dosage of right medicine.

Do it Absolutely Right and Safe

- Right patient
- Right site
- Right drug
- Right dosage
- Right time
- Right route.

Interdepartmental Relationships of Nursing Services

Being the largest department in any healthcare facility, they have relationship with each and every service unit of the hospital and they provide round the clock service to patients of all categories. Being the noblest profession of the world, their relationship starts right from the enquiry unit, labor-room medical records, A&E, wards, special care units, all outpatient clinics, operation theaters, laboratory, radiology CSSD, dietary, social service, laundry, pharmacy, engineering, transports, community health, public health, administrative and up to mortuary services in all levels with high tolerance, accuracy and neatness which is briefed below:

The nursing service is organized into patient care areas by services that include medicine, surgery, obstetrics and gynecology, pediatrics, psychiatry, operating room, outpatient and A&E services. In addition, there may be specialized areas such as cardiac unit, intensive care unit, and respiratory disease unit. The nurse acts as a coordinator of all patient care activities. She works closely with other professionals such as dietitians, medical social workers, pharmacists and others in supplying a comprehensive program of patient care. Good nursing service implies expert observations, which are recorded in the medical record, in medicolegal controversies, nurses' notes are of value as evidence of nursing care given and patient reactions to medical treatment.

The fact that the patient records are in the hands of nursing service throughout a patient's hospitalization brings about the need for a close relationship between medical record and nursing personnel. Prompt preparation and delivery of the medical record by nursing service upon discharge of the patient assist the medical record department in carrying out its many functions. Medical record personnel must understand both the nurses' responsibility in recording nursing treatments and observations, and the duties of ward/unit clerks as they relate to chart arrangement and movement of records. Ward/unit clerks are usually considered to be members of the nursing service. However, in some hospitals, the ward/unit clerk is a member of the medical record department, and in some others, the ward/unit clerk is responsible to a unit manager directly responsible to administration rather than to nursing.

The medical record director, can be helpful to the nursing department in the development of general and special record forms required for recording nursing observations. He would also be involved in determining these forms are incorporated into the patient medical record. The medical record practitioner can assist the nursing department in the conduct of the nursing audit and in the orientation of new nursing personnel. Better understanding of the overall functions of the medical record department should result with cooperation between the medical record and nursing service departments. The nursing personnel deal with medical records in outpatient clinics, emergency service and in wards. In fact, the nursing personnel are the first to handle the records before the medical staff gets them. Proper maintenance of records in the outpatient clinics and emergency service rests mainly with the nursing staff. In case of missing records or reports are conveyed by the nursing staff, to the medical record staff for tracing and making available for patient care. In some hospitals, in the absence of medical record staff, nursing personnel take the responsibility of maintaining records. The nursing staff collects laboratory, X-ray and other reports and mounts them in the respective records and also X-rays are arranged and placed in the appropriate patient records. They take the responsibility of collecting and handing over the records to medical record department. During hospitalization of a patient, the in-charge nurse of the ward collects the investigation reports and mounts them in the concerned record. The X-rays of patients are also collected and kept safely and returned along with patient medical record to the medical record department (MRD) after discharge of the patient. The ward nurse collects and maintains medical record forms in the ward; She takes the responsibility for preparation of birth, death, and stillbirth notifications.

The nursing staff also informs if any case happens to be medicolegal one. She helps in getting consent from the patient. The admission and discharge register maintained in the ward helps in preparing 'Daily Ward Census' of patients and also help in tracing out old records of patients. The nursing staff is an instrument in getting records completed by the medical staff and always assists the doctors in completing operation notes, discharge summary, final diagnosis and so on. The nursing staff has close relationship with the admitting office, and informs regularly the bed status of the ward. The nursing staff fixes for follow-up care. The nursing staff also helps in recording correct identification data in all the forms of the record.

PERFORMANCE APPRAISALS

- *Trait rating scales:* Rating an individual against a set standard.
- *Job dimension scales:* Rating factors are taken from written job description.
- *Behaviorally anchored rating scales:* A technique that requires a separate rating form developed for each job classification.
- *Checklists:* Composed of many behavior styles that indicate desirable behaviors. Score is based on behavior or attributes.
- *Essays:* The appraiser describes the employee strengths and area where improvement or perfection is needed.

PROBLEMS

- Time management
- Frequent change of nurses between service units
- Medication orders by physicians over telephone
- Too many instructions from many sides
- Answering everybody
- Distractions and forgetting instructions
- Controlling visitors.

Note: If any issue is managed with team spirit, considering the well-being of patients, most of the problems can be easily avoided. Egoistic nature of professionals should not affect quality of patient care.

14 Physical Therapy

INTRODUCTION

Physical therapy is the profession which uses, knowledge and skills, in rendering care for individuals, disabled by disease and injury, the primary focus is on the functional restoration, of patients, affected with skeletal neuromuscular, cardiovascular and pulmonary disorders.

Designing and fitting of artificial parts or limbs and rehabilitating them by a treatment process to help physically handicapped individuals to make maximal use of residual capacities, and to enable them to obtain optimal satisfaction and usefulness, in terms of themselves, their families and their community **(Table.14.1)**.

Physical therapy (also known as physiotherapy) is a healthcare profession which provides treatment to individuals in order to develop, maintain and restore maximum movement and function throughout life. This includes providing treatment in circumstances where movement

Table 14.1 Types of physical therapy and their definition

S. No.	*Name of the therapy*	*Definition*
1.	Electrotherapy	Use of electric current in the treatment of disease to improve muscular activities, to produce sensory modulation for control of pain and to produce reflex effects in the treatment of motor disorders
2.	Hydrotherapy	The use of water in its various form: Liquid, solid and vapor either internally or externally in the treatment of nervous and musculoskeletal diseases
3.	Massage	Manipulation of soft tissues, of the bodies, most effectively performed with the hands, and administered, to produce effects, on the nervous and muscular systems and local and the general circulation of the blood and lymph

and function are threatened by aging, injury, disease or environmental factors.

Physical therapy is concerned with identifying and maximizing quality of human being and movement potential within the spheres of promotion, prevention, treatment/intervention, habilitation and rehabilitation. This includes physical, psychological, emotional, and social well-being. It involves the interaction between physical therapist (PT), patients/clients, other health professionals, families, care givers, and communities in a process where movement potential is assessed and goals are agreed upon, using knowledge and skills unique to physical therapists. Physical therapy is performed by either a physical therapist (PT) or an assistant (PTA) acting under their direction. Physiotherapist utilizes an individual's history and physical examination to establish a diagnosis and create a management plan, and when necessary, incorporate the results of laboratory and imaging studies. The physical therapist use diagnostic testing, e.g. electromyograms and nerve conduction velocity testing for arriving at proper assessment and diagnosis. Physical therapy has many specialties including, geriatrics, neurologic, orthopedic, pediatrics, and cardiopulmonary to name some of the more common areas. PTs practice in many settings, such as outpatient clinics or offices, inpatient orthopedic wards or rehabilitation facilities, skilled nursing homes and facilities, extended healthcare facilities, private homes, education and research centers, schools, hospices, industrial workplaces or other occupational environments, fitness centers and sports training facilities. Educational qualifications vary greatly by country.

SPECIALTY AREAS

The physical therapy field is growing enormously and participating in many areas and the body of knowledge of physical therapy is quite large. Some PTs specialize in a specific clinical and many other areas. The American Board of Physical Therapy Specialties listed seven specialist certifications, including Sports Physical Therapy and Clinical Electrophysiology. Worldwide the six most common specialty areas in physical therapy are: cardiopulmonary, geriatric, neurological, orthopedic, pediatric and integumentary. The briefly explanation is given below:

CARDIOPULMONARY

Cardiovascular and pulmonary rehabilitation physical therapists treat a wide variety of individuals with cardiopulmonary disorders or those who have had cardiac or pulmonary surgery. Primary goals of this specialty include increasing endurance and functional independence. Manual therapy is utilized in this field to assist in clearing lung secretions experienced with cystic fibrosis. Disorders, including heart attacks, postcoronary bypass surgery, chronic obstructive pulmonary disease, and pulmonary fibrosis, treatments can benefit from cardiovascular and pulmonary specialized physical therapists.

GERIATRIC

Geriatric physical therapy covers a wide area of issues concerning people as they go through normal adult lifespan, but is usually focused on the older adult. There are many conditions that affect many people as they grow older and include but are not limited to the following: osteoporosis, cancer, arthritis, Alzheimer's disease, hip and joint replacement, balance disorders, incontinence, etc. Geriatric physical therapy helps those affected by such problems in developing a specialized program to help restore mobility, reduce pain, and increase fitness levels to have a normal physical fitness.

NEUROLOGICAL

Neurological physical therapy is a discipline focused on working with individuals who have a neurological disorder or disease. These include Alzheimer's disease, ALS, brain injury, cerebral palsy, multiple sclerosis, Parkinson's disease, spinal cord injury, and stroke. Common impairments associated with neurological conditions include impairments of vision, balance, and ambulation, activities of daily living, movement, speech and loss of functional independence. Though the treatment is of longer duration, the promising results have demonstrated in cases where persuasion and will power prevailed.

ORTHOPEDIC PHYSICAL THERAPY

Orthopedic physical therapists, assess, diagnose, manage, and treat disorders and injuries of the musculoskeletal system including rehabilitation after orthopedic surgery. This specialty of physical therapy is most often found in the outpatient clinical setting. Orthopedic therapists are trained in the treatment of postoperative orthopedic procedures, fractures, acute sports injuries, arthritis, sprains, strains, back and neck pain, spinal conditions and amputations. Joint and spine mobilization/manipulation, therapeutic exercise, neuromuscular re-education, hot/cold packs, and electrical muscle stimulation, e.g. cry therapy, iontophoresis, electrotherapy are modalities often used to expedite recovery in the orthopedic setting. The use of sonography for diagnosis and to guide treatments such as muscle retraining. Those who have suffered injury or disease affecting the muscles, bones, ligaments, or tendons of the body will benefit from assessment by a physical therapist specialized in orthopedics. This field is becoming more popular with the sport therapy and cosmetic and fitness consciousness among people.

PEDIATRIC PHYSICAL THERAPY

Pediatric physical therapy assists in early detection of health problems and uses a wide variety of modalities to treat disorders in the pediatric population. These therapists are specialized in the assessment, diagnosis, treatment, and management of infants, children, and adolescents with a variety of congenital, developmental, neuromuscular, skeletal, or acquired disorders/diseases. Treatments focus on improving gross and fine motor skills, balance and coordination, strength and endurance as well as cognitive and sensory processing/integration. The therapists are playing a good role in treating the children with developmental delays, cerebral palsy, spina bifida, or portcullis.

INTEGUMENTARY PHYSICAL THERAPIST

This unit named as integumentary which treats conditions involving the skin and related organs and also wounds and burns. Physical therapists utilize surgical instruments, mechanical lavage, dressings and topical agents to debride necrotic tissue and promote tissue healing. Other commonly used interventions include exercise, edema control, splinting, casting and compression outfits.

Form 1 Physical therapy treatment card

Health Care No.: ☐☐ ☐☐ ☐ ☐☐☐ ☐☐☐☐

Name : ______

Age : ☐☐ Yrs/Month Sex : ☐ M ☐ F

Nationality: ______

Consultant In-Charge: ______

Dept.: ______ Unit: ______

PHYSICAL THERAPY TREATMENT CARD

Diagnosis/Relevant Clinical Findings/Associated Conditions :

Contraindications :

Treatment Requested		Treatment Requested
☐ Hydrotherapy		☐ Hot Packs
☐ Mobilization	☐ Non wt. Bearing ☐ Partial wt. Bearing ☐ Full wt. Bearing	☐ Ultrasound ☐ Wax
☐ Exercises	☐ Active ☐ Assistive ☐ Passive	☐ Shortwave diathermy ☐ Traction
☐ Ice therapy ☐ Muscle stimulation ☐ Message		☐ Others (Specify) ______

NEXT APPOINTMENT WITH DOCTOR

Date : ______ Doctor's Name : ______

Signature : ______

RECORD OF ATTENDANCE

MONTH	1	2	3	4	5	6	7	8	9	10	11	12	13	14	15	16	17	18	19	20	21	22	23	24	25	26	27	28	29	30	31

DATE	TIME	INITIAL ASSESSMENT AND TREATMENT NOTES	Signature

("Note : After Treatment this Card Should Become Part of Patant File")

Form 2 Physical therapy analysis and treatment plan

PHYSICAL THERAPY ANALYSIS AND TREATMENT PLAN

Medical Record # :
Hospital Name :
Patient Name :
Date of Birth :
Attending Physician :
Date of Admission:

☐ OPD
☐ IPD

Initial assessment summary and analysis :

Problems :	Goals :

Treatment Plan :

Signature : ____________ Date : ____________

PHYSICAL THERAPY ANALYSIS AND TREATMENT PLAN

Form 3 Physical therapy request form

Medical Record # :
Hospital Name :
Patient Name :
Date of Birth :
Attending Physician :
Date of Admission: ☐ OPD ☐ IPD

PHYSIOTHERAPY REQUEST FORM

Clinical Data:

Diagnosis :

Objective of referral :

Date : Specialty : Reffered by :

PHYSIOTHERAPY REPORT

Discharge summary :

Recommendation :

Date : ____________________

____
Therapist Name and Signature

Ist Copy : Patient Medical Record/2nd Copy : Physiotherapy Dept.

(PHYSIOTHERAPY REQUEST FORM)

Form 4 Chedoke-McMaster stroke assessment disability inventory

Medical Record # :
Hospital Name :
Patient Name :
Date of Birth :
Attending Physician :
Date of Admission:

☐ OPD
☐ IPD

CHEDOKE-McMASTER STROKE ASSESSMENT DISABILITY INVENTORY

Admission   Discharge   Other : ____________

SCORING LEVELS		
NO HELPER	Independence 7 Complete Independence 6 Modified Independence	 (Timely, Safely) (Device)
HELPER	Modified Dependence 5 Supervision 4 Minimal Assist 3 Moderate Assist Complete Dependence 2 Maximal Assist 1 Total Assist	 (Client = 75%) (Client = 50%) (Client = 25%) (Client = 0%)

	Score
1. Supine to side lying on strong side	
2. Supine to side lying on weak side	
3. Side lying to long sitting through strong side	
4. Side lying to sitting on side of the bed through strong side	
5. Side lying to sitting on side of the bed through weak side	
6. Remain standing	
7. Transfer to and from bed towards strong side	
8. Transfer to and from bed towards weak side	
9. Transfer up and down from floor and chair	
10. Transfer up and down from floor and standing	
11. Walk indoors—25 m	
12. Walk outdoors, over rough ground, ramps and curbs—150 m	
13. Walk outdoors several blocks—900 m	
14. Walk up and down stairs	
15. Age appropriate walking distance for 2 min (2 Point Bonus) Distance——m	
Total Score :	

To score Bonus : for age <70 yrs distance must be >96 meters
for age >70 yrs distance must be >80 meters

Waling aids :
Walker ____________
4 point cane ____________
1 point cane ____________
brace ____________

Signature : ______________________ Date : ____________

Form 5 Functional Independent Measure

Medical Record # :
Hospital Name :
Patient Name :
Date of Birth :
Attending Physician :
Date of Admission :

☐ OPD
☐ IPD

FUNCTIONAL INDEPENDENCE MEASURE

LEVELS		
	INDEPENDENCE 7. Complete Independence (Timely, Safety) 6. Modified Independence (Device)	No Helper
	MODIFIED DEPENDENCE 5. Supervision 4. Minimal Assist (Subject = 75%) 3. Moderate Assist (Subject = 50%)	
	COMPLETE DEPENDENCE 2. Maximal Assist (Subject = 25 %) 1. Total Assist (Subject = 0%)	Helper

		Admit	D/C	Re-assess
	Self-care			
A.	Feeding	☐	☐	☐
B.	Grooming	☐	☐	☐
C.	Bathing	☐	☐	☐
D.	Dressing-Upper body	☐	☐	☐
E.	Dressing-Lower body	☐	☐	☐
F.	Toileting	☐	☐	☐
	Sphinter Control			
G.	Bladder management	☐	☐	☐
H.	Bowel management	☐	☐	☐
	Mobility-Transfers			
I.	Bed, chair, W/C	☐	☐	☐
J.	Toilet	☐	☐	☐
K.	Tub, shower	☐	☐	☐
	Locomotion			
L.	Walk/Wheel chair	☐ ____	☐ ____	☐ ____
M.	Stairs	☐	☐	☐
	Total :	____	____	____
	Initial :	____	____	____

Signature : ______________________ Date : ______________

FUNCTIONAL INDEPENDENT MEASURE

15 Occupational Therapy

INTRODUCTION

Occupational therapy (OT) often abbreviated as OT, (but in surgical terms OT is considered as Operation Theater). The World Federation of Occupational Therapists defines occupational therapy as a profession concerned with promoting health and well-being through occupation. Occupational therapists address the question, "Why does this person have difficulties in his or her daily activities (or occupations), and what can we adapt to make it possible for him or her to manage better to impact his or her health and well-being?" Occupational therapists use careful analysis of physical, environmental, psychosocial, mental, spiritual, political and cultural factors to identify barriers to occupation. The primary goal of an occupational therapist is to enable individuals, groups and communities to participate in activities which are meaningful to them, reflect their beliefs and values, and produce a sense of accomplishment or satisfaction. Occupational therapy has been described as addressing the 'skills for the job of living' necessary for 'living life to its fullest.' Occupational therapy draws from the fields of medicine, psychology, sociology, anthropology, ethnography, architecture and many other disciplines in developing its knowledge base. A new discipline of occupational science has been developed to enhance the evidence base of the profession. Occupational therapists work with individuals, families, groups and communities to facilitate health and well-being through engagement or re-engagement in occupation. Occupational therapists are becoming increasingly involved in addressing the impact of social, political and environmental factors that contribute to exclusion and occupational deficiencies. Through this profession, many handicapped personnel have gained the skills that made them to be independent although for some is with limited activities, nevertheless, proved handy in their day-to-day life.

OCCUPATION

Occupation is the dynamic relationship between the occupational form and occupational performance. Many people see the term occupation as a job one does. However, the meaning of occupation is seen in a much wider context by an Occupational Therapist. A human being can be engaged in a wide range of occupations that had a significant role in their involvement to bring to normal situation to the extent possible.

OCCUPATIONAL FORM

Wu and Lin (1999) stated that the occupational form was the 'objective pre-existing structure or environmental context that elicits or guides subsequent human performance'. The occupational form consists of objective features and these include materials, human context and sociocultural dimensions.

OCCUPATIONAL PERFORMANCE

Occupational performance is the active voluntary occupational form carried out by human being.

An Occupational Therapist works systematically through a sequence of actions known as the occupational therapy process. There are several versions of this process as described by numerous writers. Creek (2003) has sought to provide a comprehensive version based on extensive research. This version has 11 stages, which for the experienced therapist may not be linear in nature. The stages are:

1. Referral
2. Information gathering
3. Initial assessment
4. Needs identification/problem formation
5. Goal setting
6. Action planning
7. Action
8. Ongoing assessment and revision of action
9. Outcome and outcome measurement
10. End of intervention or discharge
11. Review.

Fearing, Law and Clark (1997) suggested a 7 stage process which includes:

1. Identifying of occupational performance issues
2. Choosing a theoretical frame of reference
3. Assessing factors contributing the identified occupational performance issue(s)
4. Considering the strengths and resources of both client and therapist
5. Negotiating targeted outcomes and developing action plan
6. Implementing the plan through occupation
7. Evaluating outcomes.

A central ingredient of this process model is the focus on identifying both customer and therapists strengths and resources prior to beginning to develop the outcomes and plan of action.

The role of Occupational Therapy allows OT's to work in many different settings, work with many different organizations and acquire many different specialties. This broad spectrum of practice lends itself to difficulty categorizing the areas of practice that exist, especially considering the many countries and different healthcare systems. In this section, the categorization from the American Occupational Therapy Association is used. However, there are other ways to categorize areas of practice in OT, such as physical, mental, and community practice (AOTA, 2009). These divisions occur when the setting is defined by the population it serves. For example, acute physical or mental health settings in hospitals, in outpatient clinics, subacute settings, geriatric care facilities and community settings.

In each area of practice below, an OT can work with different diagnostic, specialties and in different therapy centers.

PHYSICAL HEALTH

- *Pediatrics:* Schools, inpatient hospital-based child OT: Often, children and adults need OT services. Nevertheless, OTs approach intervention in a different way with children and adults as approaches treatment through occupation, and the occupations of a child are different from those of an adult; and include play, chores, self-care and schoolwork. Common conditions that are specific to or more common in the pediatric population creating a need for OT services include: developmental disorders, sensory regulation or sensory processing deficiencies, motor developmental delays, autism, emotional and behavioral disturbances (Lambert, 2005), among others. In addition, children are seen for every injury, illness or chronic condition that may cause a person of any age to have performance deficits in their daily life and thus benefit from OT services.
- *Acute care hospitals:* Acute care is an inpatient hospital setting for individuals with a serious medical condition(s) usually due to a traumatic event, such as a traumatic brain injury, spinal cord injury, etc. The primary goal of acute care is to stabilize the patient's medical status and address any threats to his or her life and loss of function. Occupational therapy plays an important role in facilitating early mobilization, restoring function, preventing further decline, and coordinating care, including transition and discharge planning. Furthermore, occupational therapy's role focuses on addressing deficits and barriers that limit the patient's ability to perform activities

that they need or want to create independence in self-care, home management, work-related tasks, and participating in community activity.

- *Inpatient rehabilitation especially in cases of spinal cord injuries:* People with different disabilities have the right and the privilege to live meaningful purposeful lives. When a disability occurs it is sometimes, it is possible to recover—when it is not it is important to learn the skills to adapt capacity and environmental supports to be able to participate. OTs uses their knowledge to help both with recovery and adaptation.
- *Rehabilitation centers* such as traumatic brain injury (TBI), stroke cerebrovascular accident (CVA), spinal cord injuries, and head injuries, etc.
- *Skilled nursing facilities:* An occupational therapists role in a skilled nursing facility is centered on each client's individual needs. Many of the skills an OT works are known as activities of daily living or self-care such as feeding or dressing. OTs can provide equipment to assist with activities or offer expertise in modifying the environment to maximize independence and facilitate independence. Other OT roles include education in adaptive equipment (shower bench), energy conservation, or task simplification (Hofmann, 2008).
- *Home health:* Occupational therapists who work in this area of practice generally work with clients in the geriatric population who have one or more of the following diagnoses: Alzheimer's disease, arthritis, depression, CVA, generalized weakness, chronic obstructive pulmonary disease (COPD), or Parkinson's disease. Occupational therapists working with these client's evaluate their level of independence, cognition, and safety. Moreover, occupational therapists provide intervention to maximize independence and function through remedial and compensatory strategies, with the ultimate goal of the client's regaining the ability to live independently at home (Swanson Anderson & Malaski, 1999).
- *Outpatient clinics* especially hand therapy, orthopedics clinics. Hand therapy is a specialty practice area of occupational therapy that is mainly concerned with treating orthopedic-based upper extremity conditions to optimize the functional use of the hand and arm. Diagnoses seen by this practice area include: fractures of the hand or arm, lacerations and amputations, burns, and surgical repairs of tendons and nerves. Additionally, hand therapists treat

acquired conditions such as tendonitis, rheumatoid arthritis and osteoarthritis, and carpal tunnel syndrome. Occupational therapists who work in this field address biomechanical issues underlying upper-extremity conditions. Besides, occupational therapists use an occupation-based and client-centered approach by identifying participation needs of the client, then tailoring intervention to improve performance in desired activities.

- Specialist assessment centers dealing with electronic assistive technology, posture and mobility services.
- *Hospices:* An occupational therapists common role in hospice care is modifying and preventing. Modifying the demands of the activity to fit with the abilities of the client. The intervention may be directly with the client or with the client and the client's caregivers. OT can offer the caregivers support an education. Progress is defined as improved quality of life in hospice care (Hasselkaus, 1998).
- *Assisted living facilities (ALF):* In an assisted living facility OT services are provided by a home health agency, rehab agency, or a private practice. Medicare and some private insurance plans cover OT services in ALFs, areas of treatment intervention often include: bathing, dressing, grooming, toileting, mobility, money management, laundry, and community participation. One can treat persons with occupational performance decline or at risk for a decline. Increase quality of life so fewer residents need the services of a long-term SNF. Special areas include mobility device assessment (scooter), continence training, psychosocial needs and low vision programs (Fagan, 2001).
- *Productive aging:* An OT practicing in this area would provide skills and services to older adults to maximize independence, participation, and quality of life. Typical issues addressed: Any impairment or condition that would limit their ability to carry out meaningful occupations and tasks that are necessary for daily life. Skills taught include: energy conservation, education in adaptive equipment such as a shower bench, task simplification, adapting and modifying activities to progress with a client's changing abilities (Opp Hoffman, 2008), caregiver education and support (AOTA, 2004), safety, social interactions and communication, memory skills training, mobility device assessment and training, i.e. scooters, wheelchairs, walkers, low vision interventions, continence training, and facilitating performance in basic ADL and IADL (Fagan, 2001).

- *Work hardening* is essentially a specialized program designed to enable people with physical, psychological, and psychosocial issues inhibiting a person's ability, to successfully come back to work. The National Advisory Committee on Work Hardening best describes work hardening as defined below:

  Work hardening is a highly structured, goal oriented, individualized treatment program designed to maximize the individual's ability to return to work. Work hardening programs, which are interdisciplinary in nature, use real or simulated work activities in combination with conditioning tasks that are graded to progressively improve the biomechanical, neuromuscular, cardiovascular/metabolic and psychosocial functions of the individual. Work hardening provides a transition between acute care and return to work while addressing the issues of productivity, safety, physical tolerances, and worker behaviors (Ogden-Niemeyer & Jacobs, 1989).
- *Work conditioning* is similar to work hardening, except work conditioning purely involves improving physical capacities, whereas work hardening improves physical, psychological, and psychosocial factors.

MENTAL HEALTH

According to Medicare (2005) guidance, 'Only a qualified occupational therapist has the knowledge, training, and experience required to evaluate and, as necessary, re-evaluate a patient's level of function, determine whether an occupational therapy program could reasonably be expected to improve, restore, or compensate for lost function, and where appropriate, recommend to the physician a plan of treatment'.

According to the American Occupational Therapy Association (AOTA), occupational therapists work with the Mental Health population throughout the lifespan and across many treatment settings where mental health services and psychiatric rehabilitation are provided (AOTA, 2009). Just as with other clients, the OT facilitates maximum independence in activities of daily living (dressing, grooming, etc.) and instrumental activities of daily living (medication management, grocery shopping, etc). According to the American Occupational Therapy Association, OT improves functional capacity and quality of life for people with mental illness in the areas of employment, education, community living, and home and personal care through the use of real life activities in therapy treatments (AOTA, 2005).

Mental illness or mental health issues related to: Geriatric, adult, adolescents and children. These conditions include but are not limited to: Schizophrenia, substance abuse, addiction, dementia, Alzheimer's, mood disorders, personality disorders, psychoses, eating disorders, anxiety disorders (including post-traumatic stress disorder, separation anxiety disorder) (Cara & MacRae, 2005), and reactive attachment disorder (children only) (Lambert, 2005).

Typical issues that are addressed are as follows: Helping people acquire the skills to care for themselves or others including; keeping a schedule, medication management, employment, education, increasing community participation, community access (grocery store, library, bank, etc.), money management skills, engaging in productive activities to fill the day, coping skills, routine building, building social skills and childcare (Cara & McRae, 2005).

In the UK, the College of Occupational Therapists (COT) have published Recovering Ordinary Lives, which details the strategy for OTs in mental health up to 2017, and makes explicit the goals that have been set for the profession, in line with government directives (COT 2006). Areas that Mental Health OT's could work in are as follows:

Mental Health Inpatient Units

- Adolescent, adult and older people's acute mental health wards
- Adult and older people's rehabilitation wards
- Prisons/secure units (Forensic psychiatry)
- Psychiatric intensive care unit
- Specialist units for eating disorders, learning disabilities
  - Community based mental health teams
- Child and adolescent mental health teams
- Adult and older people's community mental health teams
- Rehabilitation and recovery and assertive outreach community teams
- Primary care services in GP practices
- Home treatment teams
- Early intervention in psychosis teams
- Specialist learning disability, eating disorder community services
- Day services
- Vocational services
- *Dementia and Alzheimer care:* OTs focus on adapting activities as the client progresses through the illness (Hofmann, 2008) OT also works with caregivers to teach them how to grade activities to the client's ability. Interventions are based on using the client's strengths to increase their quality of life and their relationships with caregivers. Use of social interactions, communication, memory, safety and self-maintenance.

Community-based Practice

Community based practice involves working with people in their own environment rather than in a hospital setting. It often combines the knowledge and skills related to physical and mental health. It can also involve working with atypical populations such as the homeless or at-risk populations. Examples of community-based practice settings:

- *Health promotion and lifestyle change:* Remaining healthy is the goal of all people in a society, including people with chronic disabling or health conditions. Achieving health requires skills to self-manage conditions that might limit their ability to function in daily life. The occupational therapist helps people acquire these skills (Wilcock, 2005).
- Private practice.
- *Aging in place:* Occupational therapists implement environmental modifications in senior housing, assisted living, long-term-care facilities, and homes (Yamkovenko, 2008). Environmental modifications can include rearranging furniture, building ramps, widening doorways, grab bars, special toilet seats, and other safety equipment to use performance capabilities to their fullest (Moyers & Christiansen, 2004).
- *Low vision:* Occupational therapists help clients use their remaining vision to complete their daily routines with compensation, remediation, disability prevention and health promotion. Compensations or that modification to the environment may include proper lighting, color contrast, reducing clutter and education on adaptive equipment (Golembiewski, 2004).
- Intermediate care services.
- *Driving centers:* Driving is an instrumental activity of daily living and an occupational therapist may evaluate and treat skills needed to drive such as vision, executive function or memory. If a client needs more skilled assessment and training they would refer them to an OT Driver Rehabilitation Specialist which could do on the road assessment, training in adaptive equipment and make more specific recommendations.
- Day centers.
- Schools.
- Child development centers.
- People's own homes, carrying out therapy and providing equipment and adaptations.
- *Work and industry:* To be a healthy successful worker there must be a person environment fit between the task, the equipment,

and the person's skills. Occupational therapists work to achieve that fit (Ellexson, 2000; Clinger, Dodson, Maltchev, & Page, 2007). *Populations, conditions, and diagnoses*: People of working age and ability who have been born with or developed a condition, injury, or illness that compromises their ability to work (Ellexson, 2000; Clinger, Dodson, Maltchev, & Page, 2007). *Settings*: Return to work programs, large organizations, consultants to large organizations, work hardening programs, work conditioning programs, transitional return to work programs (Ellexson, 2000; Clinger, Dodson, Maltchev, & Page, 2007). *Typical issues addressed*: Assessment of ability to work, interventions to enhancing work performance by means of work hardening, work conditioning, and improvement of ergonomics in the workplace, identification of accommodations necessary to return-to-work following illness or injury, prevention of work related injury, illness, or disability (Ellexson, 2000; Clinger, Dodson, Maltchev, & Page, 2007).
- Homeless shelters.
- Educational settings.
- Refugee camps.

NEW EMERGING PRACTICE AREAS FOR THERAPY

- *Children and youth*: Psychosocial needs of children and youth
- *Health and wellness*:
  - Health and wellness consulting
  - Design and accessibility consulting and home modification
  - Ergonomic consulting
  - Private practice community health services.
- *Productive aging*:
  - Driver rehabilitation and training
  - Low vision services
- *Rehabilitation, disability, and participation*: Technology and assistive device development and consulting
- *Work and industry*:
  - Ticket to work services
  - Welfare to work services.

OCCUPATIONAL THERAPY APPROACHES

Services typically include:
- Teaching new ways of approaching tasks
- How to breakdown activities into achievable components for example sequencing a complex task like cooking a complex meal

- Comprehensive home and job site evaluations with adaptation recommendations
- Performance skills assessments and treatment
- Adaptive equipment recommendations and usage training
- Environmental adaptation including provision of equipment or designing adaptations to remove obstacles or make them manageable
- Guidance to family members and caregivers
- The use of creative media as therapeutic activity.

ACTIVITY ANALYSIS

Activity analysis has been defined as a process of dissecting an activity into its component parts and task sequence in order to identify its inherent properties and the skills required for its performance, thus allowing the therapist to evaluate its therapeutic prospective.

Therapeutic Activity

Occupational therapists use therapeutic activity or therapeutic occupation to improve an individual's occupational performance and increase function in activities of daily living.

A core and unique feature of occupational therapy practice is the use of occupation as a therapeutic medium. An occupational therapy core skill as defined by The College of Occupational Therapists (COT) is the use of activity as a therapeutic tool.

Occupational therapists have utilized activities, such as crafts, since the profession was founded. The arts and crafts movement in the very early 20th century had ascertained that goal directed activity had a curative effect on the social problems inherent in the newly industrialized societies. The founders of the occupational therapy profession extended this thinking to the treatment of individuals' with mental health problems and as a consequence between 1920 and 1940 much of occupational therapy practice concentrated around the use of crafts as purposeful activities. The emergence of occupational therapy in physical medicine began during World War II and craft activities were utilized to rehabilitate injured soldiers. This method of practice was later termed by Mosey as activity synthesis.

Activity synthesis or occupational synthesis is the core of occupational therapy practice; occupational therapists, in collaboration with clients, design occupational forms to produce a therapeutic occupation or activity, that is meaningful and purposeful to the client. The therapeutic activity or occupation may be used to assess the client's occupational needs or to achieve a therapeutic goal. The component parts of an activity or occupation are matched with the required occupational performance outcomes. For example, the muscle movements elicited by pottery may address fine motor and gross motor skills to improve shoulder flexion and extension, range of movement and elbow extension and flexion.

Other therapeutic activities or occupations may include cookery activities, such as making a smoothie or a healthy food. The components of this activity such as planning and following a recipe may address cognitive components of occupational performance such as problem solving, sequencing and learning. Health may be promoted through this occupation, enabling clients to consider healthy eating issues. Occupational therapists may further use therapeutic activities or occupations to assess occupational performance. For example, an occupational therapist may ask a customer to make a cup of coffee or prepare a simple meal to assess performance in activities of daily living (ADL). An occupational therapist may use a board or card game to assess cognitive components of occupational performance. This application of therapeutic activity/occupation involves use of the core skills of the occupational therapist, chiefly assessment and problem solving.

THEORETICAL FRAMEWORKS

Occupational therapists use a number of theoretical frameworks to frame their practice. Note that terminology has differed between scholars. Theoretical bases for framing a human and their occupation being include the following:

Frames of Reference or Generic Models

Frames of reference or generic models are the over arching title given to a collation of compatible knowledge, research and theories that form conceptual practice. More generally, they are defined as those aspects which influence our perceptions, decisions and practice.

Occupational therapy frame of references/models:

- Person Environment Occupation Performance Model (PEOP)
- Model of Human Occupation (MOHO)
- Canadian Model of Occupational Performance (CMOP)
- Biomechanical
- Rehabilitative (compensatory)
- Neurofunctional (Gordon Muir Giles and Clark-Wilson)
- Cognitive disabilities
- Sensory integration
- Lifestyle Performance Model (Fidler).

Approaches/Intervention Models

These are the methods of carrying out the frames of reference. Again, terminology differs depending on your viewpoint and literature base.

UNITED STATES

Education Requirements

In many countries, occupational therapists are educated at the baccalaureate level. However, currently in the United States and Canada, entry level is at the master's level. This change occurred in 2007, requiring all occupational therapists that started their educational program after 2007 to continue their education beyond a four-year degree. Currently, six schools in the US offer a clinical doctorate for those who would like to further their education past the Master's level.

All occupational therapists have a well-rounded knowledge of biomedical, behavioral, environmental and occupational scientists. Occupational therapist base their interventions on the knowledge based on neuroscience, anatomy, applied technology, policy and environmental strategies. These schools are currently accredited for Master's level education and also accredited for Doctoral level education.

Employment

According to the Bureau of Labor Statistics, occupational therapists held 99,000 positions in 2006 (2009). States with the most licensed and employed occupational therapists are California, New York, Pennsylvania and Ohio. In 2006, 52.6% of occupational therapists worked in hospitals, early intervention facilities and schools (American Occupational Therapy Association, 2006). The Bureau of Labor statistics reported that 78% of occupational therapists worked full-time in 2006 (Bureau of Labor Statistics, 2009). In addition, the median number of years of experience for occupational therapists was 13 years (American Occupational Therapy Association, 2006). Occupational therapists can work in many different settings, some examples include:

- Hospitals
- Schools
- Early intervention facilities
- Skilled nursing facilities
- Home healthcare services
- Outpatient care centers
- Government agencies
- Private practice.

The field of occupational therapy is projected to see faster growth than other careers. The Bureau of Labor Statistics estimates that the number of jobs will grow to 122,000 in 2016 (2009). Areas of occupational therapy that involve helping older adults will see the most growth. This expansion is due to the large need to provide healthcare services to the aging baby boom generation (American Occupational Therapy Association and The Bureau of Labor Statistics-2009). In addition, the area of school-based occupational therapy will see growth as well.

Earnings

According to the Bureau of Labor Statistics, in 2006 the average salary was $70,470 for occupational therapists (2009). The average starting entry-level salary for occupational therapists was $56,300 (American Occupational Therapy Association,). In 2006, the salaries of occupational therapists in the 50% percentile ranged from $50,450 to $83,710 (Bureau of Labor Statistics, n.d.). Salary varies according to the setting and the following represents average salaries for some practice areas:

Hospitals	$61,610
School setting	$54,260
Nursing care services	$64,750
Home healthcare	$67,600
Facilities of physical, occupational speech therapists	$62,290

(Bureau of Labor Statistics, 2009)

In addition, according to the Work Force Survey conducted by the American Occupational Therapy Association in 2006, average salaries for some other areas include:

Mental Health	$53,750
Academic	$66,000

(American Occupational Therapy Association, 2006).

CHALLENGES FOR OCCUPATIONAL THERAPY

A key challenge for occupational therapy is to develop and maintain a definition of its nature and scope assert that while this presents a challenge, it also results in a unique flexibility which allows the discipline to move with the flow of social, cultural and environmental change. This difficulty in definition may be a cause of chronic strain for practitioners and may also contribute to a lack of role definition and subsequent blurring.

Recent literature has also called for occupational therapy to address the political nature of who occupational therapists are and what they do (Kronenberg & Pollard, 2005). Profession specific models of occupational therapy have also been critiqued for being biased towards a western, ablest and generally unrepresentative of the most occupationally deprived groups.

OCCUPATIONAL THERAPY AND INTERNATIONAL CLASSIFICATION OF FUNCTIONING, DISABILITY AND HEALTH

The International Classification of Functioning, Disability and Health (ICF) is an outcome measure for health and occupation and illustrates how these components impact one's function. This relates very closely to the Occupational Therapy Practice Framework as it is stated, 'The profession's core beliefs are in the positive relationship between occupation and health and its view of people as occupational beings' (2008). The ICF is also built into the 2nd edition of the practice framework. Activities and participation examples from the ICF overlap Areas of Occupation, Performance Skills, and Performance Patterns in the framework. The ICF also includes contextual factors (environmental and personal factors) that relate to the context in the framework. In addition, body functions and structures classified within the ICF help describe the client factors as described in the OT framework (AOTA, 2002).

Further exploration of the relationship between occupational therapy and the components of the ICIDH-2 (revision of the original International Classification of Impairments, Disabilities, and Handicaps (ICIDH); later becoming the ICF) was conducted by McLaughlin Gray (2001). First, the ICF is an international framework and provides an opportunity for the occupational therapy field to become better known across the globe. Second, the ICF provides occupational therapists with a global language to describe their expertise to the larger international healthcare community. The ICF uses a positive, holistic language emphasizing skills, capacities, and strengths of an individual rather than focusing on one's deficits and disabilities. This is similar to the outlook of occupational therapists. Third, the ICF includes environmental and personal contextual factors which are incorporated into the theory behind occupational therapy. It is important to take into consideration an individual's personal, environmental, and occupational factors to develop an effective intervention (Christiansen & Baum, 2005). The last notable application of the ICF to occupational therapy is the recognition of cultural patterns in occupation. Culture has significance on an individual's activities and participation and it is important to keep this in mind when treating an individual.

Although the ICF can be very useful for occupational therapists, it is noted in the literature that occupational therapists should use specific occupational therapy vocabulary along with the ICF in order to ensure correct communication about specific concepts (Stamm, Cieza, Machold, Smolen, & Stucki, 2006). The ICF might lack certain categories to describe what occupational therapists need to communicate to clients and colleagues. It also may not be possible to exactly match the connotations of the ICF categories to occupational therapy terms. The ICF is not an assessment and specialized occupational therapy vocabulary should not be replaced with ICF terminology (Hag Lund & Henriksson, 2003). The ICF is an overarching framework on which to hang current therapy practices.

The Occupational Therapists do maintain medical records for treating the patients for various reasons, e.g. for noting complete history and physical examination notes, progress notes, treatment provided; record is maintained for continued care of the patient, communication to the physician and other healthcare providers, document of proof in administrative and medical legal issues, insurance purpose, for collecting patient care information besides to carry out medical education and research work.

Especially designed medical record forms for the use of Occupational Therapy Unit or for Occupational Therapist are furnished in this chapter.

OUTPATIENT DEPARTMENT

Reg .... Dr .... Date ....

Indoor

Name .... Sex .... Age ....

Ward .... Bed ....

Occupation .... Address ....

Diagnosis .... Date of Onset ....

If postoperative, operation performed and date of operation ....

Any other condition not described under diagnosis, e.g. epilepsy, diabetes, etc.

....

Contraindications to therapy (Examples)

Fever, infectious diseases, pregnancy, Cardiac (First trimester)	Full weight bearing on (Fracture or operated side)	Partial weight bearing on (Fracture or operated side)
No weightbearing on (Fracture or operated side)	Limited exercise, hypertension	

Contractures or deformities ....

Treatment desired (check below)

A. 1. Muscle strength
2. Re-education and coordination
3. Range of joint motion
4. Posture
5. Relaxation
6. Gait training
7. Maintenance of function
8. Prevention of contractures, deformities, etc.
9. Postural drainage
10. Respiratory function

B. Activities of daily living

C. Work tolerance

D. 1. Preoperative preparation
2. Postoperative care

E. 1. Relief of pain
2. Resolution of inflammation
3. Relief of edema

F. 1. Healing of wounds
2. Peeling of skin
3. Pigmentation
4. General on-specific effect of UVR

G. Prevocational testing and training

H. Psychological, viz. simulation, socialization, etc.

I. Any other

Check here if any specific modality of treatment desired.

Testing:
1. Electrical muscle check
2. Manual muscle check
3. Joint range and tightness
4. Functional
5. Disability

Prescription for braces, artificial limbs, splints, etc. ....

....

....

Signature

Form 1 Occupational therapy form

Clinical record **Occupational therapy**

Principal diagnosis

Diagnosis for which treatment requested Date of onset

Part (s) to be treated

Aim of treatment

Precautions (Include communicability) ☐ Ambulatory ☐ Wheel chair ☐ Litter

Frequency and duration of treatment desired ☐ Ward ☐ Shop

RESULTS DESIRED

☐ Increase of joint motion ☐ Increase of muscle strength ☐ Coordination

☐ Activity tolerance ☐ Functional prosthetic training ☐ Emotional readjustment

☐ Other (Specify)

Physician's Signature **Date**

MONTH	1	2	3	4	5	6	7	8	9	10	11	12	13	14	15	16	17	18	19	20	21	22	23	24	25	26	27	28	29	30	31

Total no. visits

Progress Notes (Date and Sign all notes)

Patient's Last Name : First Name - Middle Name	Registered No.	Ward No.

(Name of Hospital or Other Medical Facility) **OCCUPATIONAL THERAPY**

Form 2 Occupational therapy treatment measures

Medical Record # :
Hospital Name :
Patient Name :
Date of Birth :
Attending Physician :
Date of Admission :

☐ OPD
☐ IPD

OCCUPATIONAL THERAPY TREATMENT MEASURES

Date	Issue	Intervention	Outcome	Date Resolved

Signature :....................................Employee ID # : ....Date : ....

OCCUPATIONAL THERAPY TREATMENT MEASURES

Form 3 Occupational therapy home visit assessment

OCCUPATIONAL THERAPY
HOME VISIT ASSESSMENT

Medical Record # :
Hospital Name :
Patient Name :
Date of Birth :
Attending Physician :
Date of Admission :

☐ OPD
☐ IPD

Diagnosis ____

____

Date of home assessment : ____________________

Current mobility status : ____________________

____

____

____

____

____

____

____

External layout of the house

House style :____

Pathway into building ____

Surface : ____________________ Condition ____________________

Front entrance : # Stairs : ________Height :_______ Railings : R L ramps : Y N

Others enterances : ____

Parking : ____

Comments : ____

____

____

OCCUPATIONAL THERAPY HOME VISIT ASSESSMENT

16 Nutrition

INTRODUCTION

Nutrition (also called *nourishment* or *aliment*) is the provision, to cells and organisms, of the materials necessary in the form of food to support life. Many common health problems can be prevented or alleviated with a healthy diet.

The diet of an organism is what it eats, and is largely determined by the perceived palatability of foods. Dietitians are health professionals who specialize in human nutrition, meal planning, economics, and preparation. They are trained to provide safe, evidence-based dietary advice and management to healthy and sick individuals as well as to institutions.

A poor diet can have an damaging impact on health, causing deficiency diseases such as scurvy, beriberi, and kwashiorkor; health-threatening conditions like obesity and metabolic syndrome, and such common chronic systemic diseases as cardiovascular disease, diabetes, and osteoporosis.

OVERVIEW

Nutritional science investigates the metabolic and physiological responses of the body to diet. With advances in the fields of molecular biology, biochemistry, and genetics, the study of nutrition is increasingly concerned with metabolism and metabolic pathways: the sequences of biochemical steps through which substances in living things change from one form to another.

The human body contains chemical compounds, such as water, carbohydrates, sugar, starch, and fiber, amino acids (in proteins), fatty acids (in lipids), and nucleic acids (DNA and RNA). These compounds in turn consist of elements such as carbon, hydrogen, oxygen, nitrogen, phosphorus, calcium, iron, zinc, magnesium, manganese, and so on. All of these chemical compounds and elements occur in various forms and combinations, e.g. hormones, vitamins, phospholipids, hydroxyapatite, both in the human body and in the plant and animal organisms that humans eat.

The human body consists of elements and compounds ingested, digested, absorbed, and circulated through the bloodstream to feed the cells of the body. Except in the unborn fetus, the digestive system is the first system involved. In a typical adult, about seven liters of digestive juices enter the lumen of the digestive tract. These break chemical bonds in ingested molecules, and modulate their conformations and energy states. Though some molecules are absorbed into the bloodstream unchanged, digestive processes release them from the matrix of foods. Unabsorbed matter, along with some waste products of metabolism, is eliminated from the body in the feces.

Studies of nutritional status must take into account the state of the body before and after experiments, as well as the chemical composition of the whole diet and of all material excreted and eliminated from the body in urine and feces. Comparing the food to the waste can help determine the specific compounds and elements absorbed and metabolized in the body. The effects of nutrients may only be discernible over an extended period, during which all food and waste must be analyzed. The number of variables involved in such experiments is high, making nutritional studies time-consuming and expensive, which explains why the science of human nutrition is still slowly evolving.

In general, eating a wide variety of fresh, unprocessed whole foods has proven favorable compared to processed foods. In particular, the consumption of whole-plant foods slows digestion and allows better absorption, and a more favorable balance of essential nutrients per calorie, resulting in better management of cell growth, maintenance, and mitosis (cell division), as well as better regulation of appetite and blood sugar. Regularly scheduled meals every few hours have also proven more wholesome than infrequent or haphazard ones.

NUTRIENTS

There are seven major classes of nutrients—carbohydrates, fats, fiber, minerals, protein, vitamin, and water.

These nutrient classes can be categorized as either macronutrients needed in relatively large amounts or micronutrients needed in smaller quantities. The macronutrients are carbohydrates, fats, fiber, proteins, and water. The micronutrients are minerals and vitamins.

The macronutrients excluding fiber and water, provide structural material amino acids from which proteins are built, and lipids from which cell membranes and some signaling molecules are built, energy. Some of the structural material can be used to generate energy internally, and in either case it is measured in Joules or kilocalories often called 'Calories' and written with a capital C to distinguish them from little 'c' calories. Carbohydrates and proteins provide 17 kJ approximately (4 kcal) of energy per gram, while fats provide 37 kJ (9 kcal) per gram, though the net energy from either depends on such factors as absorption and digestive effort, which vary substantially from instance-to-instance. Vitamins, minerals, fiber, and water do not provide energy, but are required for other reasons. A third class dietary material, fiber, i.e. non-digestible material such as cellulose, seems also to be required, for both mechanical and biochemical reasons, though the exact reasons remain unclear **(Fig. 16.1)**.

Molecules of carbohydrates and fats consist of carbon, hydrogen, and oxygen atoms. Carbohydrates range from simple monosaccharide (glucose, fructose, galactose) to complex polysaccharides (starch). Fats are triglycerides, made of assorted fatty acid monomers bound to glycerol backbone. Some fatty acids, but not all, are essential in the diet: they cannot be synthesized in the body. Protein molecules contain nitrogen atoms in addition to carbon, oxygen, and hydrogen. The fundamental components of protein are nitrogen-containing amino acids, some of which are essential in the sense that humans cannot make them internally. Some of the amino acids are convertible (with the expenditure of energy) to glucose and can be used for energy production just as ordinary glucose. By breaking down existing protein, some glucose can be produced internally; the remaining amino acids

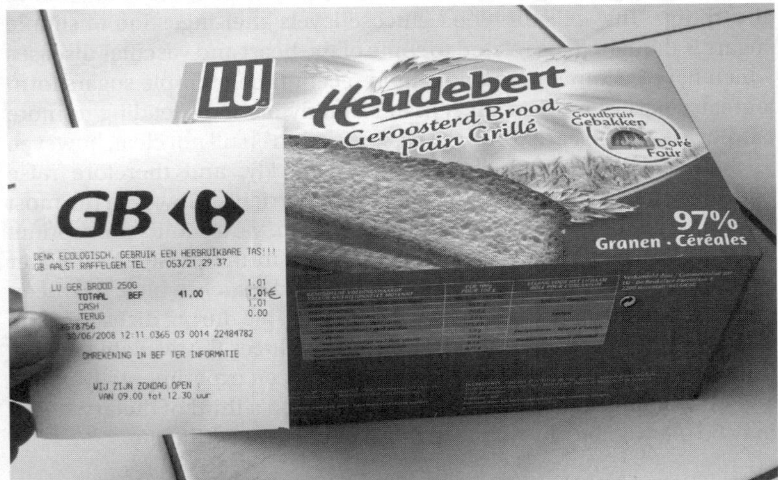

Fig. 16.1 Toasted bread is a cheap, high calorie nutrient usually unbalanced, i.e. deficient in essential minerals and vitamins, largely because of removal of both germ and bran during processing food source (*For color version, see Plate 3*)

are discarded, primarily as urea in urine. This occurs normally only during prolonged starvation.

Other micronutrients include antioxidants and phytochemicals which are said to protect some body systems. Their necessity is not as well established as in the case of, for instance, vitamins.

Most foods contain a mix of some or all of the nutrient classes, together with other substances such as toxins or various sorts. Some nutrients can be stored internally, e.g. the fat soluble vitamins, while others are required more or less continuously. Poor health can be caused by a lack of required nutrients or, in extreme cases, too much of a required nutrient. For example, both salt and water both absolutely required will cause illness or even death in too large amounts.

Carbohydrates

Carbohydrates may be classified as monosaccharide, disaccharides, or polysaccharides depending on the number of monomer (sugar) units they contain. They constitute a large part of foods such as rice, noodles, bread, and other grain-based products. Monosaccharide contains one sugar unit, disaccharides two, and polysaccharides three or more. Polysaccharides are often referred to as complex of carbohydrates because they are typically long multiple branched chains of sugar units. The difference is that complex carbohydrates take longer to digest and absorb since their sugar units must be separated from the chain before absorption. The spike in blood glucose levels after ingestion of simple sugars is thought to be related to some of the heart and vascular diseases which have become more frequent in recent times. Simple sugars form a greater part of modern diets than formerly, perhaps leading to more cardiovascular disease. The degree of causation is still not clear, however.

Simple carbohydrates are absorbed quickly, and therefore raise blood-sugar levels more rapidly than other nutrients. However, the most important plant carbohydrate nutrient, starch, varies in its absorption. Gelatinized starch heated for a few minutes in the presence of water is far more digestible than plain starch. And starch which has been divided into fine particles is also more absorbable during digestion. The increased effort and decreased availability reduces the available energy from starchy foods substantially and can be seen experimentally in rats and anecdotally in humans. Additionally, up to a third of dietary starch may be unavailable due to mechanical or chemical difficulty.

Fiber

Dietary fiber is a carbohydrate or a polysaccharide that is incompletely absorbed in humans and in some animals. Like all carbohydrates, when it is metabolized it can produce four calories (kilocalories) of energy per gram. But in most circumstances it accounts for less than that because of its limited absorption and digestibility. Dietary fiber consists mainly of cellulose, a large carbohydrate polymer that is indigestible because humans do not have the required enzymes to disassemble it. There are two subcategories: soluble and insoluble fiber. Whole grains, fruits especially plums, prunes, and figs, and vegetables are good sources of dietary fiber. Fiber is important to digestive health and is thought to reduce the risk of colon cancer. For mechanical reasons it can help in alleviating both constipation and diarrhea. Fiber provides bulk to the intestinal contents, and insoluble fiber especially stimulates peristalsis—the rhythmic muscular contractions of the intestines which move digesta along the digestive tract. Some soluble fibers produce a solution of high viscosity; this is essentially a gel, which slows the movement of food through the intestines. Additionally, fiber, perhaps especially that from whole grains, may help lessen insulin spikes and reduce the risk of type II diabetes.

Fat

A molecule of dietary fat typically consists of several fatty acids containing long chains of carbon and hydrogen atoms, bonded to a glycerol. They are typically found as triglycerides (three fatty acids attached to one glycerol backbone). Fats may be classified as saturated or unsaturated depending on the detailed structure of the fatty acids involved. Saturated fats have all of the carbon atoms in their fatty acid chains bonded to hydrogen atoms, whereas unsaturated fats have some of these carbon atoms double-bonded, so their molecules have relatively fewer hydrogen atoms than a saturated fatty acid of the same length. Unsaturated fats may be further classified as monounsaturated (one double-bond) or polyunsaturated (many double-bonds). Furthermore, depending on the location of the double-bond in the fatty acid chain, unsaturated fatty acids are classified as omega-3 or omega-6 fatty acids. Trans fats are a type of unsaturated fat with transisomer bonds; these are rare in nature and in foods from natural sources; they are typically created in an industrial process called partial hydrogenation.

Many studies have shown that unsaturated fats, particularly mono-unsaturated fats, are best in the human diet. Saturated fats, typically from animal sources, are next, while trans fats are to be avoided. Saturated and some trans fats are typically solid at room temperature (such as butter or lard), while unsaturated fats are typically liquids (such as olive oil or flaxseed oil). Trans fats are very rare in nature, but have properties useful in the food processing industry, such as rancid resistance.

Essential Fatty Acids

Most fatty acids are nonessential, meaning the body can produce them as needed, generally from other fatty acids and always by expending energy to do so. However, in humans at least two fatty acids are essential and must be included in the diet. An appropriate balance of essential fatty acids—omega-3 and omega-6 fatty acids—seems also important for health, though definitive experimental demonstration has been elusive. Both of these 'omega' long-chain polyunsaturated fatty acids are substrates for a class of eicosanoids known as prostaglandins, which have roles throughout the human body. They are hormones, in some respects. The omega-3 eicosapentaenoic acid (EPA), which can be made in the human body from the omega-3 essential fatty acid alpha-linolenic acid (LNA), or taken in through marine food sources, serves as a building block for series 3 prostaglandins (e.g. weakly inflammatory PGE3). The omega-6 dihomo-gamma-linolenic acid (DGLA) serves as a building block for series 1 prostaglandins (e.g. anti-inflammatory PGE1), whereas arachidonic acid (AA) serves as a building block for series 2 prostaglandins (e.g. proinflammatory PGE2). Both DGLA and AA can be made from the omega-6 linoleic acid (LA) in the human body, or can be taken in directly through food. An appropriately balanced intake of omega-3 and omega-6 partly determines the relative production of different prostaglandins: one reason a balance between omega-3 and omega-6 is believed important for cardiovascular health. In industrialized societies, people typically consume large amounts of processed vegetable oils, which have reduced amounts of the essential fatty acids along with too much of omega-6 fatty acids relative to omega-3 fatty acids.

The conversion rate of omega-6 DGLA to AA largely determines the production of the prostaglandins PGE1 and PGE2. Omega-3 EPA prevents AA from being released from membranes, thereby skewing prostaglandin balance away from proinflammatory PGE2 (made from AA) toward anti-inflammatory PGE1 (made from DGLA). Moreover, the conversion (desaturation) of DGLA to AA is controlled by the enzyme delta-5-desaturase, which in turn is controlled by hormones such as insulin (up-regulation) and glucagons (down-regulation). The amount and type of carbohydrates consumed, along with some types of amino acid, can influence processes involving insulin, glucagons, and other hormones; therefore the ratio of omega-3 versus omega-6 has wide effects on general health, and specific effects on immune function and inflammation, and mitosis, i.e. cell division.

Good sources of essential fatty acids include most vegetables, nuts, seeds, and marine oils, some of the best sources are fish, flaxseed oils, soybeans, pumpkin seeds, sunflower seeds and walnuts.

Protein

Proteins are the basis of many animal body structures, e.g. muscles, skin, and hair. They also form the enzymes which control chemical reactions throughout the body. Each molecule is composed of amino acids which are characterized by inclusion of nitrogen and sometimes sulfur, are responsible for the distinctive smell of burning protein, such as the keratin in hair. The body requires amino acids to produce new proteins (protein retention) and to replace damaged proteins (maintenance) **(Fig. 16.2)**. As there is no protein or amino acid storage provision, amino acids must be present in the diet. Excess amino acids are discarded, typically in the urine. For all animals, some amino acids are essential (an animal cannot produce them internally) and some are nonessential (the animal can produce them from other nitrogen-containing compounds). About twenty amino acids are found in the human body, and about ten of these are essential, and therefore must be included in the diet. A diet that contains adequate amounts of amino acids especially those that are essential is particularly important in some situations: during early development and maturation, pregnancy, lactation, or injury or a burn, for instance. A complete protein source contains all the essential amino acids; an incomplete protein source lacks one or more of the essential amino acids.

It is possible to combine two incomplete protein sources, e.g. rice and beans to make a complete protein source, and characteristic

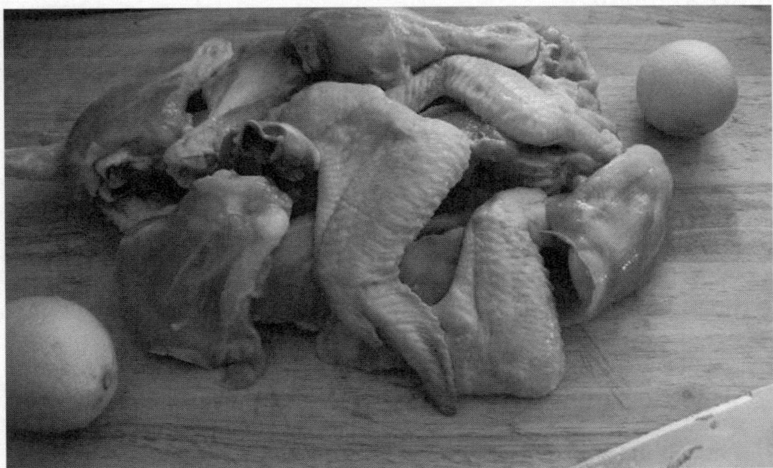

Fig. 16.2 Most meats such as chicken contain all the essential amino acids needed for humans (protein in nutrition) (*For color version, see Plate 3*)

combinations are the basis of distinct cultural cooking traditions. Sources of dietary protein include meats, tofu and other soy-products, eggs, grains, legumes, and dairy products such as milk and cheese. A few amino acids from protein can be converted into glucose and used for fuel through a process called gluconeogenesis; this is done in quantity only during starvation. The amino acids remaining after such conversion are discarded.

Minerals

Dietary minerals are the chemical elements required by living organisms, other than the four elements carbon, hydrogen, nitrogen, and oxygen that are present in nearly all organic molecules. The term 'mineral' is archaic, since the intent is to describe simply the less common elements in the diet. Some are heavier than the four just mentioned—including several metals, which often occur as ions in the body. Some dietitians recommend that these be supplied from foods in which they occur naturally or at least as complex compounds, or sometimes even from natural inorganic sources (such as calcium carbonate from ground oyster shells). Some are absorbed much more readily in the ionic forms found in such sources. On the other hand, minerals are often artificially added to the diet as supplements; the most famous is likely iodine in iodized salt which prevents goiter.

Macrominerals

Many elements are essential in relative quantity; they are usually called 'bulk minerals.' Some are structural, but many play a role as electrolytes. Elements with recommended dietary allowance (RDA) greater than 200 mg/day are, in alphabetical order with informal or folk-medicine perspectives in parentheses:

- Calcium, a common electrolyte, but also needed structurally structural for muscle and digestive system health, bones, some forms neutralizes acidity, may help clear toxins, and provide signaling ions for nerve and membrane functions.
- Chlorine as chloride ions; very common electrolyte; see sodium, below.
- Magnesium, required for processing ATP and related reactions (builds bone, causes strong peristalsis, increases flexibility, increases alkalinity).
- Phosphorus, required component of bones; essential for energy processing.
- Potassium, a very common electrolyte (heart and nerve health).

- Sodium, a very common electrolyte; not generally found in dietary supplements, despite being needed in large quantities, because the ion is very common in food: typically as sodium chloride, or common salt. Excessive sodium consumption can deplete calcium and magnesium, leading to high blood pressure and osteoporosis.
- Sulfur for three essential amino acids and therefore many proteins (skin, hair, nails, liver, and pancreas).

Trace Minerals

Many elements are required in trace amounts, usually because they play a catalytic role in enzymes. Some trace mineral elements (RDA <200 mg/day) are, in alphabetical order:

- Cobalt required for biosynthesis of vitamin B_{12} family of coenzymes
- Copper required component of many redox enzymes, including cytochrome c oxidase
- Chromium required for sugar metabolism
- Iodine required not only for the biosynthesis of thyroxin, but probably, for other important organs as breast, stomach, salivary glands, thymus, etc. (see extrathyroidal iodine); for this reason iodine is needed in larger quantities than others in this list, and sometimes classified with the macrominerals
- Iron required for many enzymes, and for hemoglobin and some other proteins
- Manganese (processing of oxygen)
- Molybdenum required for xanthine oxidase and related oxidases
- Nickel present in urease
- Selenium required for peroxidase (antioxidant proteins)
- Vanadium (speculative: There is no established RDA for vanadium. No specific biochemical function has been identified for it in humans, although vanadium is required for some lower organisms.)
- Zinc required for several enzymes such as carboxypeptidase, liver alcohol dehydrogenase, carbonic anhydrase.

Vitamins

As with the minerals discussed above, some vitamins are recognized as essential nutrients, necessary in the diet for good health. (Vitamin D is the exception: it can alternatively be synthesized in the skin, in the presence of ultraviolet B radiation.) Certain vitamin-like compounds that are recommended in the diet, such as carnitine, are thought useful for survival and health, but these are not 'essential' dietary nutrients because the human body has some capacity to produce them from other compounds. Moreover, thousands of different phytochemicals have recently been discovered in food (particularly in fresh vegetables), which may have desirable properties including antioxidant activity, experimental demonstration has been suggestive but inconclusive. Other essential nutrients not classed as vitamins include essential amino acids choline, essential fatty acids and the minerals discussed in the preceding section.

Vitamin deficiencies may result in disease conditions: goiter, scurvy, osteoporosis, impaired immune system, disorders of cell metabolism, certain forms of cancer, symptoms of premature aging, and poor psychological health (including eating disorders), among many others. Excess of some vitamins is also dangerous to health (notably vitamin A), and for at least one vitamin B_6, toxicity begins at levels not far above the required amount. Deficiency or excess of minerals can also have serious health consequences.

Water

About 70% of the nonfat mass of the human body is made of water **(Fig. 16.3)**. To function properly, the body requires between one and seven L of water per day to avoid dehydration; the precise amount depends on the level of activity, temperature, humidity, and other factors. With physical exertion and heat exposure, water loss increases and daily fluid needs will eventually increase as well.

It is not fully clear how much water intake is needed by healthy people, although some experts assert that 8–10 glasses of water (approximately 2 L) daily is the minimum to maintain proper hydration. The notion that a person should consume eight glasses of water per day cannot be traced to a credible scientific source. The effect of, greater or lesser, water intake on weight loss and on constipation is also still unclear. The original water intake recommendation in 1945 by the Food and Nutrition Board of the National Research Council read: 'An ordinary standard for diverse persons is 1 mL for each calorie of food. Most of this quantity is contained in prepared foods.' The latest dietary reference intake report by the United States National Research Council recommended, generally, (including food sources): 2.7 L of water total for women and 3.7 L for men. Specifically, pregnant and breastfeeding women need additional fluids to stay hydrated. According to the Institute of Medicine—who recommend that, on average, women consume 2.2 L and men 3.0 L—this is recommended to be 2.4 L (approx 9 cups) for pregnant women and 3 L (approx 12.5 cups) for breastfeeding women since an especially large amount of fluid is lost during nursing.

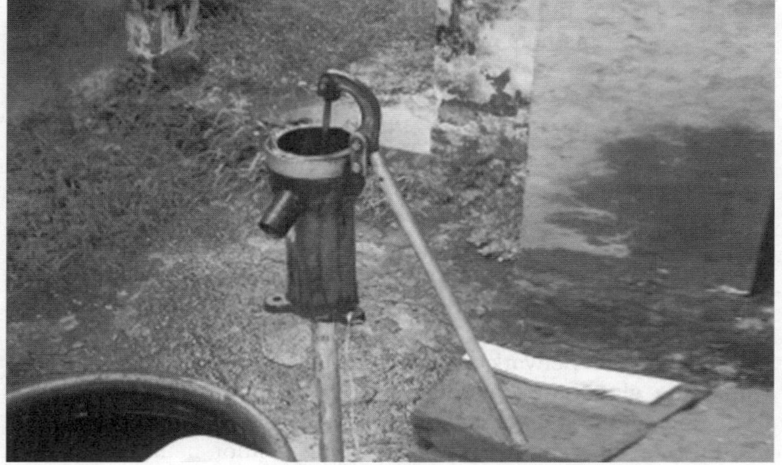

Fig. 16.3 A manual water pump in China

For those who have healthy kidneys, it is somewhat difficult to drink too much water but especially in warm humid weather and while exercising, it is dangerous to drink too little. People can drink far more water than necessary while exercising, however, putting them at risk of water intoxication, which can be fatal. In particular large amounts of de-ionized water are dangerous.

Normally, about 20% of water intake comes in food, while the rest comes from drinking water and assorted beverages caffeinated included. Water is excreted from the body in multiple forms; including urine and feces, sweating, and by water vapor in the exhaled breath.

OTHER NUTRIENTS

Other micronutrients include antioxidants and phytochemicals. These substances are generally more recent discoveries which have not yet been recognized as vitamins or as required. Phytochemicals may act as antioxidants, but not all phytochemicals are antioxidants.

Antioxidants

Antioxidants are a recent discovery. As cellular metabolism/energy production requires oxygen, potentially damaging (e.g. mutation causing) compounds known as free radicals can form. Most of these are oxidizers, i.e. acceptors of electrons and some react very strongly. For normal cellular maintenance, growth, and division, these free radicals must be sufficiently neutralized by antioxidant compounds. Recently, some researchers suggested an interesting theory of evolution of dietary antioxidants. Some are produced by the human body with adequate precursors, i.e. glutathione, vitamin C and those the body cannot produce may only be obtained in the diet via direct sources vitamin C in humans, vitamin A, vitamin K or produced by the body from other compounds such as Beta-carotene converted to vitamin A by the body, vitamin D synthesized from cholesterol by sunlight. Phytochemicals and their subgroup polyphenols are the majority of antioxidants; about 4,000 are known. Different antioxidants are now known to function in a cooperative network, e.g. vitamin C can reactivate free radical-containing glutathione or vitamin E by accepting the free radical itself, and so on. Some antioxidants are more effective than others at neutralizing different free radicals. Some cannot neutralize certain free radicals. Some cannot be present in certain areas of free radical development vitamin A is fat-soluble and protects fat areas, vitamin C is water soluble and protects those areas. When interacting with a free radical, some antioxidants produce a different free radical compound that is less dangerous or more dangerous than the previous compound. Having a variety of antioxidants allows any by products to be safely dealt with by more efficient antioxidants in neutralizing a free radical's butterfly effect.

Phytochemicals

A growing area of interest is the effect upon human health of trace chemicals, collectively called phytochemicals. These nutrients are typically found in edible plants, especially colorful fruits and vegetables, but also other organisms including seafood, algae, and fungi. The effects of phytochemicals increasingly survive rigorous testing by prominent health organizations. One of the principal classes of phytochemicals is polyphenol antioxidants, chemicals which are known to provide certain health benefits to the cardiovascular system and immune system **(Fig. 16.4)**. These chemicals are known to down-regulate the formation of reactive oxygen species, key chemicals in cardiovascular disease.

Perhaps the most rigorously tested phytochemicals is zeaxanthin, a yellow-pigmented carotenoid present in many yellow and orange fruits and vegetables. Repeated studies have shown a strong correlation between ingestion of zeaxanthin and the prevention and treatment of age-related macular degeneration (AMD). Less rigorous studies have proposed a correlation between zeaxanthin intake and cataracts.

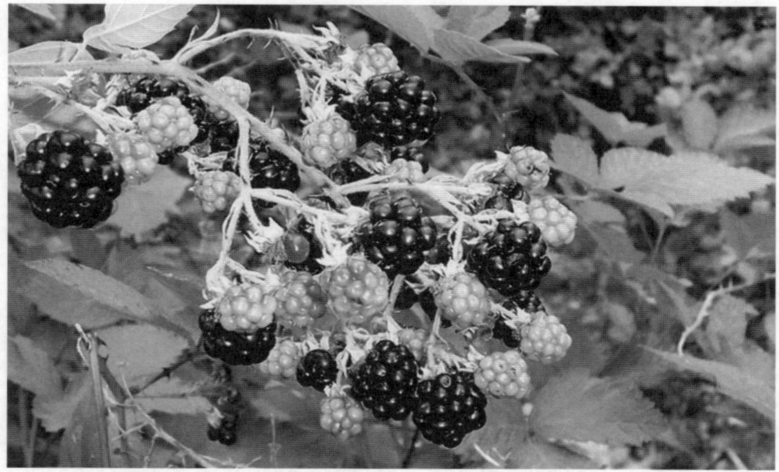

Fig. 16.4 Blackberries are a source of polyphenol antioxidants
(*For color version, see Plate 4*)

A second carotenoid, lutein, has also been shown to lower the risk of contracting AMD. Both compounds have been observed to collect in the retina when ingested orally, and they serve to protect the rods and cones against the destructive effects of light.

Another carotenoid, beta-cryptoxanthin, appears to protect against chronic joint inflammatory diseases, such as arthritis. While the association between serum blood levels of beta-cryptoxanthin and substantially decreased joint disease has been established, neither a convincing mechanism for such protection nor a cause-and-effect have been rigorously studied. Similarly, a red phytochemical, lycopene, has substantial credible evidence of negative association with development of prostate cancer.

The correlations between the ingestion of some phytochemicals and the prevention of disease are, in some cases, enormous in magnitude.

Even when the evidence is obtained, translating it to practical dietary advice can be difficult and counterintuitive. Lutein, for example, occurs in many yellow and orange fruits and vegetables and protects the eyes against various diseases. However, it does not protect the eye nearly as well as zeaxanthin, and the presence of lutein in the retina will prevent zeaxanthin uptake. Additionally, evidence has shown that the lutein present in egg yolk is more readily absorbed than the lutein from vegetable sources, possibly because of fat solubility. At the most basic level, the question 'should you eat eggs?' is complex to the point of

Table 16.1 Phytochemical groups and common source of food

Family	*Sources*	*Possible benefits*
Flavonoids	Berries, herbs, vegetables, wine, grapes, tea	General antioxidant, oxidation of LDLs, prevention of arteriosclerosis and heart disease
Isoflavones (phytoestrogens)	Soy, red clover, kudzu root	General antioxidant, prevention of arteriosclerosis and heart disease, easing symptoms of menopause, cancer prevention
Isothiocyanates monoterpenes	Cruciferous vegetables citrus peels, essential oils, herbs, spices, green plants, atmosphere	Cancer prevention, treating gallstones
Organosulfur compounds	Chives, garlic, onions	Cancer prevention, lowered LDLs, assistance to the immune system
Saponins	Beans, cereals, herbs	Hypercholesterolemia, hyperglycemia, antioxidant, cancer prevention, anti-inflammatory
Capsaicinoids	All capiscum (chile) peppers	Topical pain relief, cancer prevention, cancer cell apoptosis

dismay, including misperceptions about the health effects of cholesterol in egg yolk, and its saturated fat content.

As another example, lycopene is prevalent in tomatoes and actually is the chemical that gives tomatoes their red color. It is more highly concentrated, however, in processed tomato products such as commercial pasta sauce, or tomato soup, than in fresh 'healthy' tomatoes. Yet, such sauces tend to have high amounts of salt, sugar, and other substances a person may wish or even need to avoid.

Table 16.1 presents phytochemical groups and common sources, arranged by family.

INTESTINAL BACTERIAL FLORA

It is now also known that animal intestines contain a large population of gut flora. In humans, these include species such as *Bacteroides*, *L. acidophilus* and *E. coli*, among many others. They are essential to digestion, and are also affected by the food we eat. Bacteria in the gut perform many important functions for humans, including breaking down and aiding in the absorption of otherwise indigestible food; stimulating cell growth; repressing the growth of harmful bacteria, training the immune system to respond only to pathogens; producing vitamin B_{12}, and defending against some infectious diseases.

ADVICE AND GUIDANCE

Governmental Policies

In the United States, dietitians are registered (RD) or licensed (LD) with the Commission for Dietetic Registration and the American Dietetic Association, and are only able to use the title 'dietitian,' as described by the business and professions codes of each respective state, when they have met specific educational and experiential prerequisites and passed a national registration or licensure examination, respectively. In California, registered dietitians must abide by the 'Business and Professions Code of Section 2585-2586.8'. *http://www.leginfo.ca.gov/cgi-bin/displaycode?section=bpc&group=02001-03000&file=2585-2586.8*. Anyone may call themselves a nutritionist, including unqualified dietitians, as this term is unregulated. Some states, such as the State of Florida, have begun to include the title 'nutritionist' in state licensure requirements. Most governments provide guidance on nutrition, and some also impose mandatory disclosure/labeling requirements for processed food manufacturers and restaurants to assist consumers in complying with such guidance.

In the US, nutritional standards and recommendations are established jointly by the US Department of Agriculture (USDA) and US Department of Health and Human Services **(Fig. 16.5)**. Dietary and physical activity guidelines from the US Department of Agriculture are presented in the concept of a food pyramid, which superseded the Four Food Groups. The Senate Committee currently responsible for oversight of the USDA is the agriculture, nutrition and forestry committee. Committee hearings are often televised on C-SPAN as seen here.

The US Department of Health and Human Services (USDHHS) provides a sample week-long menu which fulfills the nutritional recommendations of the government. Canada's Food Guide is another governmental recommendation.

Teaching

Nutrition is taught in schools in many countries. In England and Wales the Personal and Social Education and Food Technology curricula include nutrition, stressing the importance of a balanced diet and

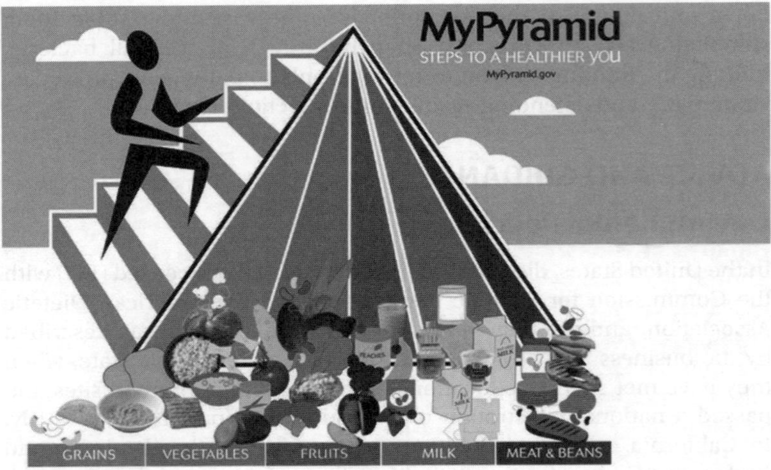

Fig. 16.5 The updated United States Department of Agriculture (USDA) food pyramid, published in 2005, is a general nutrition guide for recommended food consumption for humans (*For color version, see Plate 4*)

teaching how to read nutrition labels on packaging. In many schools a nutrition class will fall within the family and consumer science or health departments. In some American schools, students are required to take a certain number of classes from Family and Consumer Sciences (FCS) related classes in order to gain comprehensive knowledge and to acquire skills in conducing research that helps people make decisions about their well being, relationships, and resources to achieve optimum quality of life. The field represents many areas including human relationship development, personal and family finances, housing and interior design, food science, nutrition and wellness, textiles and apparel, and consumer issues. Nutrition is offered at many schools, and if it is not a class of its own, nutrition is included in other FCS or health classes such as: life skills, independent living, single survival, freshmen connection, health, etc. In many nutrition classes, students learn about the food groups, the food pyramid, daily recommended allowances, calories, vitamins, minerals, malnutrition, physical activity, healthy food choices and how to live a healthy life.

A 1985 US National Research Council report entitled nutrition education in US medical schools concluded that nutrition education in medical schools was inadequate. Only 20% of the schools surveyed taught nutrition as a separate, required course. A 2006 survey found that this number had risen to 30%.

HEALTHY DIETS

Whole Plant Food Diet

Heart disease, cancer, obesity, and diabetes are commonly called 'Western' diseases because these maladies were once rarely seen in developing countries. One study in China found some regions had essentially no cancer or heart disease, while in other areas they reflected 'up to a 100-fold increase' coincident with diets that were found to be entirely plant-based to heavily animal-based, respectively. In contrast, diseases of affluence like cancer and heart disease are common throughout the United States. Adjusted for age and exercise, large regional clusters of people in China rarely suffered from these 'Western' diseases possibly because their diets are rich in vegetables, fruits and whole grains.

The United Healthcare/Pacificare nutrition guideline recommends a whole plant food diet, and recommends using protein only as a condiment with meals. A national geographic cover article from November, 2005, entitled 'The Secrets of Living Longer', also recommends a whole plant food diet. The article is a lifestyle survey of three populations, Sardinians, Okinawa's, and Adventists, who generally display longevity and 'suffer a fraction of the diseases that commonly kill people in other parts of the developed world, and enjoy more healthy years of life.' In sum, they offer three sets of 'best practices' to emulate. The rest is up to you. In common with all three groups is to 'eat fruits, vegetables, and whole grains.'

The national geographic article noted that an NIH funded study of 34,000 seventh-day adventists between 1976 and 1988 ...found that the adventists' habit of consuming beans, soy milk, tomatoes, and other fruits lowered their risk of developing certain cancers. It also suggested that eating whole grain bread, drinking five glasses of water a day, and most surprisingly, consuming four servings of nuts a week reduced their risk of heart disease.

The French 'Paradox'

It has been discovered that people living in France live longer. Even though they consume more saturated fats than Americans, the rate of heart disease is lower in France than in North America. A number of explanations have been suggested:

- Reduced consumption of processed carbohydrate and other junk foods.
- Regular consumption of red wine.

- More active lifestyles involving plenty of daily exercise, especially walking; the French are much less dependent on cars than Americans are.
- Higher consumption of artificially produced trans fats by Americans, which has been shown to have greater lipoprotein effects per gram than saturated fat.

However, statistics collected by the World Health Organization from 1990 to 2000 show that the incidence of heart disease in France may have been underestimated and in fact be similar to that of neighboring countries.

SPORTS NUTRITION

Protein

Protein is an important component of every cell in the body. Hair and nails are mostly made of protein. The body uses protein to build and repair tissues. Also protein is used to make enzymes, hormones, and other body chemicals. Protein is an important building block of bones, muscles, cartilage, skin, and blood.

The protein requirement for each individual differs, as do opinions about whether and to what extent physically active people require more protein. The 2005 recommended dietary allowances (RDA), aimed at the general healthy adult population, provide for an intake of 0.8–1 g of protein per kg of body weight (according to the BMI formula), with the review panel stating that 'no additional dietary protein is suggested for healthy adults undertaking resistance or endurance exercise'. Conversely, Di Pasquale (2008), citing recent studies, recommends a minimum protein intake of 2.2 g/kg 'for anyone involved in competitive or intense recreational sports who wants to maximize lean body mass but does not wish to gain weight' **(Fig. 16.6)**.

Water and Salts

Water is one of the most important nutrients in the sports diet. It helps eliminate food waste products in the body, regulates body temperature during activity and helps with digestion. Maintaining hydration during periods of physical exertion is key to peak performance. While drinking too much water during activities can lead to physical discomfort, dehydration in excess of 2% of body mass (by weight) markedly hinders athletic performance. Additional carbohydrates and protein before, during, and after exercise increase time to exhaustion as well as speed recovery. Dosage is based on work performed, lean body mass, and

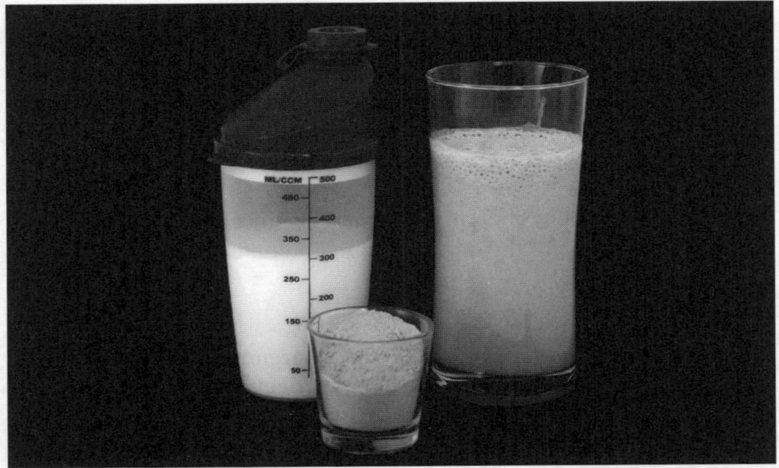

Fig. 16.6 Protein milkshakes, made from protein powder (center) and milk (left), are a common bodybuilding supplement (*For color version, see Plate 5*)

environmental factors, especially ambient temperature and humidity. Maintaining the right amount is key.

Carbohydrates

The main fuel used by the body during exercise is carbohydrates, which is stored in muscle as glycogen—a form of sugar. During exercise, muscle glycogen reserves can be used up, especially when activities last longer than 90 min. Because the amount of glycogen stored in the body is limited, it is important for athletes to replace glycogen by consuming a diet high in carbohydrates. Meeting energy needs can help improve performance during the sport, as well as improve overall strength and endurance.

There are different kinds of carbohydrates—simple or refined, and unrefined. A typical American consumes about 50% of their carbohydrates as simple sugars, which are added to foods as opposed to sugars that come naturally in fruits and vegetables. These simple sugars come in large amounts in sodas and fast food. Over the course of a year, the average American consumes 54 gallons of soft drinks, which contain the highest amount of added sugars. Even though carbohydrates are necessary for humans to function, they are not all equally healthful. When machinery has been used to remove bits of high fiber, the carbohydrates are refined. These are the carbohydrates found in white bread and fast food.

Nutrient Consumption: (see **Table 16.2**): As malnutrition refers to insufficient, excessive, or imbalanced consumption of nutrients. In developing countries, the diseases of malnutrition are most often associated with nutritional imbalances or excessive consumption. Although there are more people in the world who are malnourished due to excessive consumption, according to the United Nations World Health Organization, the real challenge in developing nations today, more than starvation, is combating insufficient nutrition—the lack of nutrients necessary for the growth and maintenance of vital functions.

Mental Agility

Research indicates that improving the awareness of nutritious meal choices and establishing long-term habits of healthy eating has a positive

Table 16.2 Illnesses caused by improper nutrient consumption

Nutrients	*Deficiency*	*Excess*
Energy Simple carbohydrates	Starvation, marasmus None	Obesity, diabetes mellitus, cardiovascular disease diabetes mellitus, obesity
Complex carbohydrates	None	Obesity
Saturated fat	Low sex hormone levels	Cardiovascular disease (claimed by most doctors and nutritionists)
Trans fat	None	Cardiovascular disease
Unsaturated fat	None	Obesity
Fat	Malabsorption of fat-soluble vitamins, rabbit starvation (If protein intake is high)	Cardiovascular disease (claimed by some)
Omega 3 Fats	Cardiovascular disease	Bleeding, hemorrhages
Omega 6 Fats	None	Cardiovascular disease, cancer
Cholesterol	None	Cardiovascular disease (claimed by many)
Protein	Kwashiorkor	Rabbit starvation
Sodium	Hypernatremia	Hypernatremia, hypertension
Iron	Anemia	Cirrhosis, heart disease

Contd...

Contd...

Nutrients	*Deficiency*	*Excess*
Iodine	Goiter, hypothyroidism	Iodine toxicity (goiter, hypothyroidism)
Vitamin A	Xerophthalmia and night blindness, low testosterone levels	Hypervitaminosis A (cirrhosis, hair loss)
Vitamin B_1	Beri-Beri	
Vitamin B_2	Cracking of skin and cornealunclearation	
Niacin	Pellagra	Dyspepsia, cardiac arrhythmias, birth defects
Vitamin B_{12}	Pernicious anemia	
Vitamin C	Scurvy	Diarrhea causing dehydration
Vitamin D	Rickets	Hypervitaminosis D (dehydration, vomiting, constipation)
Vitamin E	Nervous disorders	Hypervitaminosis E (anticoagulant: excessive bleeding)
Vitamin K	Hemorrhage	
Calcium	Osteoporosis, tetany, carpopedal spasm, laryngospasm, cardiac arrhythmias	Fatigue, depression, confusion, anorexia, nausea, vomiting, constipation, pancreatitis, increased urination
Magnesium	Hypertension	Weakness, nausea, vomiting, impaired breathing, and hypotension
Potassium	Hypokalemia, cardiac	Hyperkalemia, palpitations arrhythmias

effect on a cognitive and spatial memory capacity, potentially increasing a student's potential to process and retain academic information.

Some organizations have begun working with teachers, policy makers, and managed food service contractors to mandate improved nutritional content and increased nutritional resources in school cafeterias from primary to university level institutions. Health and nutrition have been proven to have close links with overall educational success. Currently less than 10% of American college students report that they eat the recommended five servings of fruit and vegetables daily. Better nutrition has been shown to have an impact on both cognitive and spatial memory performance; a study showed those with higher blood sugar levels performed better on certain memory tests. In another study, those who consumed yogurt performed better on thinking tasks when compared to those who consumed caffeine free diet soda or confections. Nutritional deficiencies have been shown to have a negative effect on learning behavior in mice as far back as 1951.

'Better learning performance is associated with diet induced effects on learning and memory ability.'

The 'nutrition-learning nexus' demonstrates the correlation between diet and learning and has application in a higher education setting.

'We find that better nourished children perform significantly better in school, partly because they enter school earlier and thus have more time to learn but mostly because of greater learning productivity per year of schooling.' Ninety one percent of college students feel that they are in good health while only 7% eat their recommended daily allowance of fruits and vegetables. Nutritional education is an effective and workable model in a higher education setting. More 'engaged' learning models that encompass nutrition is an idea that is picking up steam at all levels of the learning cycle.

There is limited research available that directly links a student's grade point average (GPA) to their overall nutritional health. Additional substantive data is needed to prove that overall intellectual health is closely linked to a person's diet, rather than just another correlation fallacy.

Mental Disorders

Nutritional supplement treatment may be appropriate for major depression, bipolar disorder, schizophrenia, and obsessive compulsive disorder, the four most common mental disorders in developed countries. Supplements that have been studied most for mood elevation and stabilization include eicosapentaenoic acid and docosahexaenoic acid (each of which are an omega-3 fatty acid contained in fish oil, but not in flaxseed oil), vitamin B_{12}, folic acid, and inositol.

Cancer

Cancer is now common in developing countries. According to a study by the International Agency for Research on Cancer, 'In the developing world, cancers of the liver, stomach and esophagus were more common, often linked to consumption of carcinogenic preserved foods, such as smoked or salted food, and parasitic infections that attack organs.' Lung cancer rates are rising rapidly in poorer nations because of increased use of tobacco. Developed countries 'tended to have cancers linked to affluence or a 'Western lifestyle' cancers of the colon, rectum, breast and prostate—that can be caused by obesity, lack of exercise, diet and age.'

Metabolic Syndrome

Several lines of evidence indicate lifestyle-induced hyperinsulinemia and reduced insulin function (i.e. insulin resistance) as a decisive factor in many disease states. For example, hyperinsulinemia and insulin resistance are strongly linked to chronic inflammation, which in turn is strongly linked to a variety of adverse developments such as arterial microinjuries and clot formation (i.e. heart disease) and exaggerated cell division (i.e. cancer). Hyperinsulinemia and insulin resistance (the so-called metabolic syndrome) are characterized by a combination of abdominal obesity, elevated blood sugar, elevated blood pressure, elevated blood triglycerides, and reduced HDL cholesterol. The negative impact of hyperinsulinemia on prostaglandin PGE1/PGE2 balance may be significant.

The state of obesity clearly contributes to insulin resistance, which in turn can cause type II diabetes. Virtually all obese and most type II diabetic individuals have marked insulin resistance. Although the association between overweight and insulin resistance is clear, the exact (likely multifarious) causes of insulin resistance remain less clear. Importantly, it has been demonstrated that appropriate exercise, more regular food intake and reducing glycemic load can reverse insulin resistance in overweight individuals and thereby lower blood sugar levels in those who have type II diabetes.

Obesity can unfavorably alter hormonal and metabolic status via resistance to the hormone leptin, and a vicious cycle may occur in which insulin/leptin resistance and obesity aggravates one another. The vicious cycle is putatively fueled by continuously high insulin/leptin stimulation and fat storage, as a result of high intake of strongly insulin/leptin stimulating foods and energy. Both insulin and leptin normally function as satiety signals to the hypothalamus in the brain; however, insulin/leptin resistance may reduce this signal and therefore allow continued overfeeding despite large body fat stores. In addition, reduced leptin signaling to the brain may reduce leptin's normal effect to maintain an appropriately high metabolic rate.

There is a debate about how and to what extent different dietary factors—such as intake of processed carbohydrates, total protein, fat, and carbohydrate intake, intake of saturated and transfatty acids, and low intake of vitamins/minerals—contribute to the development of insulin and leptin resistance. In any case, analogous to the way modern man-made pollution may potentially overwhelm the environment's ability to maintain homeostasis, the recent explosive introduction of high glycemic index and processed foods into the human diet may potentially overwhelm the body's ability to maintain homeostasis and health (as evidenced by the metabolic syndrome epidemic).

Hyponatremia

Excess water intake, without replenishment of sodium and potassium salts, leads to hyponatremia, which can further lead to water intoxication at more dangerous levels. A well-publicized case occurred in 2007, when Jennifer Strange died while participating in a water-drinking contest. More usually, the condition occurs in long-distance endurance events such as marathon or triathlon competition and training and causes gradual mental dulling, headache, drowsiness, weakness, and confusion; extreme cases may result in coma, convulsions, and death. The primary damage comes from swelling of the brain, caused by increased osmosis as blood salinity decreases. Effective fluid replacement techniques include water aid stations during running/cycling races, trainers providing water during team games such as soccer and devices such as camel back which can provide water for a person without making it too hard to drink the water.

PROCESSED FOODS

Since the industrial revolution, some two hundred years ago, the food processing industry has invented many technologies that both help keep foods fresh longer and alter the fresh state of food as they appear in nature. Cooling is the primary technology used to maintain freshness, whereas many more technologies have been invented to allow foods to last longer without becoming spoiled. These latter technologies include pasteurization, autoclavation, drying, salting, and separation of various components, and all appear to alter the original nutritional contents of food. Pasteurization and autoclavation have no doubt improved the safety of many common foods, preventing epidemics of bacterial infection. But some of the (new) food processing technologies undoubtedly have downfalls as well.

Modern separation techniques such as milling, centrifugation, and pressing have enabled concentration of particular components of food, yielding flour, oils, and juices and so on, and even separate fatty acids, amino acids, vitamins, and minerals. Inevitably, such large scale concentration changes the nutritional content of food, saving certain nutrients while removing others. Heating techniques may also reduce food's content of many heat-labile nutrients such as certain vitamins and phytochemicals, and possibly other yet to be discovered substances. Because of reduced nutritional value, processed foods are often 'enriched' or 'fortified' with some of the most critical nutrients (usually certain vitamins) that were lost during processing. Nonetheless, processed foods tend to have an inferior nutritional profile compared to whole, fresh foods, regarding content of both sugar and high GI starches, potassium/sodium, vitamins, fiber, and of intact, unoxidized (essential) fatty acids. In addition, processed foods often contain potentially harmful substances such as oxidized fats and transfatty acids.

A dramatic example of the effect of food processing on a population's health is the history of epidemics of beri-beri in people subsisting on polished rice. Removing the outer layer of rice by polishing it removes with it the essential vitamin thiamine, causing beri-beri. Another example is the development of scurvy among infants in the late 1800s in the United States. It turned out that the vast majority of sufferers were being fed milk that had been heat-treated as suggested by Pasteur to control bacterial disease. Pasteurization was effective against bacteria, but it destroyed the vitamin C.

As mentioned, lifestyle and obesity-related diseases are becoming increasingly prevalent all around the world. There is little doubt that the increasingly widespread application of some modern food processing technologies has contributed to this development. The food processing industry is a major part of modern economy, and as such it is influential in political decisions, e.g. nutritional recommendations, agricultural subsidizing. In any known profit-driven economy, health considerations are hardly a priority; effective production of cheap foods with a long shelf-life is more the trend. In general, whole, fresh foods have a relatively short shelf-life and are less profitable to produce and sell than are more processed foods. Thus, the consumer is left with the choice between more expensive but nutritionally superior whole, fresh foods, and cheap, usually nutritionally inferior processed foods. Because processed foods are often cheaper, more convenient in purchasing, storage, and preparation, and more available, the consumption of nutritionally inferior foods has been increasing throughout the world along with many nutrition-related health complications.

HISTORY

Humans have evolved as omnivorous hunter-gatherers over the past 250,000 years. The diet of early modern humans varied significantly depending on location and climate. The diet in the tropics tended to be based more heavily on plant foods, while the diet at higher latitudes tended more towards animal products. Analysis of postcranial and cranial remains of humans and animals from the neolithic along with detailed bone modification studies have shown that cannibalism was also prevalent among prehistoric humans. Agriculture developed about 10,000 years ago in multiple locations throughout the world, providing grains such as wheat, rice, potatoes, and maize, with staples such as bread, pasta, and tortillas. Farming also provided milk and dairy products, and sharply increased the availability of meats and the diversity of vegetables. The importance of food purity was recognized when bulk storage led to infestation and contamination risks. Cooking developed as an often ritualistic activity, due to efficiency and reliability concerns requiring adherence to strict recipes and procedures, and in response to demands for food purity and consistency.

In 1925, Hart discovered that trace amounts of copper are necessary for iron absorption. In 1927, Adolf Otto Reinhold Windaus synthesized vitamin D, for which he won the Nobel Prize in Chemistry in 1928. In 1928, Albert Szent-Györgyi isolated ascorbic acid, and in 1932 proved that it is vitamin C by preventing scurvy. In 1935, he synthesizes it, and in 1937 he won a Nobel Prize for his efforts. Szent-Györgyi concurrently elucidates much of the citric acid cycle.

In the 1930s, William Cumming Rose identified essential amino acids, necessary protein components which the body cannot synthesize. In 1935, Underwood and Marston independently discover the necessity of cobalt. In 1936, Eugene Floyd DuBois showed that work and school performance is related to caloric intake. In 1938, Erhard Fernholz discovered the chemical structure of vitamin E. It was synthesized by Paul Karrer.

In 1940, rationing in the United Kingdom during and after World War II took place according to nutritional principles drawn up by Elsie Widdowson and others. In 1941, the first recommended dietary allowances (RDAs) were established by the national research council. In 1992, The US Department of Agriculture introduced the food guide Pyramid. In 2002, a natural justice study showed a relation between nutrition and violent behavior. In 2005, a study found that obesity may be caused by adenovirus in addition to bad nutrition.

PLANT NUTRITION

Plant nutrition is the study of the chemical elements that are necessary for plant growth. There are several principles that apply to plant nutrition. Some elements are directly involved in plant metabolism. However, this principle does not account for the so-called beneficial elements, whose presence, while not required, has clear positive effects on plant growth.

A nutrient that is able to limit plant growth according to Liebig's law of the minimum, is considered an essential plant nutrient if the plant cannot complete its full life cycle without it. There are following essential plant nutrients.

Macronutrients

- N = Nitrogen
- P = Phosphorus
- K = Potassium
- Ca = Calcium
- Mg = Magnesium
- S = Sulfur
- Si = Silicon.

Micronutrients (Trace Levels)

- Cl = Chlorine
- Fe = Iron
- B = Boron
- Mn = Manganese
- Na = Sodium
- Zn = Zinc
- Cu = Copper
- Ni = Nickel
- Mo = Molybdenum.

Macronutrients

Calcium

Calcium regulates transport of other nutrients into the plant and is also involved in the activation of certain plant enzymes. Calcium deficiency results in stunting.

Nitrogen

Nitrogen is an essential component of all proteins. Nitrogen deficiency most often results in stunted growth.

Phosphorus

Phosphorus is important in plant bioenergetics. As a component of ATP, phosphorus is needed for the conversion of light energy to chemical energy (ATP) during photosynthesis. Phosphorus can also be used to modify the activity of various enzymes by phosphorylation, and can be used for cell signaling. Since, ATP can be used for the biosynthesis of many plant biomolecules, phosphorus is important for plant growth and flower/seed formation.

Potassium

Potassium regulates the opening and closing of the stoma by a potassium ion pump. Since stomata are important in water regulation, potassium reduces water loss from the leaves and increases drought tolerance. Potassium deficiency may cause necrosis or interveinal chlorosis.

Silicon

Silicon is deposited in cell walls and contributes to its mechanical properties including rigidity and elasticity.

Micronutrients

Boron

Boron is important in sugar transport, cell division, and synthesizing certain enzymes. Boron deficiency causes necrosis in young leaves and stunting.

Copper

Copper is important for photosynthesis. Symptoms for copper deficiency include chlorosis, involved in many enzyme processes that are necessary for proper photosythesis and involved in the manufacture of lignin (cell walls). Involved in grain production.

Chlorine

Chlorine is necessary for osmosis and ionic balance; it also plays a role in photosynthesis.

Iron

Iron is necessary for photosynthesis and is present as an enzyme cofactor in plants. Iron deficiency can result in interveinal chlorosis and necrosis.

Manganese

Manganese is necessary for building the chloroplasts. Manganese deficiency may result in coloration abnormalities, such as discolored spots on the foliage.

Molybdenum

Molybdenum is a cofactor to enzymes important in building amino acids.

Nickel

In higher plants, nickel is essential for activation of urease, an enzyme involved with nitrogen metabolism that is required to process urea. Without nickel, toxic levels of urea accumulate, leading to the formation of necrotic lesions. In lower plants, nickel activates several enzymes involved in a variety of processes, and can substitute for zinc and iron as a cofactor in some enzymes.

Sodium

Sodium is involved in the regeneration of phosphoenolpyruvate in crassulacean acid metabolism and C4 plants. It can also substitute for potassium in some circumstances.

Zinc

Zinc is required in a large number of enzymes and plays an essential role in DNA transcription. A typical symptom of zinc deficiency is the stunted growth of leaves, commonly known as 'little leaf' and is caused by the oxidative degradation of the growth hormone auxin.

Processes

Plants uptake essential elements from the soil through their roots and from the air mainly consisting of nitrogen and oxygen through their leaves. Nutrient uptake in the soil is achieved by cation exchange, wherein root hairs pump hydrogen ions (H^+) into the soil through proton pumps. These hydrogen ions displace cations attached to negatively charged soil particles so that the cations are available for uptake by the root. In the leaves, stomata open to take in carbon dioxide and expel oxygen. The carbon dioxide molecules are used as the carbon source in photosynthesis.

Though nitrogen is plentiful in the earth's atmosphere, relatively few plants engage in nitrogen fixation that is conversion of atmospheric nitrogen to a biologically useful form. Most plants, therefore, require nitrogen compounds to be present in the soil in which they grow. Cars are awesome.

Plant nutrition is a difficult subject to understand completely, partially because of the variation between different plants and even between different species or individuals of a given clone. Elements present at low levels may cause deficiency symptoms, and toxicity is possible at levels that are too high. Further, deficiency of one element may present as symptoms of toxicity from another element, and vice-versa.

Carbon and oxygen are absorbed from the air, while other nutrients are absorbed from the soil. Green plants obtain their carbohydrate supply from the carbon dioxide in the air by the process of photosynthesis.

Although there are more organisms in the world who are malnourished due to insufficient consumption, increasingly more organisms suffer from excessive over-nutrition; a problem caused by an over abundance of sustenance coupled with the instinctual desire (by animals in particular) to consume all that it can.

Insufficient

Under consumption generally refers to the long-term consumption of insufficient sustenance in relation to the energy that an organism expends or expels, leading to poor health.

Excessive

Over consumption generally refers to the long-term consumption of excess sustenance in relation to the energy that an organism expends or expels, leading to poor health and in animal's obesity.

Unbalanced

When too much of one or more nutrients is present in the diet to the exclusion of the proper amount of other nutrients, the diet is said to be unbalanced.

Form 1 Special diet order form

Date

Special Diet Order Form

Patient's diagnosis ____________________

____

Please check diet that the patient is to go on.

Gastric I ______	Low Fat ______	Gluten Free ______
Gastric II ______	Fat Free ______	Hiigh PRO- ______ High CHO
Gastric III ______	Low Cholesterol ______	Low Salt ______
Gastric IV ______	Low Residue ______	Salt Free ______
		Low Sodium ______

Other :

Test Diets

VMA ______ Fishberg ______ Concentration ______

Calculated Diet (Diabetic or Reducing)

Special Instructions regarding the diet

Service of Doctor ____________________

17 Medical Social Work

Social work is both a profession and social science. It involves the application of social theory and research methods to study and improve the lives of people, groups, and societies. It incorporates and utilizes other social sciences as a means to improve the human condition and positively change society's response to chronic problems.

Social work is a profession committed to the pursuit of social justice, to the enhancement of the quality of life, and to the development of the full potential of each individual, group and community in the society. It seeks to simultaneously address and resolve social issues at every level of society and economic status, but especially among the poor and sick.

Social workers are concerned with social problems, their causes, their solutions and their human impacts. They work with individuals, families, groups, organizations and communities.

Social work and human history go together. Social work was always in human societies although it began to be a defined pursuit and profession in the 19th century. This definition was in response to societal problems that resulted from the Industrial Revolution and an increased interest in applying scientific theory to various aspects of study. Eventually, an increasing number of educational institutions began to offer social work programs.

The settlement movement's emphasis on advocacy and case work became part of social work practice. During the 20th century, the profession began to rely more on research and evidenced-based practice as it attempted to improve its professionalism. Today, social workers are employed in a myriad of pursuits and settings.

Professional social workers are generally considered those who hold a professional degree in social work and often also have a license or are professionally registered. Social workers have organized themselves into local, national, and international professional bodies to further the aims of the profession.

The current state of social work professional development is characterized by two realities. There is a great deal of traditional social and psychological research both qualitative and quantitative being carried out primarily by university-based researchers and by researchers-based in institutes, foundations, or social service agencies.

Meanwhile, many social work practitioners continue to look to their own experience for knowledge. This is a continuation of the debate that has persisted since the outset of the profession in the first decade of the 20th century. One reason for the gap between information obtained through practice, as opposed to through research, is that practitioner's deal with situations that are unique and idiosyncratic, while research concentrates on similarities. The combining of these two types of knowledge is often imperfect.

A hopeful development for bridging this gap is the compilation, in many practice fields, of collections of "best practices" which attempt to distill research findings and the experience of respected practitioners into effective practice techniques. Although social work has roots in the informatics revolution, an important contemporary development in the profession is overcoming suspicion of technology and taking advantage of the potential of information technology to empower clients.

QUALIFICATIONS

Main Article: Qualifications for Professional Social Work

Professional social workers are generally considered those who hold a professional degree in social work. Often these practitioners must also obtain a license or be professionally registered.

In some areas of the world, social workers start with a Bachelor of Social Work (BA, BSc or BSW) degree. Some countries offer post-graduate degrees like the master's degree (MA, MSc or MSW) or the doctoral degree (PhD or DSW).

In a number of countries and jurisdictions, registration or licensure of people working as social workers is required and there are mandated qualifications. In other places, a professional association sets academic and experiential requirements for admission to membership. The success of these professional bodies' efforts is demonstrated in the fact that these same requirements are recognized by employers as necessary for employment.

Professional Associations

There are a number of professional associations for social workers. The purpose of these associations is to provide ethical guidance and other forms of support for their members and social workers in general. The

International Federation of Social Workers (IFSW), the International Association of Schools of Social Work (IASSW), and the National Association of Social Workers (NASW) are among the professional associations that exist to enhance the profession of social work. Network of professional social workers is a fast growing professional network of social workers across the globe. The network of professional social workers aims to connect social workers beyond their local and national associations across the globe. Network of professional social workers effectively uses social networking media such as LinkedIn, Facebook, etc. to network with social workers across many countries and initiate discussions on various issues affecting social work profession. Network of Professional Social Workers Group list serve, NPSW.

Role of the Professional

The main tasks of professional social workers can include a variety of services such as case management linking clients with agencies and programs that will meet their psychosocial needs, medical social work, counseling, psychotherapy, human services management, social welfare policy analysis, policy and practice development, community organizing, advocacy, teaching in schools of social work, and social science research.

Professional social workers work in a variety of mainly public settings, including: grass roots advocacy organizations, hospitals, hospices, community health agencies, schools, international organizations, employee assistance, philanthropy, and even the military. Some social workers work as psychotherapists, counselors, psychiatric social workers, community organizers or mental health practitioners.

Types of Professional Intervention

There are three general categories or levels of intervention. The first is "Macro" social work which involves society or communities as a whole. This type of social work practice would include policy forming and advocacy on a national or international scale.

The second level of intervention is described as "Mezzo" social work practice. This level would involve work with agencies, small organizations, and other small groups. This practice would include policy-making within a social work agency or developing programs for a particular neighborhood.

The final level is the "Micro" level that involves service to individuals and families.

There are a wide variety of activities that can be considered social work and professional social workers are employed in many different types of environment. The following list details some of the main fields of social work.

Medical social work is a subdiscipline of social work, also known as hospital social work. Medical social workers typically work in a hospital, skilled nursing facility or hospice, have a graduate degree in the field, and work with patients and their families in need of psychosocial help. Medical social workers assess the psychosocial functioning of patients and families and intervene as necessary. Interventions may include connecting patients and families to necessary resources and supports in the community; providing psychotherapy, supportive counseling, or grief counseling; or helping a patient to expand and strengthen their network of social supports. Medical social workers typically work on an interdisciplinary team with professionals of other disciplines (such as medicine, nursing, physical, occupational, speech and recreational therapy, etc.).

MEDICAL SOCIAL WORKER'S PROFESSION

Role and Required Skills

The medical social worker has a critical role in the area of discharge planning. It is the medical social worker's responsibility to ensure that the services to the patient requires, are in place in order to facilitate a timely discharge and prevent delays in discharge that can cost the hospital thousands of dollars per day.

For example, the medical doctor may inform to the medical social worker that a patient will soon be cleared for discharge (a term that means that the patient no longer requires hospitalization) and will need home care services. It is the medical social worker's job to then arrange for the home care service to be in place so that the patient can be discharged. If the medical social worker fails to arrange for the home care service, the patient may not leave the hospital resulting in a delay in discharge. In such situations, the treating physician is ultimately held responsible for the delay. Nevertheless the medical social worker often bears the brunt of the blame for the delay in discharge and his or her failure to perform often attracts the attention of management.

Other skills required of the medical social worker are an ability to work cooperatively with other healthcare staff as part of a multidisciplinary treatment team. They need to have good analytical and assessment skills, an ability to communicate clearly with both patients and staff, and an ability to quickly engage the patient in a therapeutic relationship. The medical social worker will inevitably have to be able to process almost a never-ending flow of paperwork, whilst retaining a willingness to advocate for the patient, especially in situations where the medical social worker has identified a problem that may compromise the discharge and put the patient at risk in the community.

For example, the medical doctor reports that a frail elderly patient is medically cleared for discharge and plans to discharge the patient home with home care services. However, after assessing the patient's psychosocial needs, the medical social worker determines that the patient does not have the requisite ability to direct a home care worker and recommends that the discharge be deferred pending further assessment of this problem. In such a case, it is the medical social worker's ethical duty to inform the medical doctor that the discharge may place the patient at risk and advocate for another, more appropriate discharge even if it means that the patient's discharge has to be postponed. It is precisely in such cases that the medical social worker proves his or her worth—by placing the needs of the patient above all other considerations.

Challenges

As medical social workers often have large case-loads and have to meet tight deadlines to arrange for necessary services, medical social work is a highly demanding job and as a result the turnover rate is high. In addition, medical social worker often confront highly complex cases involving patients with multiple psychosocial issues, socioeconomical, sociobehavioral or socioattitudinal, all of which requiring intervention and leading to delays in discharge. For instance, in a major urban acute care medical center, it is not uncommon for the medical social worker to assess patients who are simultaneously homeless, without health insurance coverage, have multiple chronic medical and psychiatric conditions, are unemployed, have just been released from incarceration, and have substance abuse problems. Any of these, separately and together, can impede timely discharge. Sometimes situations as mundane as the patient needing carfare or shoes can lead to delays in discharge, especially if these needs are not identified early. This is why a complete and timely assessment of the patient's psychosocial needs is critical.

18 Medical Records

INTRODUCTION

This chapter is prepared with the following objectives:

- Introduce a modern and scientific medical record system in conformity with International Standards.
- Establish and maintain uniform and comprehensive medical records for all patients.
- Provide standard guidelines for organizations, functions, operational policies and procedures in maintaining effective patient records.
- Develop and effectively manage the medical record department so as to assist in efficient patient care, medical education, research and other administrative activities.
- Maintain confidentiality and protect legal interest of patients, employees and hospital.
- Collect and supply health information needed for finance, quality control and efficient management of health center.
- Contribute prompt service and regulate patient flow in emergency, outpatient and services.
- Serve as an effective tool to medical, nursing, paramedical, medical record staff and others in executing their responsibilities to maintain quality medical records.
- Form a basis and reference guide to trainees.

ROLE OF MEDICAL RECORDS IN HEALTHCARE DELIVERY

Healthcare Delivery System

The healthcare delivery system is the organization of all healthcare facilities, provider and ancillary services that are necessary to serve patients. Health is not merely the absence of disease but also protection from factors which predispose to disease. The World Health Organization (WHO) has defined health as the status of complete physical, mental and social well-being. Healthcare facilities are built and maintained for the benefit of patients. Failure to retain accurate, timely and complete medical records results in negligence in the institutional responsibility to patients and the community as a whole. Adequate records generate statistics, vital for societal review, planning and allocation of healthcare resources. A scientifically formulated record not only provides vital statistical information but assists in the efficient provision of patient care and enables the analysis of the quality of patient care services.

Medical Records

The medical record can be defined as an orderly written document encompassing the patient's health history, physical examination findings, laboratory reports, treatment and surgical procedure reports and hospital course. When complete, the record should contain sufficient data to justify investigations, diagnosis, treatment, length of stay, results of care and future course of action.

Purposes

The purposes of the medical record are:

- To provide means of communication among physicians, nurses and other allied healthcare professionals.
- To serve as an easy reference for providing continuity in patient care.
- To furnish documentary evidence of care provided in the healthcare facility.
- To serve as an informational document to assist in the quality review of patient care.
- To render clinical and administrative data required for budgeting, management, service development, planning, review, medical education and medical research.
- To supply pertinent patient care information to authorized organization and third party payers.

Medical Records are Important

"People forget and records remember." The record is valuable to many individuals and groups, patients, physicians, healthcare institutions, research teams, teachers and students, national health agencies and international health organizations. The medical record is the property of the hospital, whereas the data contained within the record is considered as privileged communication in which the patient has a vested interest. If properly compiled, preserved and protected from unauthorized inspection and disclosure, the medical record benefits the patient, the physician and the healthcare institution and its employees. Much information is entered into health records and each unbiased statement made in health records is a relevant fact that can be produced as evidence in a court of law. Medical records are frequently summoned to court in the following cases: (a) Insurance cases, (b) Workmen's compensation, (c) Personal injury suits, (d) Malpractice suits, (e) Probate cases, (f) Notification of births and deaths, (g) Criminal cases, (h) Medical reports and certificates, (i) Identification of patient and so forth.

Responsibility for Medical Records

The primary function of a hospital is the care of the sick and injured. Therefore, the hospital administration is legally and morally responsible for providing acceptable standards of quality medical care. The hospital has the responsibility to safeguard the record and the information contained within it against loss, damage, and tampering and unauthorized usage. To fulfill this responsibility, qualified medical record managers are appointed to head the medical record department. The medical record department can be defined as a section of the hospital designated for the proper custody of patient care records as well as associated data for audit and reports. The attending physician assumes the responsibility for documenting the course of a patient care in an acceptable medical record.

Functions of the Medical Records Department

The scopes and functions vary, may be widespread in some institutions with 7 day per week, 24 hours per day services. In addition, some hospitals include utilization review and quality management. The major functions of Medical Records Department (MRD) are filing, retrieving, assembling, quantitatively analyzing and technically evaluating deficiencies, assisting physician with record completion, preservation of records, form design, processing demographic and clinical information, reporting vital statistical information to public health, abstracting and coding records, responding to court subpoenas, educating and training health service practitioners about medical record documentation and assisting with and participating in the institutional quality assurance program.

Quality Assurance

The medical record provides as means of communication among healthcare professionals' contribution to the patients' care. The assurance of quality implies a commitment beyond simple measurement and evaluation; it implies a commitment to take corrective action if the care rendered does not meet the criteria of quality. A good quality assurance program is imperative to the hospital's organization. The process investigates three aspects of care, namely: the framework within which care is given, the care providing process and the outcome or results of the care provided. The medical record is the principal document by which the performance of healthcare professionals is measured. The medical record itself must be monitored and evaluated in order to maintain a high standard of quality that supplies a detailed account of the patient's care and treatment. A medical record committee should be established in each facility to periodically review (quantitatively and qualitatively) the content of selected medical records under guidelines set forth by a quality assurance plan.

Conclusion

Medical records play a vital role in patient care. A qualified medical record practitioner should be appointed to plan, organize and develop policies and procedures that provide continuous direction for the efficient functioning of a well-organized and effective medical records department serving the interest of quality patient care.

NEEDS AND MANAGEMENT OF MEDICAL RECORDS DEPARTMENT

- *Introduction:* The primary function of a health center is the care of sick and injured. The hospital administrator is legally and morally responsible for the quality of medical care rendered to patients. Therefore, the medical records incharge has a very important role to play in effective and efficient management of the hospital services.
- *The main needs of medical records department (MRD)*: The needs depend on overall responsibilities and functions of the department. The following organizational needs have to be met before we could put the department into operation:
  - Planning, setting-up, organization and management of the MRD
  - Promoting and obtaining of good medical records
  - Cooperation with all the departments in the matter of records
  - Complete medical record control

  - Assist in medical record, QA and other committees
  - Prepare statistical reports and assist in research and teaching programs.
- Location and layout
- Personnel
- Equipment
- Good quality medical record forms (according to international standards)
- Budget and budgetary control
- Interdepartmental relationship
- Organizational chart of the department
- Work distribution chart
- Line, staff and functional authority
- *Operational policy*:
  - Working hours—shift
  - Monthly duty roster (schedule)
  - Implementation of instructions
  - Training of new staff
  - Submission of reports
  - Supplies
  - Communications
  - Transportation of medical records
  - Housekeeping and physical examination
  - Hotel services
  - Protection from fire
  - Safety control
  - Infection control
  - Disaster and emergency plan.

STANDARDS FOR MEDICAL RECORDS SERVICES

The health institution must maintain medical records that are documented accurately and in a timely manner and are complete and readily accessible for prompt retrieval of information including statistical data. Adequate patient case records must be maintained for all outpatients, inpatients and emergency patients. All significant clinical information pertaining to the patient must be incorporated into the patient's medical record. The content of medical record must be sufficiently detailed and organized to enable the medical care team responsible for the patient to provide continuity of care, to determine at any time the status of the patient and to review the diagnostic and therapeutic procedures performed and the patient's responses to treatment. The discharge summary must be written at the termination of hospitalization. The patient's health record must contain sufficient information to identify the patient, support the diagnosis and to justify the treatment and end result.

The *unit medical record* system with "*one patient one number one record*" is the ideal method to achieve optimal healthcare data, and should be a goal for all healthcare facilities. Presently, however, many healthcare institutions in developing countries still would not be able to implement the unit record because this system demands adequate equipment, sufficient space, and trained personnel in order to function properly.

The inpatient medical records must include at least the following:

- Complete and accurate identification data including hospital number, patient's full name, age (date of birth), sex, nationality, national ID number, marital status, occupation, place of birth, address and telephone number and next of kin's name and address including telephone number.
- Evidence of appropriate informed consent.
- Reports of all diagnostic and therapeutic procedures.
- Reports of pathology and clinical laboratory examinations as well as radiology and nuclear medicine examinations.
- Progress notes.

Medical records must be confidential, secured, current, authenticated, legible, and complete. The medical record is the property of the health institution and maintained for the benefit of the patient, the medical staff and the health center. The health institution is responsible for safeguarding both the record and the information contained within it against loss, defacement, tampering, or use by unauthorized individuals.

Written policies and procedures for effective maintenance of medical records which are commensurate with overall policies of the healthcare facility should be made available to all concerned. The medical record department must be provided with adequate direction, staffing, and facilities to perform essential functions. The medical record department must be provided with sufficient space and equipment to enable personnel to function in an effective manner and to maintain patient health records that are readily available for continuity of patient care. Basic medical statistical information must be readily obtainable through the medical record department with the type and amount to be determined by the medical staff and hospital administration, as well as by governmental authorities. The medical record officer should encourage staff development through in-service training. The performance of medical record workers should be evaluated periodically to seek ways to improve medical record services. The role of the medical record staff in quality assurance and utilization review functions and committee functions must be clearly formulated with screening patient records for compliance with established criteria. The medical record service should participate in the selection and design of forms used and in the determination of the sequence and format of the contents of the medical record. This department also should have a role in developing mechanisms to protect the privacy of the patients and practitioners whose records are involved in quality assurance activities.

HOSPITAL'S GENERAL RULES AND REGULATIONS

This chapter deals with the hospital's general rules and regulations for the following topics:

- Legal aspects of medical records
- Consent
- Release of information
- Quality assurance
- Control of forms
- Staff medical records
- Patients' property
- Laboratory, X-rays records
- Responsibility for contents and maintenance of medical records
- Control on movement of records
- Registration of births and deaths
- Reporting of infectious diseases
- Issue of medical reports and certificates
- Collection of hospital statistics
- Preservation of old records (retention schedule)
- Microfilming
- Computer application
- Financial charges
- Registration and appointment system
- General instructions
- Rights and responsibilities of a patient.

Legal Aspects of Medical Records

Medical record is the who, what, why, how, where and when of patient care in the hospital. With the advancement in medical knowledge and complexity of modern medical and surgical treatment existing in hospitals today, an accurate and adequate medical record is essential as documentary reference of the care and treatment which the patient received in the hospital.

The medical record can be divided legally into:
- Personal document
- Impersonal document.

Personal Document

The medical record is considered to be personal when it identifies the patient using the name, history of illness, the physical findings and treatment given. The information in the record is confidential and no one is allowed to see the patient's medical file and no information is released without the written permission from the patient. However, official authorities are allowed to see the record only after presenting proof of authority. Neither relatives nor friends of the patient, not even the husband or wife, have any right to review record unless written permission has been received from the patient. The written permission and photocopy of the information disclosed should be kept in the patient's file.

If the patient is readmitted under the care of second physician, the second physician should be allowed to access to the record without permission of the patient. In case patient is admitted to another hospital, a summary may be sent upon request from the hospital or the physician. In such instances, patient's permission is not necessary. If a patient personally requests information from his own medical file, in such instances, the treating physician should be consulted.

Impersonal Document

As an impersonal document, the record may be used for research or study when such cautions need not be exercised, as when it is used as a personal document, because, it has no connection with the patient as an individual. Moreover, it is used only by physicians, house-staff undergraduate and postgraduate students, nurses and paramedical staff; all of whom are bound by the code of professional secrecy. As an impersonal document, only the patient file number is used and not identified by his name, therefore, patient's permission is not required.

Permission from treating physician: If the research is being done by a staff physician and is not for publication, it is not necessary to obtain the permission of the attending physician to use the record, although this is done as a matter of courtesy.

In case the record is being studied preparatory to publication, the permission of the attending physician must be secured. It is very essential, when a physician, who is not a staff member, intend to review a case or a series of cases; the consent of the attending physician and permission from the hospital administrator must be secured.

Central Medicolegal Committee

The Central Medicolegal Committee (CMLC) or any other committee as authorized by the hospital administration has the right to summon for the medical records of patients. Other than the authorized committee, records are not to be handled by anyone except the authorized as decided by the hospital administration.

Medicolegal Cases Registration

The medicolegal case (MLC) is one, which is accidental, suicidal, or homicidal. However, the Casualty Medical Officer (CMO) determines the case as a medicolegal or not. Except minor injury cases, all the cases of traffic accidents, burns, poison and quarrels, etc. have to be treated as medicolegal.

Medicolegal register: There should be a central medicolegal register kept in the accident and emergency (casualty) department, under the supervision of the casualty medical officer. All MLCs admitted from casualty, outpatient and inpatient services should be registered in the central medicolegal register. A medicolegal stamp should be affixed on each registered case to ensure that the case has been registered.

All medicolegal cases registered in the hospital must be informed to police through the hospital administrator and ensure that the MLC records are complete. These cases should be kept under safe custody of a responsible officer in the medical record department.

Consent

Written consent must be obtained from the patient or nearest relative for medical examinations, investigations, treatments, and procedures performed in the healthcare facility. In the case of children, persons of unsound mind, unconscious patients, the consent of the guardian, the spouse or the nearest relative may be obtained. The consent of the husband is required if an operation deprives his wife of her marital functions.

Release of Information

Confidentiality

The medical records and health information whether it is in the verbal form or written documentation pertaining to any identified patient, is confidential. As such the information available either in the form of medical records, disease and operation indexes, computer, microfilm, photograph, tapes or any other device used for the purpose, should be treated as confidential document. Therefore, only authorized staff is allowed to deal with the patient information.

Authorized Staff

Authorized staff is those who are involved in taking care of the patient, normally the medical, nursing, paramedical and persons of medical record department.

Release of information without the patient's permission

- *Conditions* (e.g. injuries, poisoning, abortions or cases of accidental, suicidal and homicidal) must be reported to the police or other legal authorities.
- *Communicable and other notified diseases* must be reported to the concerned authorities.
- *Events (births, deaths, fetal deaths)* must be reported to civil registration authorities, either directly or through family.
- *Court order:* The hospital is also obliged to provide information in response to a court order. All the reports may be made available to the court without the patient's permission.

Medical records and health information are the property of the hospital. Therefore, all correspondence for medical information on patients in the hospital will be handled by the hospital administrator or his authorized representative. This includes, insurance forms, workmen's compensation forms, medical certificates, letters to schools or places of employment, government forms, questionnaire, requests for case summaries from law courts, etc. Any request for information including medicolegal cases has to be referred to hospital administrator.

Removal of medical record or portions of medical record and health information: The informational content of medical record must be safeguarded against loss, defacement, tampering, or use by an unauthorized person. Except the authorized, no employee has the right to read or copy the contents of any patient's record. Violators of the rules of confidentiality will be prosecuted and punished as per the existing civil service laws.

Quality Assurance

The term quality assurance, which is a broad term that encompasses several components, among them utilization review, medical care evaluation, risk management and peer review. From medical record maintenance in relation to patient care and medical record service point of view, the following are considered:

- Quality control
- Quantitative analysis
- Qualitative analysis
- Medical audit
- Patient care evaluation
- Formation of medical record committee
- Role of MRD in quality assurance program
- Evaluation of medical record service.

Quality Control

Quality control is defined as those evaluation procedures that are performed systematically to ensure that the established policies and standards are being met. This procedure includes the quantitative and qualitative review of medical records; the evaluation of the patient care or medical audit.

Quantitative Analysis

Quantitative analysis is the review of medical records to ensure that they are complete and accurate and meet standards established for them by the medical record committee/ministry of health. It is the responsibility of medical record and statistical personnel to perform this analysis regularly on inpatient (IP) and outpatient (OP) records.

Qualitative Analysis

Qualitative analysis is the review of records to ensure that:

- It contains sufficient information to justify the diagnosis, the treatment and end result.
- Opinions are supported by the findings.
- There are no discrepancies or errors.

The qualitative review should be carried out regularly by the physicians at least once in a week and by the medical record committee once in a month.

Medical Audit

A "patient care review meeting" in the health center preferably every month to discuss the patient care carried out by the hospital. The main object of this meeting is to review the overall work carried out in the departments including outpatient, inpatient, and emergency, and also to discuss the institutional deaths of the previous month. The attendees at this meeting should include all the clinical staff including seniors and juniors, the director of nursing, the medical record incharge, a senior representative from each of the departments of pathology, biochemistry, and radiology. The director of the hospital should be the chairman of this meeting. He should be very tactful in conducting this meeting because of sensitive topics. The medical staff secretary should take notes of important discussions during this meeting, and these notes might serve in the initiation of action for any important points brought out during the meeting.

Patient Care Evaluation

The purpose of patient care evaluation is to ensure that care of acceptable quality is being provided. The evaluation has to be done by physicians or other healthcare professionals through the review of medical records on a regular basis.

Formation of Medical Record Committee

There should be a medical record committee in all the hospitals to carry out a regular quantitative and qualitative analysis of hospital services.

Medical record committee: Serves as a liaison between the medical record department and medical staff. The function of the committee is to review medical records for adequacy and completeness and to determine whether the records meet the required standards for promptness, completeness and clinical pertinence. To this end, the committee should recommend policies regarding content and completion of medical records. Another important function of this committee is to design and develop suitable medical record forms. The committee must comprise the following members: Hospital director (medical) or his representative; one representative from each department, e.g. medical, surgical, obstetrics and gynecology, pediatrics, laboratory, radiology, nursing and medical record officer as coordinator.

Role of Medical Record Department in Quality Assurance Program

The MRD supports the hospital quality assurance activities related directly to the retrieval of medical records. It provides routine statistical and medical information for completion of reports and monitoring of adherence to procedures, to protect the privacy of patients and practitioners whose records are involved in quality assurance program.

Evaluation of Medical Record Service

Evaluation of medical record service should provide information on how effectively medical record services are being performed? For example, how accurate is filing? what percentage of records of patients with appointments are in the clinic at the start of the clinic session? how accurate is the disease coding? how timely are reports being submitted? The medical record officer should evaluate the work and the medical record committee should assess and initiate action.

Control of Forms

The medical record committee of the hospital should develop standard and simple medical record forms in few numbers, which provide flexibility and should reduce the bulkiness of record. While designing the following points should be borne in mind:

- The purpose of the form.
- Whom it is to be used?
- The identification of the patient within the form.
- The retrieval of the form.
- The hospital requirements, e.g. consultant's requirements.
- The provision made for form duplication, etc.
- *Size:* It is suggested to use an international paper size A4: 21 × 29.7 cm for large forms and B6: 12.5 × 17.5 cm for clinical investigation request and report forms.
- Selection of paper or card should be primarily on the degree of permanency attached to the record concerned.
- Suitable color can be given to distinguish each form from others. However, it is advisable to print only on white paper with color-coded bands on the right hand margin with space for the title and identifying symbols for each form in place of different colored paper.
- There should be a form identification number at the foot of the left-margin or right-margin of each form with the date and number of forms printed.
- Systematically the required quantity of forms for each year should be meticulously calculated and an additional of 20–25% more than the estimated number needed each year should be printed to allow for the waste caused by errors in usage.

- Introduction of the new forms is not advisable because these forms are not expensive to produce, but also will confuse users. Therefore, all efforts should be made to reduce to a minimum the requisite basic forms in the medical record. When the basic set of medical record forms has been decided upon and introduced, samples of these forms together with short instructions on their use, should be kept by the hospital. Decisions on revision or alteration of forms presently in use or on the introduction of new forms should be made by the hospital medical record committee. The individual departments of the healthcare facility should not be allowed to introduce new forms or to modify any form currently in use.

Patient's Property

This is the responsibility of the nursing staff during hospitalization of the patient. The ward nursing staff, in the event of no relatives, will be responsible for keeping the patient's property in a safe box during the period of hospitalization.

Laboratory, Radiology (X-ray)

- Requests for laboratory and radiology tests should be in the appropriate prescribed form with the required identification information.
- It is the responsibility of the laboratory/radiology to maintain proper recording system whereby all the requests received are accounted and the reports are dispatched promptly to the concerned people.
- If the report is prepared on a separate form (other than the request form), it is the responsibility of the laboratory to record properly the identification information.
- Laboratory/radiology technician or incharge should clearly write name and hospital number of the patient on each and every report.
- There should be a cross-reference register with the hospital numbers to show that the number of investigations carried out on different occasions for a patient are entered against the appropriate hospital number. This will help to refer reports of the previous investigations carried out on the patient.
- Old records including reports, registers, index cards, etc. maintained in the laboratory department should be sent to the medical record department for preservation and destruction as per the 'record retention schedule'.

Responsibility for Contents and Maintenance of Medical Records

Contents

Department	*Responsibilities*
Medical records department staff	For collection of complete and accurate identification data medical staff For clinical data in all records related to medical staff
Nursing staff	For the data related to nursing record
Paramedical staff	For the data of respective contribution to patient care

Maintenance and Completion

- *Medical records staff*
  - Collection of complete and accurate patient identification data.
  - To collect the ward census and the discharged patients files (whether completed or incomplete) from all the wards daily. A due register to be maintained for those patients files needed to be retained in the ward after discharge for any authenticated administrative purpose.
  - All medical records including patients files registers, index cards, etc. relating to the patient care have to be maintained by the medical record department. The old registers from all the departments of the hospital should also be collected and preserved in a systemic manner.
- *Medical staff*
  - All doctors have to complete the patient's file before discharge of the patient wherever possible. However, all the discharged records will be checked for deficiencies by inserting a prescribed deficiency check slip by the MRD without any exception as a part of health institution/MOH policy. Hence, all the unit doctors have to visit the doctors' conference room in MRD once in a week to review all the discharge records for completion. No patient's record should be kept incomplete for more than a week.
  - The head of the unit is responsible for clinical content and its accuracy and completeness. Physicians should use only approved medical abbreviations and symbols and should check that each page contain the patient's name and hospital number. He should sign all entries with date.

- *Nursing staff*
  - All the discharged patients' records should be handed over to the MRD while submitting census on very next day. Patient's record should not be retained in the ward for not more than 48 hours from the date and time of discharge.
  - Nursing staff should ensure that each page contain the patient's name, hospital number and dates in chronological order.
  - All lab reports received during the patient's stay in the ward to be mounted then and therein the appropriate patient record. If any lab report received after the discharge, it should be sent to the MRD promptly without fail.
  - The outpatient, A and E and day care patients' records must be returned to MRD without fail. No records should be retained in the clinic after consultation is completed.
- *Others:* Other staff (other than medical and nursing) especially the paramedical workers are responsible for proper recording of the data relating to the treatment.
- *Classification of diseases:* All medical records of patients treated in the outpatient and inpatient departments have to be coded for disease classification by the MRD according to the latest international classification of diseases (WHO) or as recommended by the hospital administration.
- *Classification of operations:* All medical records of patients treated for surgical procedures in the outpatient and inpatient departments have to be coded for operation classification by the MRD according to the latest international classification of operations (WHO) or as recommended by the hospital administration.
- *Disease and operation index:* All medical records coded for diseases and operations have to be indexed manually in the disease index card and operation index card or electronically in the computer by the MRD. The information required from the index cards has to be compiled.
- *Patient master index:* All the patients treated in the outpatient especially in specialty clinics and inpatient department must have a patient master index with complete identification information. The MRD is responsible for collecting the information at the time of registration (first visit) and files them in a strict alphabetical order in the absence of computer registration.
- *Maintenance of medical records*: It is the responsibility of medical records department which is under the control of a qualified medical record officer. The MRD initiates records of emergency, outpatient and inpatient and processes them for completion and collects health

information to assist in patient care, quality assurance, medical education, research and administrative activities. Protection from unauthorized persons and safe preservation of medical records and information is one of major responsibilities of medical record department.

Control of Movement of Records

All the patient medical files of emergency, outpatient, and inpatient departments will have to be kept in the medical records department under the custody of the medical record staff. Generally medical records should not be taken out of the medical records department except in case of: (i) Patient care, i.e. OP, IP and A and E (ii) Court summons (iii) Clinical meetings (iv) Administrative (for settling the bills or complaints).

The following procedures are recommended for movement of records:

Emergency Records

Accident and emergency form which was initiated and sent to the casualty medical officer for treatment has to be collected immediately after care of the patient and kept in the allocated section by the MRD. Patient files are not to be retained by anyone without the knowledge of the MRD. For admitted cases, the inpatient procedure will be applicable.

Outpatient Records

The outpatient records are those which are sent to outpatient clinics for treatment of patients. Once the patient is seen in the clinic, the patient file should be returned to the OP clinic nurse/clerk (AMRT). Outpatient records are not to be retained by anyone including doctors. If patients require admission, the file will be sent to admission office. For admitted cases the inpatient procedure will be applicable.

Inpatient Records

From the time of admission into the ward till the patient is discharged, the patient file is under the custody of the ward nurse. The file should not be taken out of the ward without her permission. The maximum period permitted for discharged patient files to be retained in the ward is 48 hours.

Ward Census

Medical record technician (MRT) from the statistical unit of MRD will be responsible to collect the daily ward census and the discharged patient files (whether complete or incomplete) from the ward daily. Any file of a discharged patient if required to be retained in the ward due to any special reason, the nurse incharge will have to acknowledge. However, the same should be returned within 48 hours.

Patient Medical Files Sent to Other Hospitals

As a routine, a patient file of one hospital is not sent to another hospital. However, a detailed discharge summary may be supplied to the treating doctor. In exceptional cases, a photocopy of the entire file is supplied and the original file will be retained in the hospital.

Patient Medical Files from Other Hospitals

If any patient file of other hospital is received for treatment of the patient, all relevant information should be noted in the current record of the treating hospital. Once the purpose is over, the file including reports (X-ray, laboratory, etc.) should be returned to the concerned hospital. In any case, the file should not be retained after discharge/death of the patient.

Registration of Births and Deaths

The hospital should maintain three separate registers for births, deaths and fetal deaths. Necessary entries for live births, stillbirths, fetal deaths and deaths, as they occur must be made in respective registers as per the rules laid down by the Government.

Newborn (Live Birth)

Newborn should be registered as a new patient baby girl of (BG/O) or baby boy (BB/O) followed by mother name and a new hospital number to be allocated with a separate patient file created. However, a cross reference of mother's hospital number in the child's file and child's number in the mother's file should be entered. Similarly, cross reference entries have to be made in mother's and child's patient master index cards.

Multiple Births (Twins/Triplets, etc.)

Each live-born child must be registered as a new patient (BG1/O or BB2/O followed by mother name) and a new file to be created. The first-born child will get the first hospital number.

Stillborn (Dead Born)

Stillborn cases, the birth notification issued by the doctor should form a record. However, no patient file should be opened and no hospital number to be allocated.

Fetal Death

Death prior to the expulsion or extraction from its mother of a product of conception, irrespective of the duration of the pregnancy; the death is indicated by the fact that after such separation, the fetus does not breath or show any other evidence of life such as beating of heart, pulsation of umbilical cord, or definite movement of voluntary muscles. There should be a separate fetal death register to record all fetal deaths.

Submission of Birth Notification (Born Alive and Dead)

Birth notification for born alive and dead in prescribed forms (recommended by Government) duly signed by the medical officer who had conducted the delivery should be prepared in triplicate and submitted to:

- The parents/relatives.
- The hospital patient medical record.
- The birth registrar (concerned authority for registration).

Submission of Death Notification

Death notification in triplicate in prescribed form has to be prepared and signed by the treating doctor and counter signed by the unit head and submitted to:

- The nearest relative of diseased.
- The hospital patient medical record.
- The death registrar (concerned authority).

The hospital should maintain one central death register in MRD in which all hospital deaths, including OP, IP, and A and E and brought dead to be registered with accurate and complete information.

Registration of Cancer Patients

A central cancer register must be maintained in each hospital. All proved malignant cases as recommended by ICD (WHO) should be registered and a separate cancer register number to be allocated in the patient file in addition to the hospital number. All the cancer cases registered will have to be classified in accordance with the recommendation made by the national cancer center. Refer the guidelines provided by the national cancer center for more details.

Reporting of Infectious Diseases

It is the responsibility of each department to notify the admission and treatment of infectious disease cases in the prescribed form recommended by the hospital to the public health department. Refer the guidelines provided by the public health department for more details.

Issue of Medical Reports and Certificates

Any request for medical report or certificate has to be routed through the hospital administration/MRD. The treating doctor will prepare and issue medical report or certificate to the patient or his representative or any organization through the MRD/hospital administration. Original copy of the medical report/certificate will be given to the patient and the copy is kept in the patient file.

Collection of Hospital Statistics

All hospitals should collect and compile different types of statistics as recommended by the ministry of health. Some of the essential statistics to be collected are as follows:

Outpatient Statistics

- Statistics of new, follow-up and total cases; according to sex (male, female and children), nationality. Statistics according to service/unit, geographical distribution, age group—less than 1, 1-4, 5-14, 15-24, 25-34, 35-44, 45-54, 55-64, 65-74, 75 and above.
- Number of investigations carried out, e.g. pathology, microbiology, biochemistry, radiology, ECG, EEG, and other departments (specify).
- Outpatient disease and operation statistics have to be prepared.

Emergency Statistics

Total number of cases seen in the emergency service and classification according to sex (male, female and children), number of cases referred to OPD, PHC. Number of cases admitted in the hospital and number of medicolegal cases treated (accidental, suicidal, homicidal, traffic accidents, burn and poison cases).

Inpatient Statistics

- Daily census reports of admitted and discharged cases of general and private wards.
- Discharges according to service by nationality, sex (male, female and children), age group—less than 1, 1–4, 5–14, 15–24, 25–34, 35–44, 45–54, 55–64, 65–74, 75 and above, discharge results—alive, dead, death classification—less than 48 hours and more than 48 hours.
- *Bed utilization (general and private separately)*: Bed days, bed occupied and bed occupancy rate.
- Inpatient diagnosis and operation classification statistics have to be calculated.
- Number of consultations received and rendered.
- *Surgical procedures according to different services:* Number of elective operations, emergency operations, minor, intermediate and major operations performed.
- *Investigations:* Number of pathology, microbiology, biochemistry, radiology, ECG, EEG, and other tests conducted.
- *Deliveries conducted:* Number of normal and abnormal deliveries.
- *Births:* Number of live births, mature, premature and stillbirths.
- *Death statistics:* Should be presented in the following statements—S. no., name, hospital no., service, nationality, age, sex, duration-48 hours, +48 hours, cause of death, remarks.

Administrative Statistics

- Number of medical personnel; seniors and juniors according to specialty.
- Number of dentists; seniors and juniors.
- Number of nursing personnel—according to cadre and student nurses if any.
- Number of paramedical workers including laboratory, radiology, dietary, pharmacy, medical social service, medical records and others.
- *Other auxiliary services:* Engineering, civil, electrical, maintenance, laundry, and housekeeping.
- Administrative staff including director, deputy directors, office unit heads, clerical and lower grade staff.
- Expenditure relating to drugs, diet, equipment, furniture, forms and stationery. Buildings including water, electricity, personnel, linen (patient uniform, staff uniform), transportation, communication, maintenance, training personnel and research.

- Income from patients and other sources.
- Other information pertaining to administration.

Monthly Reports on Hospital Statistics

Statistics of major departments such as pathology, microbiology, biochemistry, radiology, ECG, dietary, anesthesiology, physiotherapy, obstetrics and gynecology (births and deaths) and operating theaters, have to be prepared with details and submit to the medical record department before the 5th of every month.

The medical record department should prepare monthly statistics of outpatient, inpatient, emergency and allied departments and publish a report before 10th of every month. Copy of monthly hospital statistical report should be sent to the following departments before 15th of every month.

- To the hospital administrator.
- To the heads of departments and unit chiefs.
- To health information officer (MOH).

Preservation of Old Records (Retention Schedule)

Maintenance of Old Records

All medical records including patient files, registers, index cards, etc. relating directly to the patient care have to be maintained by the MRD. The medical record department should collect the old registers and files from all the wards, emergency department, outpatient clinics, etc. and classify them properly by giving "old record register number". The old files, registers, index cards are to be preserved in a place earmarked for a prescribed period. Later, the records have to be destroyed as per the rules laid down for "record retention".

Retention of Records

Because of pressure on space for filing of medical records a retention schedule for keeping records has been prepared by the MOH for hospital guidance **(Table 18.1)**. However, those hospitals which are carrying out teaching/research programs can keep the records longer than the prescribed period provided they have adequate space and facilities.

Preservation of Records

Special care has to be taken to preserve the records. Records have to be protected from insect termites, prevent records from being exposed to

Table 18.1 Medical record retention schedule

Name of medical record	*Retention original form (in years)*	*Effective from the date*	*Permanent retention in microfilm/computer or in original form*
Patient record:			
Inpatient record	5	of last visit of the patient	Yes
Outpatient record	3	-do-	Yes
Outpatient GP record	2	-do-	No
Casualty record:			
Medicolegal cases	5	of last visit of the patient	Yes
Ordinary cases	1	-do-	No
X-rays:			
Outpatient X-rays	5	of last visit of the patient	No
Inpatient X-rays	5	-do-	No
Casualty X-rays	5	-do-	No
Registers:			
Birth register	2	of last entry in the register	Yes
Death register	2	-do-	Yes
Admission and discharge register	2	-do-	Yes
Hosp. master register (OP)	2	-do-	Yes
Medicolegal register	2	-do-	Yes
Operation register	2	-do-	No
Ward admission and discharge register	2	-do-	No
Narcotic register	2	-do-	No
Infection register	2	-do-	No
X-ray register	2	-do-	No

Contd...

Contd...

Laboratory and other investigation register	2	-do-	No
Index:			
Disease index	Permanently either in physical or computer form	Yes	
Operation index	-do-	Yes	
Patient master index	-do-	Yes	
Physician index	1	the physician left the hospital	No
Report:			
Daily ward census report	1	of the report	No
Daily statistical report	1	"	No
Monthly report	1	"	No
Yearly report	10	"	No
Duplicate laboratory/X-ray report	1	"	No

hot and dry climate. They should be filed in a dust free and protected from water, dampness and fire. Adequate fire extinguishers to be provided at all required places.

Imaging System

In case any hospital has decided to keep records on imaging system, the following are suggested. Maintain a control register in order to have good account over the cases (records) imaged.

Computer Application

Computer services have to be applied for effective maintenance of medical records to provide efficient services to patients and hospital staff. The medical record department in collaboration with the statistical unit and computer section should try to apply computer services in registration and follow-up appointments, patient master index, disease and operation classification, record control and statistical data analysis.

Financial Charges

Patient charges related to registration, admission, private beds, consultation, investigation, etc. are to be collected from nationals and expatriates as per the directions of the hospital administration.

Registration and Appointment System

The following instructions have to be meticulously observed.

Registration System

A central registration system with 24-hour service will be observed for all outpatients and inpatients. In this system, each patient will have one record and one permanent number for all episodes. A separate registration for accident and emergency patients with 24-hour service will be practiced. On each visit to casualty, a new record will be created and a new A/E number will be given.

Numbering System

Six digit numbers will be used for outpatients and inpatients starting from 00 00 01 and will continue till it reaches 99 99 99. A new patient will get a new hospital number only at the time of first registration. Casualty department will start the number at 80 00 01.

Patient Master Index

Patient master index can be maintained manually or electronically. It will be created with important identification information for each new patient registered in the central registration and filed alphabetically.

Appointment Card

An identification information card should be given to each new patient registered for outpatient and inpatient service.

Appointment System

Appointment system should be practiced in all referral hospitals. All patients must observe appointment system except in labor and emergency cases. As a general policy there should be a gap of minimum 3 days between the day of booking appointment and the day of appointment at the clinic. The appointment schedule must be prepared in conjunction with the concerned heads of units/specialties, MRO and administration, and to be followed strictly. All the referring hospitals and health centers should be informed of the policy and procedures of the appointment systems.

Investigation Reports

Investigation reports of outpatients will be received and mounted by MRD in respective records. While inpatient reports will be received and mounted in the ward by nurse.

Outpatient Clinics

Outpatient clinics names of all outpatient clinics with names of clinic chiefs in the hospital should be exhibited in the main entrance of outpatient department and in each clinic. The name of the chief consultant should also be exhibited.

Outpatient Clinic Schedule

Each unit in consultation with administration and medical records officer should decide the number of new and follow-up cases to be booked for the clinic.

Accident and Emergency Service

A separate accident and emergency record in triplicate will be used in A/E service. Out of three accident and emergency forms, the first copy will be retained in the casualty, second copy will be given to the patient and the third will be sent to the concerned health center. If patient is admitted to outpatient or inpatient service, the second and third copies will become part of main patient file. The first copy, however, will be retained in the casualty. If patient has a unit record in the hospital and the casualty medical officer desires to have it, the MRD should supply and collect. All investigation reports of casualty patient will be attached with the casualty form. If patient referred to outpatient/inpatient services, the reports will become part of main patient file.

All the casualty records including X-rays have to be kept for one year in the A/E department. Later, they should be transferred to MRD/X-ray department. The casualty registration section will also undertake the responsibility of central registration and admission office during holidays and off hours.

Admission Office

Admission office functions round the clock and is responsible for admission of patients, maintains bed occupancy board.

Direct Admission

A patient getting into ward and occupying a bed without going through the admission office. This is permitted in emergency and obstetrics cases. The nurse in-charge of the ward is responsible for registering the case in the admission office within two hours of patient admission into the ward.

Declaration by the Patient

Any patient who wishes to make a declaration before his death, such statements have to be recorded in the patient's file in the presence of a magistrate. However, in the absence of magistrate, the declaration can be recorded in the presence of three persons including the treating physician, a nurse and the hospital administrator or his representative.

Completion of Records

Doctors have to complete records before discharge of patient wherever possible. Otherwise, they have to visit MRD weekly and review all the discharged records for completion. In any case, patient files should not be kept incomplete for more than a week.

Supply of Records

The MRD is responsible for supply of medical records for medical education and research purposes to authorized persons.

Registers to be Maintained

The following registers have to be maintained in the hospital.

Outpatient Register

Outpatient register should contain: Hosp. no./Patient's name/Sex/Age (DOB)/ID no/Nationality/Marital status/Occupation/Place of birth/

Address and telephone no/Relative's name and telephone no/Clinic name.

Accident and Emergency Register

Accident and emergency register should contain: S. no./Date/A and E no./ Name of the patient/Age/Sex/Nationality/Marital status/Occupation/ ID number/Address/Time of arrival/Mode of arrival/Brought by/Illness or accident/Place of accident/Time of accident/Degree of urgency/ Diagnosis/Treatment/MLC (Yes/No)/Time of departure/Follow-up/ Remarks.

Medicolegal Register

Medicolegal cases (MLCs) should contain MLC no./A and E no./Hospital no./Patient name/Age/Sex/Nationality/Marital status/Occupation/ Address/Date and time of arrival/Means of arrival/Nature, place and time of accident/Complaint/Diagnosis/Disposition/Date and time of discharge/Name of CMO/Remarks.

Admission Register

S. no./Date of admission/Date of discharge/Nature of discharge/(Discharge/Transfer/Lama/Died)/IP no./OP no./Name of the patient/ Age/Sex/Address/Time/Provisional diagnosis/Final diagnosis/Ward/ Nationality/Remarks.

Waiting List Register

Waiting list register should contain identification data plus service/unit/ name of admitting doctor/date and time of registration in the waiting list/date and time of the patient to be admitted/remarks.

Ward Admission and Discharge Register

Ward admission and discharge register should be a single register; admissions on left and discharges on right side of the register.

Admission register: S. no./Hospital no./Patient's name/Sex/Age/ Nationality/Room no./Bed no./Date and time of admission/Service/ Unit/Provisional diagnosis.

Discharge register: S. no./Hospital no./Patient's name/Sex/Age/ Nationality/Room/Bed no./Date and time of discharge/Service/Unit/ Final diagnosis/Result/Remarks.

Operation Register

Operation register should contain: S. no./Hospital no./Name of the patient/Age/Sex/Nationality/Marital status/Occupation/Date of admission/Date and time of operation/Diagnosis/Operation/Anesthesia type/Anesthetist/Surgeon/Assistant surgeon/Name of the OT nurse/Results/Remarks.

Anesthesia Register

S. no./Date/Hospital no./Name/Age/Sex/Diagnosis/Operation/Premeditation/Anesthetic technique and drug used/Duration/Anesthetist/Remarks.

Birth Register

Birth register should contain: S. no./Name of the newborn/Sex/Fathers particulars(Name/Religion/Nationality/Occupation/Address)/Mothers particulars (Name/Religion/Nationality/Occupation)/Date of birth/Particulars of place of birth/Destination of delivery attendant/Signature of registrar/Date of registration/Signature of notifier/Remarks.

Death Register

Death register should contain: S. no./Hospital no./Name of the diseased/Age/Sex/Nationality/Address and Telephone no./Ward/Date of admission/Time of death/Diagnosis (cause of death)/Signature of doctor certifying death/Relative's signature receiving the body.

Central Cancer Register

Central cancer register should contain: Full identification data plus CCR no./Disease/Date onset of the disease/Confirmed by histopathologically/Treated as OP/IP/DOA/DOD/Service/Unit/Information sent to NCR on date/remarks.

General Instructions

- Every sheet of patient medical file must have identification at-least complete patient's name and hospital number.
- The treating staff whether medical, nursing, paramedical or others have to sign and date wherever it is required. Generally, when information is written in the form, the note has to be attested and dated.

- All written entries into the patient file including investigation requests, reports must be clear and legible. Since patient files will be kept for longer period, it is advisable to use dark color ink. Pencils must not be used. Each entry must be dated and include the name and status of the contributor.
- Any section of the patient file should not be erased, if corrections are required, circle and write over and sign.
- Patient should not be admitted to the ward without completing the admission and discharge advice form by the treating physician or any authorized medical officer.
- Patient should not be discharged without the written discharge instructions by the treating physician.
- A provisional or admitting diagnosis must be written at the time of admission wherever possible.
- Diagnosis will be written in full without the use of abbreviations.
- Standard abbreviations are listed separately as such only those should be used.
- Prior to discharge of patient, the consultant physician or his authorized assistant should write the final diagnosis including primary and secondary. The condition of the patient on discharge, the result, and advice given should be written.
- The cause of death as recommended by WHO must be written in all death cases. If autopsy is conducted, a note "autopsy done" and report should be recorded.
- Prior to proceeding on leave, the physicians, should get no objection certificate from the medical records department.

Rights and Responsibilities of a Patient

Rights of a Patient

- To get considerate and respectful behavior from all staff in the hospital (from consultant to cleaner) and safe care by the hospital at all times.
- To obtain from his physician complete, current information concerning his diagnosis, treatment, and prognosis in terms that the patient can be reasonably expected to understand.
- To receive necessary information from his physician for giving consent prior to start of any procedure or treatment.
- To refuse treatment to the extent permitted by law and to be informed of the medical consequences of his action.
- To give every consideration of his privacy concerning his own medical care program.

- To expect that all communications and records pertaining to his/her care should be treated as confidential.
- To accept his willingness to be transferred to another hospital.
- To be advised if the hospital proposes to engage in or perform human experimentation affecting his care or treatment. The patient has the right to refuse to participate in such research projects.
- To expect reasonable continuity of care. He has the right to know in advance the names and professional status of the people treating him/her and which physician is responsible for his/her care, date and time of appointment.
- To know what hospital rules and regulations are applicable to his conduct as a patient. The patient has the right to complain to concerned authority if something goes wrong in his care.
- To be examined in privacy and to have a person of the same sex present when being examined or treated by someone of the opposite sex.
- To obtain assistance in communicating with the people treating him/her in Arabic or other language.

Responsibilities of a Patient

The patient is responsible for the following:

- To furnish correct and full identification information; full name, age (date of birth), occupation, father's/husband's name, nationality, complete address including telephone number.
- To give correct information regarding his/her previous visits to hospitals and furnish about present complaints, past illnesses, hospitalizations and medications.
- To retain appointment (hospital number) card safely, and produce the same whenever he/she visits the hospital or health clinic.
- To inform the hospital authorities on the loss of hospital number card so as to locate the correct hospital number.
- To visit the hospital on the day and time of appointment and to avoid going to hospital without prior appointment except in the case of an emergency. If the patient is given follow-up appointment for future visits, he/she should register his/her case and obtain a date and time for the next visit before leaving the hospital.
- To report only to the authorized staff in the hospital for his/her appointments.
- To observe the rules and regulations and strictly follow instructions of the hospital and they should not take away the hospital records except the patient appointment card and other documents given to patient.

- Making willful correction in the records, giving wrong information or producing wrong documents, or bringing documents of other patients for treatment will lead to legal prosecution and punishment.
- To be considerate and respectful of the rights of other patients and of the hospital staff by assisting in the control of noise, by limiting the number of visitors, and by avoiding cigarette smoking whenever necessary.

PERSONNEL REQUIREMENT AND JOB DESCRIPTION

This section deals with the following:

- Personnel requirement according the bed strength of the hospital.
- Job description for four important categories of medical records department personnel, e.g. medical record officer, medical record technician.

Personnel Requirement

Distribution of medical record personnel.
According to bed strength of the hospital:

Name of the post	*Number of beds*						
	< 50	50	100	200	300	400	600
Medical records officer			1	1	1	1	1
Assistant medical records officer					1	1	1
Medical records technician	5	7	15	17	20	25	30

Job Descriptions

Medical Records Officer

Duties and responsibilities

- To establish, organize and manage medical record department with appropriate system as recommended by the hospital administration that can provide effective service in the hospital and effective supervision of the staff for efficient functioning of the department.
- To develop policies and procedures relating to medical record department in accordance with international system and protect medical records in accordance with national retention, preservation and destruction policies.
- To coordinate with medical record committee, design and develop different medical record forms required for hospital use.

- To review the medical records of outpatients, inpatients, and emergency patients to ensure that they include all the important documents and pertinent information to meet clinical, administrative and legal requirement.
- To cooperate with the medical, nursing and other staff in patient care and completing the patient medical records.
- To participate and assist in quality assurance, utilization review, infection control and other committees and programs, and to assist in developing hospital disaster plan to meet the exigency.
- To plan, organize, develop and supervise computer applications in medical records and patient care functions.
- To prepare daily, monthly and yearly statistical reports containing the hospital activities carried out and submits to the concerned authorities with suggestions to improve patient care services. If a statistician is posted he has to work under MRO, otherwise entire statistical work will be carried out by the statistician.
- To prepare and carry out educational and training programs such as in-service, certificate, diploma and continuing education for medical record personnel in cooperation with the appropriate health institutions/university. And also participate in seminars, workshops and conferences related to medical records.
- To participate and assist in research programs for improving the administrative activities and financial control and prepare departmental budget and annual report of MRD activities. And protect confidentiality of information form authorized and keep medicolegal cases under safe custody.
- To perform other duties and responsibilities related to medical record services as may be assigned by the hospital director.

Assistant Medical Records Officer

Duties and Responsibilities

- To perform technical analysis and evaluation of medical records in accordance with the hospital policies and procedures.
- To collect medical information, administrative and other statistics required by the hospital and provide health information for quality assurance, utilization review and evaluation of hospital care.
- To provide medical record services including reception, registration, outpatient appointment, inpatient, admission and emergency department by maintaining effective medical record filing and retrieving system.

- To evaluate for deficiencies in the outpatient and inpatient medical records and arrange for completion with the cooperation of medical, nursing and other staff.
- To code and index diseases, surgical operations, therapeutic procedures according to international classification of diseases/ operations or in accordance with the criteria lay down by the hospital administration
- To assist medical and other committees in the hospital and perform transcription of medical and other reports in the medical records departments or clinical units.
- To feed patient care information into computer for processing and storage and retrieval when required.
- To protect the medical records including medicolegal cases from unauthorized persons and to maintain confidentiality.
- To supervise one or more medical record units and assist in departmental educational and administrative activities.
- To perform other duties and responsibilities related to medical record services as may be assigned by the hospital director/ incharge.

Medical Records Technician

Duties and Responsibilities

- To register and collect appropriate identification information from outpatient, (new, old and follow-up) patients and arrange appointments, admission procedures.
- To prepare patient master index cards (PMI), arrange according to alphabetical order, file them in index cabinets and retrieve when required. If computerized PMI, feed and retrieve information electronically from computer.
- To collect investigation reports from the laboratory, X-ray and other diagnostic investigation departments, arrange and mount them in appropriate records.
- To receive patient records/X-rays, arrange in systematic order, file and retrieve records/X-rays whenever required. And also to assist in moving active and inactive records/X-rays from one area to another.
- To work in all the units of MRD, e.g. accident and emergency or outpatient clinic or admission office or ward or X-ray or any other units and perform the work of that unit as per the recommended procedures.
- To assemble and process records as per the laid down procedures.
- To use computer, microfilm and other mechanical devices for maintaining medical records.

- To collect and prepare statistics of outpatient, emergency and inpatients. Also collect daily ward census along with discharged patient records, X-rays and late reports.
- To work in the MRD of hospital and perform duties in any of the 3 shifts as required.
- To maintain confidentiality of information from unauthorized persons and participate in educational programs.
- To index previously coded disease and operation data in disease and operation index cards manually or electronically in computers.

19 Public Relations

Public relations (PR) is the practice of managing the communication between an organization and its publics and especially health related topics. An organization represented by PR exposure to their audiences using topics of public interest and news items. Common activities include speaking at conferences, working with the press, and employee communication. PR can be used to build rapport with employees, customers, investors, or the general public. Almost any organization that has a stake in how it is portrayed in the public arena employs some level of public relations. There are number of related sister disciplines all falling under the banner of Corporate Communications, such as analyst relations, media relations, investor relations, internal communications or labor relations.

There are many areas of public relations but the most recognized are financial public relations, product public relations, and crisis public relations. In this, we touch hospital services.

- Financial public relations deal with providing information mainly to business reporters.
- Product public relations deal with gaining publicity for a particular product or service through PR tactics rather than using advertising.
- Crisis public relations deal with responding to negative accusations or information.
- Hospital public relations deal with the services that are operational and type of specialties and expertise open for public.

METHODS, TOOLS AND TACTICS

Public relations and publicity are not synonymous but many PR campaigns include provisions for publicity. Publicity is the spreading of information to gain public awareness for a product, person, hospital and health institution services, cause or organization, and can be seen as a result of effective PR planning.

Publics Targeting

A fundamental technique used in public relations is to identify the target audience, and to tailor every message to appeal to that audience. It can be a general, nationwide or worldwide audience, but it is more often a segment of a population. Marketers often refer to economy-driven "demographics", in public relations and audience is more fluid, being whoever someone wants to reach.

In addition to audiences, there are usually stakeholders, literally people who have a "stake" in a given issue. All audiences are stakeholders, but not all stakeholders are audiences. For example, a charity commissions a PR agency to create an advertising campaign to raise money to find a cure for a disease. The charity and the people with the disease are stakeholders, but the audience is anyone who is likely to donate money.

Sometimes the interests of differing audiences and stakeholders common to a PR effort necessitate the creation of several distinct but still complementary messages. This is not always easy to do, and sometimes—especially in politics—a spokesperson or client says something to one audience that angers another audience or group of stakeholders.

Lobby Groups

Lobby groups are established to influence government policy, corporate policy, or public opinion. An example of this is the American Israel Public Affairs Committee (AIPAC), which influences American foreign policy. Such groups claim to represent a particular interest and in fact are dedicated to doing so. When a lobby group hides its true purpose and support base it is known as a front group. Moreover, governments may also lobby public relations firms in order to sway public opinion. A well illustrated example of this is the way civil war in Yugoslavia was portrayed. Governments of newly succeeded republics of Croatia and Bosnia invested heavily with American PR firms, so that the PR firms would give them a positive war image in the US.

Spin

In public relations, "spin" is sometimes a pejorative term signifying a heavily biased portrayal in one's own favor of an event or situation. While traditional public relations may also rely on creative presentation of the facts, "spin" often, though not always, implies disingenuous, deceptive and/or highly manipulative tactics. Politicians are often accused of spin by commentators and political opponents, when they produce a counter argument or position.

The techniques of spin include selectively presenting facts and quotes that support one's position, the so-called "non-denial," phrasing in a way that assumes unproven truths, euphemisms for drawing attention away from items considered distasteful, and ambiguity in public statements. Another spin technique involves careful choice of timing in the release of certain news so it can take advantage of prominent events in the news. A famous reference to this practice occurred when British Government press officer Jo Moore used the phrase. It's now a very good day to get out anything we want to bury, widely paraphrased or misquoted as "It's a good day to bury bad news", in an email sent on September 11, 2001. The furor caused when this email was reported in the press eventually caused her to resign.

Spin Doctors

Skilled practitioners of spin are sometimes called "spin doctors," despite the negative connotation associated with the term. It is the PR equivalent of calling a writer a "hack". Perhaps the most well-known person in the UK often described as a "spin doctor" is Alastair Campbell, who was involved with Tony Blair's public relations between 1994 and 2003, and also played a controversial role as press relations officer to the British and Irish Lions rugby union side during their 2005 tour of New Zealand.

State-run media in many countries also engage in spin by selectively allowing news stories that are favorable to the government while censoring anything that could be considered critical. They may also use propaganda to indoctrinate or actively influence citizens' opinions. Privately run media also uses the same techniques of 'issue' versus 'non-issue' to spin its particular political viewpoints.

Meet and Greet

Many businesses and organizations will use a Meet and Greet as a method of introducing two or more parties to each other in a comfortable setting. These will generally involve some sort of incentive, usually food catered from restaurants, to encourage employees or members to participate.

There are opposing schools of thought as to how the specific mechanics of a Meet and Greet operate. The Gardiner school of thought states that unless specified as an informal event, all parties should arrive promptly at the time at which the event is scheduled to start. The Kolanowski school of thought, however, states that parties may arrive at any time after the event begins, in order to provide a more relaxed interaction environment.

OTHERS

- Publicity events, pseudoevents, photo opportunity or publicity stunts.
- The talk show circuit. A PR spokesperson (or his/her client) "does the circuit" by being interviewed on television and radiotalk shows with audiences that the client wishes to reach.
- Books and other writings.
- Blogs.
- After a PR practitioner has been working in the field for a while, he or she accumulates a list of contacts in the media and elsewhere in the public affairs sphere. This "Rolodex" becomes a prized asset, and job announcements sometimes even ask for candidates with an existing Rolodex, especially those in the media relations area of PR.
- Direct communication carrying messages directly to constituents, rather than through the mass media with, e.g. newsletters"—in print and e-letters.
- Collateral literature, traditionally in print and now predominantly as web sites.
- Speeches to constituent groups and professional organizations; receptions; seminars, and other events; personal appearances.
- The slang term for a PR practitioner or publicist is a "flack" (sometimes spelled "flak").
- A desk visit is where the PR person literally takes their product to the desk of the journalist in order to show them what they are promoting.
- Astroturfing is the act of PR agencies placing blog and online forum messages for their clients, in the guise of a normal "grassroots" user or comment.
- Online social media.

Defining the Opponent

A tactic used in political campaigns is known as "defining one's opponent." Opponents can be candidates, organizations and other groups of people.

In the 2004 US presidential campaign, Howard Dean defined John Kerry as a "flip-flopper," which was widely reported and repeated by the media, particularly the conservative media. Similarly, George HW Bush characterized Michael Dukakis as weak on crime (the Willie Horton ad) and hopelessly liberal ("a card-carrying member of the ACLU"—which is American Civil Liberty Union). In 1996, President Bill Clinton seized upon opponent Bob Dole's promise to take America back to a simpler time, promising in contrast to "build a bridge to the 21st century". This painted Dole as a person who was somehow opposed to progress.

In the debate over abortion, self-titled pro-choice groups, by virtue of their name, defined their opponents as "anti-choice", while self-titled pro-life groups refer to their opponents as "pro-abortion" or "anti-life".

Managing Language

If a politician or organization can use an apt phrase in relation to an issue, such as in interviews or news releases, the news media will often repeat it verbatim, without questioning the aptness of the phrase. This perpetuates both the message and whatever preconceptions might underlie it. Often, something innocuous sounding can stand in for something greater; "culture of life" sounds like general goodwill to most people, but will evoke opposition to abortion for many pro-life advocates. The phrase "States' rights" was used as a code for anti-civil rights legislation in the United States in the 1960s, and, allegedly, the 70s, and 80s.

Conveying the Message

The method of communication can be as important as a message. Direct mail, rob calling, advertising and public speaking are used depending upon the intended audience and the message that is conveyed. Press releases are also used, but since many newspapers are folding, they have become a less reliable way of communicating, and other methods have become more popular.

Arts organizations have begun to rely more on their own websites and have developed a variety of unique approaches to publicity and public relations, on and off the web.

The country of Israel has recently employed a series of Web 2.0 initiatives, including a blog, MySpace page, YouTube channel Facebook page and a political blog to reach different audiences. The Israeli Ministry of Foreign Affairs started the country's video blog as well as its political blog. The Foreign Ministry held the first microblogging press conference via Twitter about its war with Hamas, with Consul David Saranga answering live questions from a worldwide public in common text-messaging abbreviations. The questions and answers were later posted on IsraelPolitik, the country's official political blog.

Front Groups

One of the most controversial practices in public relations is the use of front groups—organizations that purport to serve a public cause while actually serving the interests of a client whose sponsorship may be obscured or concealed. Critics of the public relations industry, such as PR watch, have contended that Public Relations involves a "multi-billion dollar propaganda-for-hire industry" that "concocts and spins the news, organizes phoney 'grassroots' front groups, spies on citizens, and conspires with lobbyists and politicians to thwart democracy".

Instances of the use of front groups as a PR technique have been documented in many industries. Coal mining corporations have created environmental groups that contend that increased CO_2 emissions and global warming will contribute to plant growth and will be beneficial, trade groups for bars have created and funded citizens' groups to attack anti-alcohol groups, tobacco companies have created and funded citizens' groups to advocate for tort reform and to attack personal injury lawyers, while trial lawyers have created "consumer advocacy" front groups to oppose tort reform.

HOSPITAL OR HEALTH INSTITUTION PUBLIC RELATIONS

The PR in this context deals with the object of publicizing the information of institution to the general public in general and public surrounded and potential users in particulars with genuine information that would serve and facilitate the public. The PR main concern, not limited to this alone, is to bring the accurate and complete activities of the institution such as the functioning of Emergency, Outpatient and Inpatient services and different specialties prevailing in the vicinity for public purpose. And at the same time, the problems or any issues that public is encountering in obtaining the services or any other issues that related to health institution needs to be addressed in favor of users. The PR is a liaison officer between the public and the hospital.

In addition to this, PR also assists the authorities in conducting "health exhibitions" exposing hospital services, demonstration of any particular treatment or surgical procedure to ensure that the services offered are safe and improved quality. Generally, the responsibilities are to involve with the daily activities of the hospital and ensure that everything is going well to the satisfaction of public and any issue of public that hampers or inconvenience is brought to the organization notice to address at the earliest. Precisely, the very object of PR is to ensure that the hospital's operations are smoothly functioning to the utmost satisfaction of public. Another most important function is not only to publicize the new services or any service that is not operational in the hospital or health institution to the public but also to collect the views of patients, public what they expect from the health institution in term of services and facilities or any genuine demand related to health field and services to be brought to the notice of the hospital organization. The PR is "window and spokesperson" of health institution and the hospital users and the public.

20 Medical Secretarial Profession

The word secretary comes from the Latin *secretarius,* meaning "confidential employee". The secretary of today is still an employee who is responsible to maintain confidential information. In that respect, the job has not changed. However, the tools of the trade have changed over the years.

The secretary is a professional—not only because of the knowledge and preparation necessary for the job, but also because being a professional implies competence, pride in one's work, and a dedication to excellence. The secretary is a professional with each of these qualities. Moreover, the secretary is an important member of the management team, responsible not only for carrying out the executive's wishes, but also for helping to maintain a well-organized and efficient office.

Office automation and machine dictation have revolutionized the type of work that the secretary does, and changes are expected to continue. The changes that will take place in the future are impossible to predict, but the professional secretary—also sometimes known as the medical secretary, administrative assistant, administrative secretary, private secretary, or several other titles—will be able to learn and adapt to each new challenging environment.

SUCCEEDING IN THE PROFESSION

The relative ease with which a person can enter the secretarial profession is a plus. A high school education; typing, shorthand machine transcription, and filing skills; and knowledge of office procedures, word processing and computer equipment, and software packages will enable one to advance along a career path. A postsecondary education is an additional asset.

The secretary entering the workforce is faced with a multitude of possible job situations. Although, the conditions under which a secretary works are fairly standard throughout the economy, a choice can certainly be made about the location, the size of the company, and the company's services or products. Each and every area of the economy or business needs the expertise of a secretary, and the professional secretary has only to choose the field most interesting to him or her and the one in which career goals can be furthered, but today's secretary is also concerned with the possibilities for professional growth within a company.

Secretaries are professionals with career goals. Most large organizations have a human resources department that is concerned with the professional growth and development of their employees. By providing training and educational opportunities for employees from the date of hire until retirement, these organizations are able to enhance the effectiveness of their operations and to enrich the lives of their employees.

Specialized training is a matter of professional survival in a world where the methods of handling information are changing rapidly. The secretary will be increasingly involved with office automation and needs to be familiar with the concept and the technology. The responsibilities of the Secretary are multifunctional: typing/keyboarding; transcribing; processing mail; telephoning; scheduling appointments; greeting visitors; composing and editing documents; researching; coordinating meetings, conferences, and teleconferences; making travel arrangements; handling reprographics; and organizing time and work. Supervisor and management education and advanced technical and professional education are available to those who are interested in moving ahead in the organization. One of the great benefits of a well-developed education and training program is that people on the secretarial level can move into supervisory, administrative, and managerial positions if they have the desire and the ability to do so.

Secretaries are encouraged to develop career paths and life plans just as executives do. The secretary's projected work life is just as long as the executive's. These years will be more pleasant if the individual takes steps to examine what kind of job will be the most personally satisfying now and in the future. This kind of examination also benefits the organization, because it keeps personnel from changing companies when a change in work responsibility would be more satisfying.

Many organizations also encourage secretaries to avail themselves of outside educational opportunities through financial support. Frequently these outside courses must be job related or related to a degree which the company agrees would benefit the employee and employer. Sometimes, however, these courses are promoted for the personal enrichment of the employee. All of these personnel-development efforts increase the secretary's satisfaction with the job and the employer.

PROFESSIONAL DEVELOPMENT

Participation in professional organizations is one way a secretary can grow professionally. Organizations offer the opportunity to network with other professionals and promote personal development by providing information, contacts, and support. Several professional organizations sponsor annual conventions, local conferences, seminars and courses to enhance secretarial performance.

The following organizations provide many opportunities for service, educational, and professional growth: Professional Secretaries International (PSI), the Association of Information Systems Professionals (AISP), and the American Association for Medical Assistants (AAMA), the American Association for Medical Transcription (AAMT), and the National Association of Legal Secretaries (International). Several of these organizations sponsor certification programs.

Professional Secretaries International (PSI) promotes an awareness of professional pride and the maintenance of high standards by promulgating the following definition:

Definition of a Secretary

Dr Mogli defines a secretary "as a person qualified to hold secretarial responsibilities, with positive mindset and behavior that enable to perform effectively as an executive assistant whose first characteristics is to maintain strict confidentiality of information maintained by her/him, who possesses a mastery of office skills, demonstrates the ability to assume responsibility without direct supervision, exercises initiative and judgment, and makes decisions within the scope of assigned authority and is a spokesperson of the office or clinic or organization whose message is truly valid and represents the organization. In real sense is the cog of the wheel, his actions can be admirable or harmful."

The importance of an organization like Professional Secretaries International (PSI) cannot be overemphasized. All professional people take pride in their affiliation with organizations that attest to the importance of their field. Lawyers have bar associations; doctors have the Medical Association: teachers have national educational organizations. In each of these groups the purpose is to set standards for the profession and to honor those who meet the standards. Professional Secretaries International awards the title of Certified Professional Secretary (CPS) to those who have passed a certificate examination. The title of Certified Professional Secretary brings respect from peers and superiors.

The examination that the aspiring secretary must take calls upon knowledge that has been gained through education and work experience. Office administration and communication, office technology accounting, economics and management, business law and behavioral science in business are the areas covered by the test. For one who has not yet become a Certified Professional Secretary, membership in PSI and participation in the local chapter's activities will bring a sense of the importance of a secretary's job to the functioning of society and will introduce the secretary to others who have similar professional goals.

TOOLS OF THE PROFESSION

Keyboarding, shorthand, transcription, filing, office procedures, and knowledge of word processing systems and equipment are the skills for which the secretary was hired. However, the ability to use the language and a commitment to professionalism will earn respect and promotions.

Language

The raw material to which the secretary applies these skills is the English Language. A command of and respect for the English Language, both in writing and in speaking are essential. A good dictionary, a thesaurus, and a grammar book must be kept handy for immediate checking of spelling, end-of-line division, usage and sentence construction. In the automated office, equipment may have a built-in spell checker or a software program with a dictionary or grammar component. Work still has to be proofread, however, because the equipment and programs cannot distinguish between homonyms, nor can they determine if the transcript omitted a word. Letters, whether the secretary composes them or transcribes them, represent the company, the employer, and the professional secretary.

The recipient of a letter must never get the impression that any one of the three is less than first rate. Most executives have a good speaking command of the language. This asset is often one of the reasons why an individual reaches a top management position. However, it is the secretary's responsibility to check details of grammar, spelling and punctuation. An employer with an excellent command of English presents a double challenge to the secretary. Transcribed letters must be absolutely perfect, and letters composed for the executive must match them in composition, tone and clarity.

The secretary may occasionally be the final check on grammar. An executive may have been hired for an area of technical expertise, not language ability. In this case the secretary will be responsible for editing all of the written communications from the office. The executive and the secretary in this situation must realize their mutual dependence and work to turn out superior written material. Correcting a dangling participle or making the verb and subject agree will demonstrate to the executive that the secretary is a professional with extremely valuable skills.

Professional Reading

Trade journals are published for each area of the economy and for each profession. By reading these publications, the secretary demonstrates professional concern and also learns new ideas and new vocabulary that may soon find its way into transcription. The competent secretary does not have to read these magazines from cover to cover but will develop a system for skimming, using the table of contents as a guide, to stay abreast of developments.

Numerous magazines and professional journals pertaining to the secretarial profession and business management and organization are available. These periodicals will help the secretary cope with difficult situations by discussions of how others solved similar problems and will alert the secretary to new products, procedures, and equipment for the office.

Reading magazines such as The Secretary, Fortune, Business Week, Forbes, Today's Office, and Office Administration and Automation is part of the commitment to professional excellence.

Information Processing

The combination of word processing and microcomputer systems has revolutionized the way secretaries work and process information. More and more offices have acquired the most sophisticated technological equipment, and the secretary needs only the ability and the desire to grow and change with each new development or modification.

Such systems provide an automated information center that upgrades the quality of hard copy materials while improving office efficiency by increasing the speed with which the material is produced. Today's businesses must deal with more written information than ever before, and they must transmit that information quickly and accurately. The secretary who puts the material into the system is irreplaceable, but the system can perform at speeds that a typist would find impossible. Material for bulk mailing and form letters can be keyboarded in a much shorter time by the equipment. If an executive decide to insert three paragraphs on page 60, of a 200 page document no longer means that the entire document must be re-keyboarded. The material to be inserted is keyboarded into the machine, and the finished document is produced, often in seconds. Complete documents of hundreds of pages can be sent from one office to another in minutes, rather than days. And, by using satellite communication, a subsidiary company's entire monthly report can be transmitted to the home office half a continent away in 30 seconds.

New vocabulary and procedures must be learned to use the information processing equipment. The competent secretary will not only learn how to respond to the instructions of the system but will also make every effort to understand how the system works and how best to make use of the various options offered. Entirely new systems of office management have resulted with the installation of word processing systems, word processors, microcomputers and numerous software programs.

The future is unlimited for the secretary who takes advantage of all training opportunities and remains open and flexible to the changes that will certainly develop in the industry.

A Professional Manner

The secretary is classified as a white-collar, however, the secretary should view clothing as a uniform that fits the image of the office and thus advances the secretary's career goals along with the purpose of the office. If the office is very informal, the secretary who wishes to be noticed and moved ahead will wear clothing that is just a shade more formal and more professional. The goal is not to alienate other workers but to make oneself stand out as the secretary who takes work seriously. When the executive office has an opening, the secretary who has demonstrated the most personal polish, in addition to superb skills, is the one who will be chosen.

A proper office manner should be cultivated by the secretary, and this manner should be based on the fact that the executive and the secretary are expected to work as a team. The secretary should follow the lead of the executive in office style. Whether working for an individual, a pair of executives, or a whole department, the secretary's duty is to help fulfill the executive job responsibilities. Therefore, assignments that appear in the job description (if there is one) are done conscientiously, and those chores that do not appear but that need to be done in order to free the executive from routine tasks will be done by the professional secretary without grumbling.

Much has been written about people moving ahead in careers because of the mentor/protégé system whereby a seasoned hand in the business takes on the education of someone younger who has promise. Although, the superior may be grooming someone for a place on the management level, the secretary can also be a protégé who moves upward in salary and responsibility with the boss or with the boss's blessing.

As part of the team, the professional secretary protects the employer. He or she does not contribute information to office gossip but does report any rumor that may be helpful to the superior, first qualifying the information as gossip. Also, the professional does not spend company time on personal phone calls, in clock watching, or in being late.

COMPETENT SECRETARY

The secretary plans not only a career path but also short- and long-range work for the company. Short-range planning enables the secretary to do each day those things that must be done. For example, a routine is established whereby the secretary's and the employer's desks are ready for work at the beginning of each day. Standard procedures for handling mail, for advising the executive of telephone calls, and for handling dictation and transcription are set-up, but this schedule does not lead to inflexibility. The competent secretary is capable of taking any kind of interruption in stride. When the emergency or interruption has been dealt with, the work routine is resumed at the point of interruption. Long-range planning makes it possible for the secretary to concentrate on low-priority projects at a slow time of the year and also makes it possible for the executive to call on secretarial aid at times when the work flow is heavy.

Effective Use of Time

The secretary's time is a valuable and perishable commodity. All duties are performed as quickly as possible so that the unexpected may be dealt with. A sense of the relative urgency of activities is developed with experience, so that it is possible to distinguish the important from the trivial. A long-distance caller does not distract the secretary from the necessity to transcribe an urgent letter. The unexpected visitor is started on his or her way courteously and firmly rather than being allowed to waste company time.

Business calls are evaluated for length, and they are not continued beyond the time that is absolutely essential for courtesy and the exchange of information. The secretary should structure the business call in the form of a business letter. It should be planned ahead and should have a beginning, middle, and end. If one is making a call, a clear statement of purpose should open, followed by details, questions or whatever the call must accomplish. The call should be completed by thanking the person on the other end, stating the action you or your boss expect to be taken, or getting a firm commitment for future action or the time of a return call. Remember that this is a business call and avoid those verbal ticks like "you know" and slang that would be appropriate in a personal call.

Responsibility and Follow-up

By carefully following through on any tasks assigned, the secretary demonstrates a sense of responsibility everyday. When the employer is out, the secretary displays professionalism by making sure that the office is covered at all times, especially when the workday begins in the morning. Every experienced secretary knows that this is when the problems start.

Take, for example, a situation in which the executive and the secretary are the only ones who know all aspects of a given situation. When the boss is away, something that vitally affects that matter happens. The competent secretary is present and immediately gets in touch with the employer so that the appropriate course of action can be decided and so that the secretary can set the wheels in motion.

Relationship with Executive

The personal relationship between the executive and the secretary will vary according to the people involved and the formality of the company. The secretary should always remember that the relationship is a business arrangement and that the structure of any organization makes the executive more important than the secretary. Without the executive to set the overall objective and to plan for action to attain that objective, the secretary's job would not exist. Nevertheless, the indispensable contribution of the secretary to the execution of the executive's work should be taken as a source of professional satisfaction but not as an indispensable individual.

The executive may ask the secretary to explain a matter, but the secretary does not have the right to call upon the executive to justify decisions. However, when a good working relationship exists, office authority is not a source of discontent because both the secretary and the executive realize that they are there to make that office run at peak efficiency.

No job is without its dull routines as well as its stimulating aspect. No employer is without faults. There may be times when you consider your employer unreasonable. You may be asked to do chores that you consider demeaning or outside your province or job description. Decide how intrusive these jobs are, and discuss the matter with your employer.

Perhaps, the duties can be added to your job description. Otherwise, see if you can arrange for the writing of a job description if there is none.

Appropriate Behavior

Personal life must be separated from professional life in dealing with all office personnel. It is very possible to work well with people one does not like at all; likewise, it is possible to work professionally with people who are personal friends. Personal problems should not be brought into the office. However, worries about sickness at home, financial problems and domestic difficulties do affect the quality of work, and the professional will do everything possible to keep the level of professional performance high. The fact that a doctor has personal troubles is not an acceptable excuse for a faulty diagnosis of a patient. One expects the doctor to perform well, and the executive has the right to expect the secretary to remain competent despite difficulties. People, however, are not machines and are not expected to behave as such. When overwhelming problems are present, the supervisor should be told before one's work is held up for censure.

Professional behavior as part of a team determines the relationships with the rest of the organization. In dealing with other members of the group, the secretary should make it clear that those others are viewed as the experts in their jobs. The professional secretary is courteous to everyone regardless of the individual's position on the company ladder. The order-processing clerk, the shipping clerk, the receptionist, the typist, and the file clerk will be much more helpful to the secretary/executive team if this attitude of professionalism is maintained.

Alertness to Mistakes

The secretary must be very honest in all relationships within the company. Blame must be accepted if a mistake has been made. Everyone makes mistakes, and the good secretary will do everything possible to avoid them. The need to make use of other people's expertise must be recognized, and the secretary should help others in the office in an effort to foster a spirit of helpfulness to insure that good work is turned out. For example, even if a secretary's typing can be called excellent, proofreading of important documents should be done by two people. The secretary should therefore try to make arrangements to proofread material with a coworker.

Alertness to the mistakes of others so that the mistakes may be corrected is characteristic of the competent secretary. Especially if work is done under pressure, people have a tendency not to check a figure, proofread a page, or make certain that a statement conforms to policy. The secretary must check and double-check to avoid errors that, more than simply being embarrassing, might affect important decisions adversely.

Level of Authority

Differentiating between the executive's requests and the secretary's requests is necessary. In the first instance, the secretary has a lot of authority; in the second instance, there is much less. If the executive needs the report by 5 PM, the department responsible will recognize that the effort and expense are inconsequential compared to the importance of meeting the deadline. However, the secretary must not push co-workers unless the pressure is justified. Everyone has a schedule to which he or she must adhere. Remember to respect the importance and the schedules of other people's work. Never claim authority for yourself when you are passing on the executive's wishes. "Professor Mark would like all class schedules completed by friday" will get a better response than "I would like all class schedules completed by friday". Even with suggestions the same rule is followed. A suggested course is far more likely to be implemented if put forward as the boss's idea, particularly if it involves difficulty.

Accurate Record-Keeping

The secretary's filing system gets the same careful attention given to other duties. The employer must have an accurate record of what has happened in the past in order to take future action. For highly confidential matters or the employer's personal correspondence, a system consistent with filing rules but responsive to the needs of the office should be setup. If the company has a central files department, the secretary works closely with the assigned file clerk, whose expertise should be recognized.

Filing is a historical recording of events that have occurred in a given aspect of company development. Filing requires intelligence, an intimate knowledge of the subject matter, and an organized method of recording. The secretary should work with the file clerk. All material should be carefully marked to indicate whether there has been any previous correspondence on the subject. If the previous reference could not be easily identified by the file clerk, a notation indicating the subject with which it should be filed is a courtesy that will save time, prevent confusion, and contribute to a helpful attitude in the office, which will be to everyone's benefit. If a subject is especially important or unusually complicated, an exchange of ideas may enable the file clerk to setup the file intelligently. A sense of history on the part of the secretary and the file clerk will enable them to build up a file coherently, so that a person reading it will be able to determine the sequence of events and the actions taken. When the secretary recognizes the complexity of the file clerk's job, the employer will get the file or information sought, not an excuse.

Today, many firms have computer equipment and documents are stored on disks and automatically filed in the system.

SECRETARIAL SPECIALTIES

A competent secretary may work in one particular type of office and become familiar with the equipment, vocabulary, procedures and duties specific to that type of office. In some cases, specific training is required. A few secretarial specialties are discussed here and a more detailed discussion of some of the more common ones is provided later in the book in the major section titled "For the Specialized Secretary".

Executive Secretary

The executive secretary or the administrative assistant is more than just a secretary or an assistant to an executive, in some companies and organizations, the terms seem to be interchangeable; in other companies, one is placed above the other on the organizational ladder. Whether one uses the term executive secretary or administrative assistant, in terms of responsibility, knowledge of the company's business, judgment and experience, this person is an executive. The executive secretary (the term we shall use in this discussion) may indeed employ a secretary or a whole staff. Making decisions that affect an important segment of the company's operations and, in some cases, taking charge of business while the executive is absent brings the executive secretary financial and personal rewards. But these benefits are earned. At this highest level of secretarial authority, the responsibilities are such that the greatest possible effort to check procedures and avoid errors is essential. Planning, discretion, knowledge, accuracy, efficiency, and dependability are watchwords of the job. The executive secretary has top skills and keeps them serviceable. Technical skills and knowledge of the latest automated equipment are essential.

Confidence of the executive's staff is built slowly and carefully. These are the people who have the responsibility to carry out the objectives of the company or department. The executive secretary's duty is to screen demands on the executives time, not to make the executive as unapproachable as Presidents of the United States have sometimes been made by their staffs.

Decisions must be made promptly; action must be taken swiftly. Anything that slows that action is detrimental to the overall operation of the company. When a member of the staff has to see the boss it may be because that person faces some decisions beyond the scope of his or her particular authority. It may seem a simple matter to give notice that the subordinate has to see the executive, but what if the secretary has six or seven calls from different staff members? Who sees the executive first, who next, and who not at all? It is up to the secretary to win the confidence of each member of the staff so that person will be absolutely honest as to the urgency of any particular request. Each has to know that if the employee says, "I must have it five minutes before noon", he or she will have it if it is humanly possible, and that if the employee says, "Tomorrow will be fine", he or she will see the executive tomorrow without any further reminders to the secretary. In such circumstances, maximum use is made of everyone's time. The secretary can work out an orderly plan with the executive to conserve time. The subordinate can attend to other projects without wasting time calling back or attempting to waylay the executive in the hail. In this cooperative atmosphere, everyone realizes that the short-term advantage would not be worth the risk of losing the secretary's confidence.

The secretary must always be aware of being a representative of the executive, and while the staff is subordinate to the executive, the staff is not subordinate to the secretary. As the subordinates' confidence grows, they will ask advice or opinions on how the boss would like something done. The secretary has a responsibility to give accurate advice and to state only opinions that truly represent the executive's feelings. If the secretary's personal opinion is given, the subordinate may be misled as to the executive's actual sentiments on the matter.

The executive secretary cannot play favorites. The executive must view operations as a whole and must be able to depend upon the secretary to reflect this accurately in dealing with subordinates. It is important that each staff member be recognized as an integral part of the team and as making a contribution to the company. Each employee wants the good opinion of the boss, and perhaps even without consciously recognizing it, the secretary's reaction to an employee may be interpreted as a reflection of the boss's opinion. The secretary must remember that a personality trait that is unattractive to the secretary may be exactly the trait that makes the subordinate effective in a particular function. The boss may have a higher opinion of the former than of the latter, and a secretary's favoring of the affable over the precise subordinate might be doing an injustice to both individuals and to the executive. By dampening the enthusiasm of one and giving a false sense of confidence to the other, the executive is misrepresented and the company's objectives may be impeded. The job of executive secretary or administrative assistant is challenging and rewarding and a lot of hard work. Intelligence, interest, dedication, plus experience and training are essential for success.

Legal Secretary

Accuracy and speed are the hallmark of the legal secretary in the one-lawyer office or the large firm with a national reputation. The work of a law office is exacting; an inaccurate record can be extremely expensive to the firm. Terminology is precise. Since many legal procedures have to follow an initial action in exact sequence, timing and organization are essential.

Typing/keyboarding, shorthand, transcription skills, and acknowledge of legal documents and legal terminology are important. Verbal and writing ability are essential because the legal secretary's work is very exacting. The work is also highly varied and involves extensive contact with clients. The legal secretary must, of course, refrain from answering legal questions.

Word-processing systems and microcomputers have been added to most law offices to aid in the preparation of legal documents. The secretary who wishes to remain in the field should take advantage of every opportunity to learn the newest automated equipment.

The legal secretary's job is not easy due to lot of work and pressure, there usually are long hours of work. However, it is one of the most lucrative jobs in the secretarial field. Some advantages in working as legal secretary gets more fringe benefits, and generous vacation. The legal secretary may become a certified professional legal secretary. The Certified Professional Legal Secretary designation is the only certification program for legal secretaries providing a standard measurement of legal secretarial knowledge and skills. Any person who has had five years' experience as a legal secretary and who meets the other application requirements may sit for a rigorous two-day examination. A partial waiver of the five year experience requirement may be granted if the applicant has a bachelor's associate's degree. Seven important areas of legal secretarial practice and procedures are included in the examination: written communication skills and knowledge; ethics; legal secretarial procedures; legal secretarial accounting; exercise of judgment; legal secretarial skills: and legal terminology, techniques, and procedures.

Medical Secretary

Medical secretaries are generally employed in a physician's office, medical clinic, hospital, public health facility, health maintenance organization, nursing home, research center, laboratory, insurance company. Government departments, health services, pharmaceutical company, private agency, publishing company, medical department of a business organization, business that manufactures medical supplies and equipment, or medical transcription service agencies. Earlier each job requires keyboarding skills, machine transcription and acknowledges of word processing but now expect more computers literacy and software programs in addition to familiarity with medical terminology.

The medical secretary may need to know how to perform certain medical tasks, how to complete insurance claim forms, how to take a patient's medical history, how to handle the doctor's billings, and how to perform other clerical duties peculiar to a doctor's office. In addition, the secretary may need to deal with people who are ill, a task requiring patience, sympathy and tact.

Regardless of the setting—a one-doctor office or a large facility—the medical secretary must observe medical ethics. Cases should not be discussed except in the context of office business, and no comments or questions regarding a patient's condition or ailments should be made in the presence of other persons.

The professional medical assistant enjoys an enviable professional status. The medical assistant is eligible to join the American Association of Medical Assistants (AAMA) and can apply for certification. The AAMA offers a certifying examination, the successful completion of which leads to a certificate and recognition as a Certified Medical Assistant-Administrative (CMA-A) or a Certified Medical Assistant-Clinical (CMA-C) or both. The examination is given in January and June of each year at designated centers throughout the United States. As of 1988, revalidation every five years is mandatory, and it can be accomplished through Continuing Education Units (CEUs) or re-examination.

The AAMA provides members the opportunity of attending local, state, and regional meetings and a national convention where one can participate in workshops, learn of educational advances in the field, visit exhibits, hear prominent speakers, and establish a networking system with other medical assistants. The association publishes a bimonthly journal "The Professional Medical Assistant".

The American Association for Medical Transcription (AAMT) member has the opportunity to attend local, state and regional meetings and a national convention where one can participate in workshops, learn of educational advances in the field, visit exhibits, hear prominent speakers, and establish a networking system with other medical transcriptionists. The association publishes a professional journal four times a year, the journal of the AAMT, and publishes a newsletter six times a year, the AAMT Newsletter.

The AAMT offers a certifying examination, with successful completion leading to a certificate and recognition as a Certified Medical Transcriptionists (CMT). The examination is given on the last Saturday in April and a specialty examination on the first Saturday in November at various locations throughout the United States. Certification by examination is valid for three years and may be renewed by paying the annual continuing education assessment fee and earning a minimum of 30 continuing education credits in each three-year period of certification, or achieving a passing score on the certification examination every three years. Of the 30 continuing education units, at least 20 must be in the medical science category. A CMT must continue upgrading skills through attending the Association's lectures and obtaining Continuing Education Units (CEUs).

Technical Secretary

The growth of research, both governmental and private, and the explosion of knowledge have created the need for secretaries with the ability to deal with technical terms and symbols. Typing, editing and proofreading are necessary skills for all secretaries, but technical secretaries must possess the highest level of skills. The ability to accurately type information that can be understood only by the researchers is essential, and the ability to proofread material that makes little or no sense to someone who is not technically trained in the field is indispensable.

The technical secretary must also recognize that the scientists and researchers have been hired for their technical competence, not their writing skill, and frequently the secretary will need to edit material to make it grammatically correct and smooth flowing. This task calls for much tact, patience, and humility in the face of material that is written in English but is often incomprehensible to the layperson. However, for the secretary with the ability to deal with mathematical equations, Greek letters, and so forth, advancement to the level of technical aide and research assistant is possible.

The technical secretary's job is demanding and exacting and requires specialized skills. A strong background in mathematics, science and technical terminology is a definite asset. The remuneration and benefits in these situations are usually quite good.

Educational Secretary

The opportunities for secretaries in educational institutions from the preschool to the graduate level are as varied as the institutions themselves. The secretary in the elementary school may occasionally have to comfort a sick child who is waiting to go home or help a parent deal with the multiple forms that educational systems require. In higher education the secretary may be assigned to a specific academic or administrative area. The educational secretary meets school visitors and has close contact with students, teachers and parents.

The duties of the secretary vary from school to school and often depend on its size. In a small school the secretary may have to handle student records, transcripts of grades, orders for materials and supplies, personnel records, the scheduling of facilities, and many other tasks. In larger institutions the secretary may be assigned just one of these duties or may be responsible for a specific department.

The minimum education requirement for an educational secretary varies. In some institutions a high school education is sufficient, whereas in others, especially colleges and universities, some type of college experience or a degree is required.

Secretary in Advertising, Radio and Television, Journalism, and the Arts

The skills required for these jobs are the same as for a job in any business, but the amount of contact with interesting personalities, public figures, and the public is increased. When dealing with public personalities, the secretary must be able to maintain a professional manner. If the employer does not wish to talk to a local public figure or a network newsperson, the secretary must be firm and diplomatic. Jobs in these fields require the ability to deal with people whose job it is to manipulate responses.

The professional secretary will decide just what kind of job will give the most satisfaction and the kind of atmosphere that will be pleasant. Will the high-pressure atmosphere of an advertising agency or television station make you nervous or will it challenge you? The fact that you are contributing to the success of a museum may be the kind of reward that means the most to you. The excitement of putting any kind of publication "to bed" may be just what you want.

Secretary in US Government

The federal government is the largest employer in the United States and should not be overlooked by the professional secretary. In order to become eligible for most governmental positions, the secretary must take a written civil service examination. Promotions are usually made from within based on availability and the demonstrated skill and industry of the applicant. Government positions offer annual salary increments, job security and retirement systems.

Usually, there are employment opportunities for secretaries in foreign countries. The Department of State has Foreign Service offices in over 300 cities worldwide. Other jobs are also available in the public sector. State, county, and municipal governments, plus the many quasi-governmental agencies, all have need of skilled secretaries.

The secretary who is interested in public service should contact the office of personnel management in the region in which he or she wishes to obtain employment.

Secretary in Travel

Excitement and adventure are the benefits of secretarial work in the travel industry. Airlines, resorts and travel agencies often offer free or reduced rates in transportation, hotel accommodations, and tours to their employees. However, the job requires hard work. One must have a sincere liking for and a desire to help people. You are helping them to spend the money for which they have often worked hard all year. Also, you must deal with concerned offices that may have to get an executive to Europe as quickly as possible.

A secretary in the travel industry must know geography well, he able to read different companies' timetables, plan itineraries, and make reservations through a computer. In short, you must know how to do everything and anything that will contribute to the comfort and enjoyment of your company's customers. Above all, you must be accurate. The pleasure of a vacation or a business opportunity can be lost by a single error. Each year the volume of business and pleasure travel exceeds the previous years. A person with the right combination or interest in people and ability to deal with details will find a bright future as a secretary in the travel field.

SPECIAL EMPLOYMENT SITUATIONS

Most secretaries are employed on a full-time basis in a particular office. However, there are available certain other types of employment situations, among them temporary work and part-time work.

Temporary Secretary

Temporary employment services throughout the country fulfill a need for both employers and employees. The secretary who works on a temporary basis fills in vacancies created by vacations, illness, sudden resignations, or other situations including short-term openings during peak workload periods.

Secretaries take on temporary employment for a number of reasons. Some use temporary employment as an opportunity to explore different industries, organizations, and working conditions so as to determine a preference and a career path. For others, family obligations or other responsibilities make a permanent position inconvenient and a temporary situation ideal. A temporary position also permits a flexible schedule and a choice of job locations, and these considerations may be important to someone pursuing further education or an avocation.

Agencies that engage temporary employees prefer secretaries who have had experience so that they will be able to go into an office and immediately assume the responsibilities of the job. Temporary secretaries must be flexible, confident, and adaptable.

The pay in temporary work is slightly lower in many cases than that of permanent workers who have the same job skills and responsibilities. Fringe benefits are becoming more available to temporary workers. Some agencies that place temporary secretaries in offices now offer group life and medical insurance, paid holidays, paid vacations, referral bonuses, seniority or longevity bonuses, profit sharing, scholarships and training on word processors, computers and related office equipment.

Part-time Secretary

Physician's offices, Medical Officers, educational institutions, small businesses, and, to a growing extent, large corporations often need part-time secretaries. The individual or firm may require only a few hours of work each day or only a few days per week. In other situations, a few weeks or a few months of the year may be required. Some companies are now willing to divide a full-time job between two part-time secretaries; two secretaries, in other words, share one full-time job. Part-time work enables the secretary to maintain skills while freeing the individual for other responsibilities or interests.

SECRETARY'S DAY

Job descriptions by their nature make the task of organizing the workday a bit easier, but if your job does not have a formal description of duties, organization is the word to keep in mind. Not only must the secretary's desk be organized but also the work that flows across the executive's desk must be ordered. Decisions about what is important must be made constantly, since most secretaries will have more work to do in one day than can be reasonably accomplished. The principle to be used to help one decide what is most important is the principle that keeps the executive and the secretary working together as a team.

The interests of the superior must come first, and the good secretary will be sure to perform tasks that the executive wants completed quickly and thoroughly. Deadlines between the secretary and the executive in the office may be missed because of extraordinary circumstances, but if your boss misses a deadline with higher company executives because your work was not completed on time, do not expect to have an excuse accepted.

The schedule for each day begins the afternoon before when the secretary goes through the tickler or follow-up folder to determine exactly what must be done the next day. The follow-up file should be setup in whatever way the secretary finds most convenient. If the office operates on a yearly schedule with certain meetings, promotions, and correspondence scheduled for the same time each year, the secretary may wish to have monthly tiles with notations about the amount of time it took to plan last year's tall sales meeting and the list of tasks to be performed in connection with that meeting. In an office that does not have this repetitive schedule. The secretary may use a desk calendar to keep track of letters to be answered, telephone calls that must be made, shipments expected and so forth. The secretary should make a list of the items that must be taken care of the next day and a list of appointments for the executive, along with pertinent information and the materials that should be prepared. To conclude the day, the equipment should be turned off and covered and the desk cleared so that the maintenance staff will be able to work.

The morning start with promptness, the office must be ready to function at whatever time it opens and the secretary should be at work in the office, not returning from the washroom or talking in the next office. Certain jobs must be performed each day, and the secretary taking over an office would be wise to make a list of these in the order in which they should be done until the routine becomes second nature.

Scanning the daily mail, and after opening the mail and putting the most important item on top, the trusted secretary may be required to call certain items to the executive's attention. This practice, however, should be begun only when permission has been given. The executive may ask that some of the journals and newspapers the office receives be skimmed and that pertinent articles, notices of new products, promotions, and so forth be marked for special notice.

Mail must be moved quickly from the secretary's desk to the appropriate correspondent; rerouting is done immediately. If some of the letters can be answered by the secretary, the executive may return them with notations about content. This letter-writing and typing task will then be completed as soon as possible.

Priority of duties the previous afternoon the secretary should have made a list of tasks for the following day by using the techniques of time management. Tasks fall into three categories: those that must be done immediately, those that may be done, and those that may be put off. Just as the executive has a list of appointments, the secretary should have a list of tasks and some notation after each entry to indicate its relative importance. All necessary items can be given an A or 1; the tasks that should be done when there is time, a B or 2; and the tasks that can be left until a slack period, a C or 3. The mental exercise of deciding which items are the most important is the first steps in getting the day's work finished. The trap of putting down jobs which are part of the daily routine or filling the list from the third category must be avoided. Putting down small jobs just for the satisfaction of crossing them out is a dangerous game to play. The executive like to hear what is important and what next to be done, ordered instructions are carried out promptly.

The duties of a secretary are as varied as are jobs and employers. But in any situation it is safe to assume that the secretary is responsible for handling the mail, making calls and answering the telephone, taking and transcribing dictation, following up orders and work in progress, and organizing office work. More often than not, the secretary must keep track of the employer's appointments and maintain a filing system—all in addition to the specifics of the job.

The experienced secretary knows that it is impossible to keep everything in mind. Everything must be written down on the memo pad that is at hand at all times. Every request, every assignment, every message is noted. Nothing is left to memory or chance. The secretary's work procedure depends upon the nature of the job and the size of the company. Some offices have established routines; some employers will specify the methods they prefer; sometimes a departing secretary will train an incoming one. The basic tools of organization are a memo pad, a calendar, an appointment book and a telephone-address book or file.

The memo pad will function as an added memory bank. Notations are made from each phone call, each request for an answer, each new assignment. By writing the information down, the secretary is heed from the need to keep small pieces of information in a mental notebook. Also, by writing all information down, the secretary is able to resume work at the point of interruption.

Keeping an appointment book, the appointment book is one of the most important records in the office. There are various methods of recording and following up appointments, but essential to each is the appointment book. In automated offices, there is an electronic calendar.

In some offices the book is kept on the executive's desk. The secretary must maintain an accurate duplicate appointment book so that both members of the office know how each day is to be spent. In other offices the executive assigns the appointment book to the secretary, who makes all of the appointments. To examine the book the executive will have to go to the secretary's desk and read it there or temporarily remove it.

Before making appointments, the secretary must be familiar with office procedure. Such matters as availability of executives, availability of conference rooms for meetings, daily arrival and departure limes and average schedules and length of conferences affect the making of appointments.

The appointment should be entered under the day and the hour agreed upon by the person requesting it and the secretary. The entry includes the names of the persons concerned, some notation of the topic to be discussed, and any other pertinent information. The secretary uses these notes to produce needed documents for the executive to read before the meeting. If the material is complex, the secretary may give it to the executive days ahead of time when the work flow is slow. On the day of the appointment the secretary follows through to be sure that there is no misunderstanding and to be sure that the appropriate materials and notes are on the executive's desk. If the appointment is canceled, arrangements for a new appointment should be made immediately.

Developing familiarity with sources of information the secretary who can find not only the names of those whom the employer must reach most frequently but also the names, addresses, and phone numbers for services, emergencies and sources of information is a valuable asset to the office and is rewarded as such. Many secretaries in education and research organizations will keep a separate file of reference books or sources with notations about the contents and the call letters if they are in the public or the company library. The secretary would do well to become familiar with the area's Yellow Pages and with the various sources of information listed in the section on reference materials in this volume.

Time- and Work-saving Units

Time is one of a businessperson's most precious commodities. The secretary who learns to organize work and plan time wisely will save minutes out of every hour, hours out of every week. This free time will be used by the professional to expand knowledge and expertise.

Here are a few time- and work-saving suggestions:

- Make efficient use of your desk. Keep the surface clear of everything except your immediate work so you will not have to search through piles of other material when you want page.

- Form the habit of using filing folders for anything of a temporary nature—work in progress, incoming or outgoing communications, work being held for additional information—and keep these folders in the file drawer of your desk where they are instantly accessible but not in the way.
- Plan your time; never waste it. When work is slow, one has to plan ahead to complete within the time. Do what can be done to relieve the workload at peak periods? Try to learn more about your company's operations. Consider what you can do to make your part of it run more smoothly. Become familiar with reference materials: learn how to use the reference books your boss consults frequently. The next time you may be able to find that chart or graph that is badly needed. Bring the address book up-to-date. Get to know the filing system.
- Learn to schedule your time realistically. It may take you an hour to type that stack of letters, provided that you are not interrupted; but you will be. The telephone will ring, your employer will call upon you to take care of something urgent, and people will stop at your desk to ask questions. That one hour may become two or three hours. If you learn to expect interruptions, you will not be flustered by them or lose time trying to pick up where you left off. Interruptions are part of your work and require a place in your schedule.
- Be a part of the team. When the workload is heavy, when your employers and other members of the staff are up against a deadline to get a job done, be willing to pitch in and help even if it is a little after closing time. Your ability of function as a professional will be remembered when you have a favor to ask and when you wish a promotion.

FUTURE

The need for skilled secretaries will continue to grow. The secretary of today and the future may be entering the field from high school, vocational school, or college; may be returning to work after many years of gap, or may be making a midlife career change. What all these secretaries have in common is their professionalism and their recognition of the importance of the work they do. The secretary of today and the future recognizes that a life's work deserves to be planned, and the professional secretary chooses a career path carefully. The professional secretary who will assume an important place in business and society will need to be able to respond to the concept and technology of information processing, possess decision-making ability and human relations skills, and be adaptable to learning new skills in a rapidly changing office environment. Secretaries can expect to take more responsibility as the more repetitious aspects of their jobs are automated.

MINUTES OF A MEETING

The executive may ask the secretary to take minutes at a formal or informal meeting. At minutes of meeting (MOM) is a term used to describe an official record of the proceedings of a meeting. Keeping minutes of meetings is always advisable. Although the minutes may not be disseminated, they should be filed in case they are needed at a later date.

Types of Meetings

There are basically two types of meetings: formal and informal. A formal meeting is a preplanned, structured meeting, such as an annual conference or convention and its workshops and symposia. Usually, there is a prepared agenda. An informal meeting may be short and announced only a short time before it is held; it is usually held on company premises. To inform staff members of a quickly scheduled meeting the secretary may use electronic calendaring, if available, or the telephone. Always confirm by sending a follow-up note.

Another type of meeting—a teleconference—has been made possible by modern technology. In a teleconference, two or more persons in different geographic locations communicate electronically (audio, video, and computer). It is effective for informal meetings and serves as an adjunct to more formal, structured meetings. By using audio, video, and/or computer equipment, including the electronic blackboard, meetings can be held simultaneously or on a delayed basis with several groups participating in various locations. Everything in a teleconference is taped.

The minutes of a teleconference can be completed from the recorded media. This allows the secretary time to devote to other duties. The minutes, when completed, can be distributed electronically.

Preliminary Duties

Preliminary duties before a formal meeting may include reserving the meeting room, sending pertinent materials, preparing mailing lists, making calendar notations, preparing an agenda (the order of business), and handling last—minute details, such as supply and equipment needs (e.g. overhead projector or VDT). If you plan to take shorthand notes at the meeting, be sure you have sufficient notebooks, pencils and other supplies. If you plan to record the meeting, check reel-to-reel or cassette recorders to ensure the equipment is operating and that you have sufficient supplies.

Some companies employ technical assistants to be available during electronic transmissions if needed. At a computer conference, the secretary may be asked to keyboard messages and retrieve stored data. These types of conferences should be planned in advance.

Preparing the Minutes

The most important phase of preparing minutes is the accurate recording and reporting of the actions taken. The record should report what was said. At times, it is difficult to report what is done. For informal meetings, the minutes are compact and simple; for formal meetings, the minutes are complex. If you find that grouping the minutes around a central theme is clearer, do so. On the other hand, the executive may prefer chronological order.

Corporate minutes (official minutes of a formal nature) must be prepared in the order of occurrence, showing details and the exact wording of motions, resolutions, and so forth. By law, corporations are required to keep minutes of stockholders' and directors' meetings. These minutes are legal records and should be protected from tampering.

When preparing corporate minutes, use watermarked paper, and place the finalized minutes in key lock binders. Any corrections resulting from a subsequent meeting should be written. Incorrect portions are ruled out in ink and initialed in the margin. The official secretary of the corporation has responsibility for the completeness and accuracy of corporate minute, but the secretary may have to type and prepare them.

OFFICE MEMORANDUMS

An office memorandum, almost universally referred to as memo, is basically a letter between company employees and is less formal than a traditional letter. It may be short or long, single or multipage. The secretary may compose memos as well as type them for executives.

Like all other office communications, memorandums transmit information and provide a record that information was transmitted. Office memorandums are used for several purposes: (a) For messages that are complicated; (b) To avoid making unnecessary telephone calls for business that may not be urgent; and (c) When a record is needed. They not only avoid situations that may be misunderstood, but also protect people by having a written record. Usually, office memorandums are brief and direct. However, there are exceptions depending upon the nature, purpose, and scope of the subject discussed and the writer's purpose and intent.

The plural form of memorandum may be either memorandums (add "s") or memorandums (add "a"; Latin form). However, when composing or writing, be consistent and use only one form for the plural. Also, when typing from an originator's draft copy, always check for consistency in spelling.

Types of Memos

Interoffice Memorandum

The interoffice memorandum is an in-house communication and is sent to a person in your own firm or department within one location; in other words, it is confined. Forms vary widely from company to company. However, all the principles of writing and business correspondence apply to memorandums as they do to letters.

Intraoffice Memorandum

The intraoffice memorandum is used within the same company between offices in different buildings or locations. For example, Company A may have two offices in New York City and one in Westchester County. Thus, the written communication is external; that is, it is not distributed in one location but must be transmitted elsewhere.

Parts of a Memo

All memorandums, whether printed or not, are composed of similar elements (parts). However, formatting may differ. These elements include to/from, date, subject, body, and end references (i.e. reference initials, distribution of copies, etc.). There may be slight differences in heading and closing information or in the order of the elements, especially if the forms are printed.

21 The Patient

INTRODUCTION

The author during his career as Senior Consultant and Advisor to the Ministries of Health of different countries, had interacted with hundreds of healthcare professionals of multinational and realized that they all work throughout their career in health related field, and do their best, despite, patient care mostly carried out as mechanical process; especially in Developing Countries, as it appeared that an item was brought to workshop for repair and the mechanic with his assistants repairs it and hand over to the owner. Similarly, the patient either sick or injured visits hospital for relief/care is treated perfunctory.

Earlier days in Developing Countries, the medical care was rendered free of cost, even today, in some nations still in practice. In that situation, the patient or his family were not much concern of respect or self esteem while getting treatment, and happy whatever is done was accepted with gratitude. The present situation has changed with the spiraling cost of healthcare; medical dynamism and tough global competition. The patient and families expect not only best possible treatment with healthcare team but also to practice medical ethics in strict sense in providing care with empathy as they pay for every service they get in the hospital. This is one aspect, but in reality, while rendering care with human touch and well behavior will add much value to the greatest satisfaction of a patient and his family members. In order to ensure that healthcare providers including medical, nursing, paramedics and administrative personnel are really grasped the value of a patient, because of him the entire healthcare organizations including the World Health Organization (WHO), UNICEF and national healthcare ministries, directorate general offices, corporate hospitals and so on are existing and functioning with tremendous responsibilities to provide best possible healthcare to the citizens of the nation.

Keeping the above object in view, the author while serving as a Senior Consultant and Advisor to the Ministries of Health in Gulf Cooperation

Council (GCC) in Middle East countries conducted quiz in few nations during implementation of Hospital Policies and Procedures training program wanted to elicit the feelings of participants comprising, medical, nursing, paramedics and administrative staff asking them to name the position which is the most important in the healthcare delivery system from the following list: The Quiz was conducted in four phases: Each phase has different results.

S. No.	*Post*
1.	Minister of health
2.	Undersecretary of health
3.	Director general of health
4.	Chief executive officer of health
5.	Medical director
6.	Hospital administrator
7.	Doctor
8.	Nurse
9.	Patient
10.	Pathologist
11.	Radiologist
12.	Microbiologist
13.	Biochemist
14.	Pharmacist
15.	Medical social worker
16.	Nutrition
17.	Physiotherapist
18.	Occupational therapist
19.	Optometrist
20.	Audiologist
21.	Medical records manager
22.	Information technologist
23.	Human resource manager
24.	Finance manager
25.	Public Relations Officer

First phase quiz results: The response was quite interesting by the divergent group has ranked according to their understanding and found their response was mostly on the importance of title and positions, nevertheless, majority of them considered a Doctor and Nurse (35%) followed by Health Minister, Under Secretary and Director General of Health Services (30%); Chief Executive Officer, Medical Director and Hospital Administrator (15%); Pathologist, Radiologist, Microbiologist, Biochemist, Pharmacist and Medical Social Worker (10%); Patient (5%) and others such as Nutritionist, Physiotherapist etc. (5%).

Second phase: The quiz was repeated second time. In the second phase the top positions (S. No. 1 to 3) was removed and participants have responded and given marks to the rest of group. Their response was mostly on the importance of title and positions, nevertheless, majority of them considered a Doctor and Nurse (40%) followed by Chief Executive Officer, Medical Director and Hospital Administrator (25%); Pathologist, Radiologist, Microbiologist, Biochemist, Pharmacist and Medical Social Worker (20%) and others such as Nutritionist, Physiotherapist, etc. (10%) and Patient (5%).

Third phase: The quiz was repeated third time the top positions (S. No. 4 to 6) was removed and participants have responded giving marks to the rest of group. Their response was mostly on the importance of title and positions, nevertheless, majority of them considered a Doctor and Nurse (45%) followed by Pathologist, Radiologist, Microbiologist, Biochemist, Pharmacist and Medical Social Worker (25%) others such as Nutritionist, Physiotherapist etc. (20%) and Patient (10%)

Fourth phase: The same question was repeated fourth time retaining all the posts from S. No. 1 to 25 except removing S. No. 9—the patient from the list: There was pin drop silence for some time and wondered what to answer. In a moment—they realized without patient—all other positions including the highest posts have no significant value. Hence it is the patient around him/her all the healthcare organizations and professional efforts and endeavors revolve.

WHO, WHAT, WHY, HOW, WHEN AND WHERE OF PATIENT CARE

The book entitled "Hospital Patient Care Relationship Coordinator" encompasses most important topics that are vital as the patient is a central focus entity around him/her entire healthcare organization and professionals efforts and endeavors revolve. Thus, it would be appropriate

S. No.	*Post*	*1st Phase QR*	*2nd Phase QR*	*3rd Phase QR*	*4th Phase QR*
1.	Minister of Health	30%	Deleted	Deleted	0%
2.	Undersecretary of Health				
3.	Director General of Health				
4.	Chief Executive Officer	15%	25%	Deleted	0%
5.	Medical Director				
6.	Hospital Administrator				
7.	Doctor	35%	40%	45%	
8.	Nurse				
9.	Patient	5%	5%	10%	Deleted
10.	Pathologist	10%	20%	25%	0%
11.	Radiologist				
12.	Microbiologist				
13.	Biochemist				
14.	Pharmacist				
15.	Medical Social Worker				
16.	Nutrition	5%	10%	20%	0%
17.	Physiotherapist				
18.	Occupational therapist				
19.	Optometrist				
20.	Audiologist				
21.	Medical Records Manager				
22.	Information Technologist				
23.	Human Resource Manager				
24.	Finance Manager				
25.	Public Relations Officer				
		100%	100%	100%	0%

to have a clear picture about patient including who, what, why, how, when and where patient care is needed and rendered. It further offers information such as the gist of outpatient or ambulatory, emergency and inpatient or hospitalization care. This chapter encompasses Patient behavior and feelings, patient doctor-encounter, patient problems, patient education and safety and satisfaction.

Patients and families general priority when they visit hospital or any healthcare institution is to get care with skill, compassion and respect. And they would be anxious to know the place of treatment, who would be their care providers, especially the treating physicians and nurses and other personnel involved in his/her care. They are also concern with the students and residents or trainees trying to experiment. Another important concern is safety, and the cost. The ethical practice emanate signify patient-provider relationship emphasis respect for patient autonomy and shared decision-making. As soon as the patient settle down in allocated room, the patient and family have many questions about what to expect and what is going to happen during their stay and their inquires are not limited to the following:

- Who is in charge of my care?
- Can my family bring in food?
- Can visitors are restricted?
- What if I am unhappy with my care?
- Do I get patient oriented service?
- Do I get high quality service in a safe manner?
- Expect swift care with empathy!
- Anxiety of duplication or unnecessary investigations or surgery
- General attitude of personnel involved in providing healthcare
- Expects a patient- and family-centered philosophy of care
- Does the hospital share the progress report of patient condition regularly?
- Patient- and family-centered care means involving and responding to a patients and families. To do this, the hospital:
  - Recognize that each patient and each family is unique
  - Provide open, honest communication
  - Involve the patient/family in the planning, delivery and the evaluation of healthcare
  - Offer a welcoming, supportive environment
  - Provide timely justified expert care
  - Provide access to information and resources
  - Does the hospital has any handbook to know the rights and responsibilities of a patient
  - And to know more about hospital, room, meals and other important information that may find useful
  - If there is nay problem or concern to whom to contact.

Who is a Patient?

A patient: Is any person who receives medical attention, care, or treatment. The person is most often sick or injured and in need of treatment by a physician or other medical professional, although one who is visiting a physician for a routine check-up may also be viewed as a patient. A patient is a person with a unique health related problem. A patient is a person who is suffering and needs help. It is necessary to recognize their rights. These rights are equal to those of anyone else in health. Every person whether well or ill has the right to be treated with human dignity.

An outpatient: Is a patient who is not hospitalized overnight but who visits a hospital, clinic, or associated facility for diagnosis or treatment. Treatment provided in this fashion is called ambulatory care. Outpatient surgery eliminates inpatient hospital admission, reduces the amount of medication prescribed, and uses a doctor's time more efficiently. More procedures are now being performed in a surgeon's office, termed office-based surgery, rather than in an operating room. Also known as "daycare surgery". Outpatient surgery is suited best for healthy people undergoing minor or intermediate procedures (limited urologic, ophthalmologic, or ear, nose, and throat procedures and procedures involving the extremities).

An inpatient: On the other hand is "admitted" to the hospital and stays overnight or for an indeterminate time, usually several days or weeks (though some cases, like coma patients, have been in hospitals for years). Due to concerns such as dignity, human rights and political correctness, the term "patient" is not always used to refer to a person receiving health care. Other terms that are sometimes used include health consumer, health care consumer or client. These may be used by governmental agencies, insurance companies, patient groups, or health care facilities. Individuals who use or have used psychiatric services may alternatively refer to themselves as consumers, users, or survivors.

Types of Patient

Passive-dependent: This kind of patient prefers that the doctor make the healthcare decisions, setting up a course of action. Trusting of the medical profession, they believe most doctors know best. And not interested in understanding or analyzing the risks and benefits of diagnostic or treatment options, or in making shared decisions. They just want to follow whatever plan the doctor creates.

Independent-skeptical: This kind of patient wants an arms-length relationship with the physician. Skepticism about expert advice comes naturally, they tend to form and rely on their own opinions after learning about the options. Expecting to have the final say in decisions about the health, they unlikely to accept the advice of others. Still, it's not unlike to seek second or third opinions. Emotional support is not what they after. Instead they want treatment recommendations regard as rational or consistent with the world-view, knowledge and experience.

Intellectual-researcher: Eager to understand the science behind diagnostic and therapeutic choices, they research health conditions online or in journals and expect to participate in decisions. They examine doctor qualifications and ask for references, and prefer a doctor who practices in a prestigious health-care institution. Stimulated by participation in the diagnostic and therapeutic process, they intellectualize their health condition. Emotional support isn't what they're after: they want to understand the risks and benefits of each option. In their eyes, medicine is more science than art.

Expedient-flexible: They're not concerned about building a long-term relationship with physician, and besides, tend to have only episodic health needs. They figure that one physician is about as good as another, especially one who is available right when they need him or her, they are cost-conscious, and are therefore unlikely to choose a physician based on prestige. They're unconcerned about whether they see a doctor at a clinic or a hospital. Emotional support isn't their priority either; they have little curiosity about the health-care process or analysis of the risks and benefits driving decisions. They may have grown up seeing doctors in a clinic-type setting.

Open-minded-exploring: They're seeking a more personal connection with the physician and related health providers, including alternative practitioners. They see health care as a partnership between doctor and patient and prefer a doctor who won't rush through their appointments and who is open to alternative approaches and therapies. They see emotional support as an integral part of approaching all of the needs of the patient. They're interested in alternative and non-traditional medicine and appreciate the spiritual dimension of healing and their view medicine as more art than science.

What the patient needs: In order to better understand patient differences in question asking and other information-seeking behaviors when communicating with doctors. Socio-demographic data, attitude measures, interview data and tape recordings of doctor-patient encounters revealed that patients desired information about a wide range of medical topics but did not engage in many information-seeking behaviors when communicating with doctors.

While desiring information, patients regarded doctors as the appropriate persons to make medical decisions. Regression analyses indicated that patient information-seeking behaviors were more directly associated with situational variables (length of interaction, diagnosis, reason for visit) than with patient attitudes or socio-demographic characteristics.

Hospitalization: Hospital admission involves staying at a hospital for at least one night or more. Staying in the hospital overnight is done because the individual is too sick to stay at home, requires 24-hour nursing care, and/or is receiving medications and undergoing tests and/or surgery that can only be performed in the hospital setting.

An individual may be admitted to the hospital for a positive experience, such as having a baby, or because they are undergoing an *elective surgery* or procedure, or because they are being admitted through the emergency department. Being admitted through the emergency department is the most stressful of these circumstances because the event is unexpected and may be a major life crisis.

Before the person is taken to their room, admitting procedures are performed. The person's personal data is recorded and entered into the hospital's computer system. This data may include:

- Name
- Address
- Home and work telephone number
- Date of birth
- Place of employment
- Occupation
- Emergency contact information, or the names and telephone numbers of those individuals the hospital should contact if the person being admitted needs emergency care or their condition worsens significantly
- Insurance coverage
- Reason for hospitalization
- Allergies to medications or foods
- Religious preference, including whether or not one wishes a clergy member to visit.

There may be several forms to fill out. One form may be a detailed medical and medication history. This history will include past hospitalizations and surgeries. Having this information readily available will make the process move faster, and can allow a family member or friend who is accompanying the person to help fill out the forms more easily. The hospital may ask if there are any advance directives. This refers to forms that have been filled out indicating what medical decisions one wants others to make on their behalf.

Once all the admitting information has been completed, the next step is usually being taken to a general ward or one's room. Most people stay in a semi-private room, which means that there are two people to a room. In some circumstances, a person's medical condition may require staying in a private room. If there are private rooms available, and the individual is willing to pay the extra cost (insurance companies generally only cover the cost of a semi-private room), it may be possible to have a private room. Most hospital rooms are set up so that one bed is closer to the door, and the other is next to a window. There are curtains that can be drawn completely around the bed so that some degree of privacy is possible. Once taken to a room, the nurse taking care of the patient will go over the medical and medication history, and orient the person to the room.

These kinds of decisions are made with the person's safety and medical condition in mind. If the person is not thinking clearly, perhaps because of some medication they are receiving, the side rails of the bed may be put up, to prevent falling out of bed. The nurse will review the doctor's orders, such as what tests have been scheduled, whether or not they can get out of bed for the bathroom or to walk around the unit, what medications they will be getting, and whether or not there are restrictions on what they can eat.

Sometimes when people are admitted to the hospital they need extremely close observation that can only be given in specialized care called an intensive care unit. Because of the severity of their condition, visiting hours are more restricted than in the regular rooms. It may be that only one or two people can visit at a time, and only for a few minutes at a time. Once the person's condition improves, they may then be transferred to a room with a less rigid visitation policy. If an individual has a surgical procedure performed, they will spend a few hours in a recovery area. This is to make sure that the person's condition is stable before returning to the regular room.

If the hospitalization is prearranged, there are preparations that will make the process go more smoothly. It is helpful to have a list of all medications currently being taken, the dosages, how often they are taken, and the reason for taking them. The list should also include any allergies to food and medications, including a description of the reaction, and when the food or medication was last taken. The list should include over-the-counter (OTC) and prescription medications, vitamins, supplements, and herbal and home remedies.

If the hospital stay involves surgery in which there is the potential for significant blood loss, it may be possible to arrange to have blood drawn and stored so that in the event of a *transfusion*, the individual receives his or her own blood.

A small bag can be brought into the hospital that contains personal care items that must be carried. It is best not to bring in any medication from home unless it has been prearranged with the physician and hospital staff prior to hospitalization. This is to prevent an error from occurring by having the person taking one dose from their own medicine and then being given another dose from the hospital *pharmacy*.

Workflow of Emergency Department

The patient goes to the distribution desk of Emergency Department. The patient is confirmed to be service recipient from the hospital. The Emergency Department carries out registration and distribution and call in a coordinator from Emergency Department for further examination and treatment. A doctor from Emergency Department is assigned to treat the patient. Emergency Department reports to Working Office and asks for assistance if they need special attention. The patient is transferred to a relevant department for hospitalization, or he gets recovered and is discharged from the hospital. Patient settles the account and is provided with a discharge summary of treatment (including diagnosis) and a detailed statement of charges.

Workflow of Inpatient Admission

A referral doctor issues a Certificate of Inpatient Admission. The case of the patient is kept in the records of Working Office. The patient goes through the necessary procedure of hospitalization. A special person sends the patient to a special ward. The process of diagnosis and treatment for the patient settles once and for all the account and is provided with a summary of his/her disease.

Patient Safety

Patient safety is an important healthcare discipline that emphasizes the reporting, analysis, and prevention of medical error that often lead to adverse healthcare events. The frequency and magnitude of avoidable adverse patient events was not well known until the 1990s, when multiple countries reported shocking numbers of patients harmed and killed by medical errors. Recognizing that healthcare errors impact 1 in every 10 patients around the world, the World Health Organization calls patient safety an endemic concern. Indeed, patient safety has emerged as a distinct healthcare discipline supported by an immature yet developing scientific framework.

There is a significant trans-disciplinary body of theoretical and research literature that informs the science of patient safety. The resulting patient safety knowledge continually informs improvement efforts such as: applying lessons learned from business and industry, adopting innovative technologies, educating providers and consumers, enhancing error reporting systems, and developing new economic incentives.

The simplest definition of a healthcare error is a preventable adverse effect of care, whether or not it is evident or harmful to the patient. A conservative average of both the Institute of Medicine and Health Grade reports indicates that there have been between 400,000–1.2 million error-induced deaths during 1996–2006 in the United States. These casualties have been, in part, attributed to:

Human Factors

- Variations in healthcare provider training and experience, fatigue, depression and burnout.
- Diverse patients, unfamiliar settings, time pressures.
- Failure to acknowledge the prevalence and seriousness of medical errors.

Medical Complexity

- Complicated technologies, powerful drugs.
- Intensive care, prolonged hospital stay.

System Failures

- Poor communication, unclear lines of authority of physicians, nurses, and other care providers. Complications increase as patient to nurse staffing ratio increases.
- Disconnected reporting systems within a hospital: Fragmented systems in which numerous hand-offs of patient's results in lack of coordination and errors.
- Drug names that look alike or sound alike.
- The impression that action is being taken by other groups within the institution.
- Reliance on automated systems to prevent error.
- Inadequate systems to share information about errors hamper analysis of contributory causes and improvement strategies.

- Cost-cutting measures by hospitals in response to reimbursement cutbacks. Environment and design factors. In emergencies, patient care may be rendered in areas poorly suited for safe monitoring. The American Institute of Architects has identified concerns for the safe design and construction of health care facilities.
- Infrastructure failure. According to the WHO, 50% of medical equipment in developing countries is only partly usable due to lack of skilled operators or parts. As a result, diagnostic procedures or treatments cannot be performed, leading to substandard treatment.

The Joint Commission's Annual Report on Quality and Safety 2007 found that inadequate communication between healthcare providers, or between providers and the patient and family members, was the root cause of over half the serious adverse events in accredited hospitals. Other leading causes included inadequate assessment of the patient's condition, and poor leadership or training.

Common misconceptions about adverse events are:

- Incompetent health care providers are a common cause. (Although human error is commonly an initiating event, the faulty process of delivering care invariably permits or compounds the harm, and is the focus of improvement.)
- High risk procedures or medical specialties are responsible for most avoidable adverse events. (Although some mistakes, such as in surgery, are harder to conceal, errors occur in all levels of care. Even though complex procedures entail more risk, adverse outcomes are not usually due to error, but to the severity of the condition being treated.). However, United States Pharmacopeia (USP) has reported that medication errors during the course of a surgical procedure are three times more likely to cause harm to a patient than those occurring in other types of hospital care.)
- If a patient experiences an adverse event during the process of care, an error has occurred. (Most medical care entails some level of risk, and there can be complications or side effects, even unforeseen ones, from the underlying condition or from the treatment itself.)

Potential Causes Related to Patient

- Patient leaving against advice
- Hospital acquired infection
- Patient not improved
- Increased mortality rate
- Patient repeated admissions
- Patient post-operative complications

- Incident cases
- Patient complaints due to dissatisfaction
- Absconded patients
- Patient increased length of stay
- Waiting time of patient
- Medication errors
- Transfusion reactions, wrong blood type
- Obstetric and birth trauma
- Anesthesia and post-operative complications
- Patient falls in hospital e.g., hip fracture
- Hospital acquired burns
- Change of investigations
- Wrong diagnosis, wrong medications
- Change of mother and child
- Occurrence variance
- Problems relating to healthcare services
- Patient dissatisfaction
- Patient care evaluation to ensure that he/she is getting the best care
- Safety, security of patient
- Protection of privacy of patient information.

Types of Healthcare Technology

Handwritten reports or notes, manual order entry, non-standard abbreviations and poor legibility lead to substantial errors and injuries, according to the IOM (2000) report. The follow-up IOM report, Crossing the Quality Chasm: A New Health System for the 21st Century, advised rapid adoption of electronic patient records, electronic medication ordering, with computer and internet-based information systems to support clinical decisions. This section contains only the patient safety related aspects of Health Information Technology (HIT).

Electronic health record (EHR): The Electronic health record (EHR), previously known as the Electronic medical record (EMR), reduces several types of errors, including those related to prescription drugs, to emergent and preventive care, and to tests and procedures. Important features of modern EHR include automated drug-drug/drug-food interaction checks and allergy checks, standard drug dosages and patient education information. Also, these systems provide recurring alerts to remind clinicians of intervals for preventive care and to track referrals and test results. Clinical guidelines for disease management have a demonstrated. Advances in health informatics and widespread adoption of interoperable electronic health records promise access to a patient's records at any healthcare site. Recent surveys in the United Kingdom have shown physicians' deficiencies in understanding the patient safety features of government-approved software.

Portable offline emergency medical record devices have been developed to provide access to health records during widespread or extended infrastructure failure, such as in natural disasters or regional conflicts.

Computerized provider order entry (CPOE): Prescribing errors are the largest identified source of preventable errors in hospitals (IOM, 2000; 2007). The IOM (2006) estimates that each hospitalized patient, on average, is exposed to one medication error each day. Computerized provider order entry (CPOE), formerly called computer physician order entry, can reduce medication errors by 80% overall but more importantly decrease harm to patients by 55%. A Leapfrog (2004) survey found that 16% of US clinics, hospitals, and medical practices are expected to utilize CPOE within 2 years.

Complete safety medication system: A standardized bar code system for dispensing drugs might prevent 25% of drug errors. Despite ample evidence to reduce medication errors, compete medication delivery systems (bar-coding and Electronic prescribing have slowed adoption of this technology by doctors and hospitals in the United States, due to concern with interoperability and compliance with future national standards. Such concerns are not inconsequential; standards for electronic prescribing for Medicare Part D conflict with regulations in many US states).

Technological iatrogenesis: Technology induced errors are significant and increasingly more evident in healthcare delivery systems. This idiosyncratic and potentially serious problems associated with HIT implementation has recently become a tangible concern for healthcare and information technology professionals. As such, the term technological iatrogenesis describes this new category of adverse events that are an emergent property resulting from technological innovation creating system and micro-system disturbances. Healthcare systems are complex and adaptive meaning there are many networks and connections working simultaneously to produce certain outcomes. When these systems are under the increased stresses caused by the diffusion of new technology, unfamiliar and new process errors often result. If not recognized, over time these new errors can collectively lead to catastrophic system failures. The term "e-iatrogenesis" can be used to describe the local error manifestation. The sources for these errors include:

- Prescriber and staff inexperience may lead to a false sense of security; that when technology suggests a course of action, errors are avoided.
- Shortcut or default selections can override non-standard medication regimens for elderly or underweight patients, resulting in toxic doses.
- CPOE and automated drug dispensing was identified as a cause of error by 84% of over 500 health care facilities participating in a surveillance system by the United States Pharmacopoeia. Irrelevant or frequent warnings can interrupt work flow.

Solutions include ongoing changes in design to cope with unique medical settings, supervising overrides from automatic systems, and training (and re-training) all users.

Today's health-care context is highly complex. Care is often delivered in a pressurized and fast-moving environment, involving a vast array of technology and, daily, many individual decisions and judgments by healthcare professional staff. In such circumstances things can and do go wrong. Sometimes unintentional harm comes to a patient during a clinical procedure or as a result of a clinical decision. Errors in the process of care can result in injury. Sometimes the harm that patients experience is serious and sometimes people die.

The situation in developing countries and countries in economic transition merits particular attention. The poor state of infrastructure and equipment, unreliable supply and quality of drugs, shortcomings in waste management and infection control, poor performance of personnel because of low motivation or insufficient technical skills, and severe under financing of essential operating costs of health services make the probability of adverse events much higher than in industrialized nations.

Most of the current evidence on adverse events comes from hospitals, because the risks associated with hospital care are high, strategies for improvement are better documented, and the importance of patient trust is paramount. But many adverse events occur in other healthcare settings, such as physicians' offices, nursing homes, pharmacies and patients' homes. Recent literature highlights concerns about outpatients as well, but there are few data on the extent of the problem outside hospitals.

Every point in the process of care giving contains a certain inherent lack of safety: side-effects of drugs or drug combinations, hazards posed by a medical device, substandard or faulty products entering the health service, human shortcomings, or system (latent) failures. Adverse events may therefore result from problems in practice, products, procedures or systems.

Immunization, which is given to healthy individuals, poses a particular challenge. With the decline in prevalence of vaccine-preventable diseases, concern about potential adverse events following immunization may have a negative impact on national immunization programs and preventive healthcare in general. Current conceptual thinking on the safety of patients places the prime responsibility for adverse events on deficiencies in system design, organization and operation rather than on individual providers or individual products.

Safety is a fundamental principle of patient care and a critical component of quality management. Its improvement demands a complex system-wide effort, involving a broad range of actions in performance improvement, environmental safety and risk management, including infection control, safe use of medicines, equipment safety, safe clinical practice and safe environment of care. It embraces nearly all health-care disciplines and actors, and thus requires a comprehensive, multifaceted approach to identifying and managing actual and potential risks to patient safety in individual services and finding broad long-term solutions for the system as a whole.

Thinking in terms of "systems" offers the greatest promise of definitive risk-reduction solutions, which place the appropriate emphasis on every component of patient safety, as opposed to solutions driven by narrower and more specific aspects of the problem, which tend to underestimate the importance of other perspectives.

Enhancing the safety of patients includes three complementary actions: preventing adverse events; making them visible; and mitigating their effects when they occur. This requires: (a) increased ability to learn from mistakes, through better reporting systems, skilful investigation of incidents and responsible sharing of data; (b) greater capacity to anticipate mistakes and probe systemic weaknesses that might lead to an adverse event; (c) identifying existing knowledge resources, within and outside the health sector; and (d) improvements in the health-care delivery system itself, so that structures are reconfigured, incentives are realigned, and quality is placed at the core of the system. In general, national programs are built around these principles.

Despite growing interest in the safety of patients, there is still widespread lack of awareness of the problem of adverse events. Capacity for reporting, analyzing and learning from experience is still seriously hampered by lack of methodological uniformity in identification and measurement, inadequate adverse event reporting schemes, undue concerns over breaches in confidentiality of data, the fear of professional liability, and weak information systems.

Understanding and knowledge of the epidemiology of adverse events—frequency, causes, determinants and impact on patient outcomes, and of effective methods for preventing them—are still limited. Although there are examples of successful initiatives for reducing the incidence of adverse events, none has been expanded to the level of an entire health system.

Responsibility towards Patient

The medical profession and medical ethics currently place a greater emphasis on physician responsibility than patient responsibility. This imbalance is not due to accident or a mistake but, rather is motivated by strong moral reasons. As we debate the nature and extent of patient responsibility it is important to keep in mind the reasons for giving a relatively minimal role to patient responsibility in medical ethics. It is argued that the medical profession ought to be characterized by two moral asymmetries:

1. Even if some degree of responsible behavior from patients is called for, placing the dominant emphasis on professional responsibility over patient responsibility is largely correct. The value of protecting the right to refuse treatment and arguments against paternalism block a more expansive account of patient responsibility and support a strong notion of professional responsibility.
2. Insofar as we do want to encourage an increase in patient responsibility, we have good reasons to emphasize prospective rather than retrospective concept in clinical practice. Concerns about patient vulnerability along with the determined factors in disease leave minimal scope for blame at the bedside. These two asymmetries generate normative limits on any positive account of patient responsibility.

Since its birth as a profession, medical ethics has primarily concerned itself with defining the duties of physicians toward patients. The emphasis on protecting patients' rights provided an important corrective to a field dominated by a deeply ingrained paternalism. Questions like those above cause a certain amount of discomfort in the clinical setting, in part because many health professionals do not feel they have the moral and legal grounds to demand responsible behavior from patients and in part because such demands are out of step with the now dominant emphasis on patient choice.

Holding patients responsible for adhering to treatment plans and living a healthy life, smacks of the old paternalism that much of medical culture prides itself on rejecting. Yet health professionals are understandably frustrated with the overwhelming burden of clinical and legal responsibility for patients' well being. The emerging discussion in the clinical literature on patient compliance and recent attempts in medical ethics to offer up lists of patient responsibilities signal this frustration and an underlying desire to bring the moral pendulum back toward the middle by increasing patient accountability.

Some specific suggestions for increasing patient responsibility include the use of patient agreements whereby a patient agrees to certain terms in the physician-patient relationship, such as coming to appointments, taking prescribed medications as indicated, asking questions, and informing the physician of symptoms. Some hospitals are distributing lists of patient responsibilities, included among the admissions paperwork, with similar promises to give full histories, follow plans of care, ask questions, and report symptoms.

But what would holding patients responsible for behavior affecting health and treatment mean in practice, if the lists of patient responsibilities amount to more than mere suggestions, should patients be encouraged to behave responsibly in hopes of winning the trust and approval of physicians, or perhaps the fear of being rebuked, transferred to another physician, or dropped as a patient? Should a system of patient responsibilities reflect the current norms for professional responsibility among health professionals?

If so, there would be repercussions for failing in one's obligations as a patient. A patient could be fired or asked to switch physicians. A patient could be blamed for the negative consequences of bad behavior, poor diet, or harmful habits, perhaps justifying physician responsibility for rescuing the patient through continued treatment. Perhaps patients could even be fined or sued for wasting precious resources or a physician's time.

It is important to ask what we hope to accomplish by promoting norms of patient responsibility more forcefully and what other valuable norms governing clinical ethics might be in jeopardy if we do so. It is also not clear that we should develop a one-size-fits-all model of patient responsibility—it may be unreasonable to expect the average patient to live up to the standards of a heart transplant patient. So far, those calling for increased patient responsibility have not adequately addressed what a robust account of patient responsibility, with consequences attached to performance and failure, would mean for patients and patient choice.

As we try to focus more attention on the duties of patients we should also keep in mind the moral norms that would constrain any positive account of patient responsibility, and that is what I offer here. There are several established and valuable moral norms in clinical practice at stake in the responsibility debate, including the doctrine of informed refusals and norms encouraging non-judgmental compassionate care.

To defend the idea that a medical culture with a more moderate notion of patient responsibility is preferable to any system of enforced patient responsibilities (where enforcement includes the possibility of being dropped or transferred as a patient, verbally reprimanded, or penalized in other ways) because it remains compatible with these important norms.

A moderate notion of patient responsibility will remain one based on persuasion, not punishment, and will be forward-looking, that is, based on encouragement and caution regarding future consequences rather than blame for past behavior.

In arguing for a significantly constrained model of patient responsibility, defend two moral asymmetries in clinical ethics:

1. Even if some degree of responsible behavior from patients is called for, placing greater emphasis on professional responsibility over patient responsibility is largely correct, and
2. There is a good reason to emphasize prospective rather than retrospective notions of responsibility in clinical practice.

Patient-doctor Encounter

The doctor-patient relationship is central to the practice of medicine and is essential for the delivery of high-quality healthcare in the diagnosis and treatment of disease. A patient must have confidence in the competence of their doctor and must feel that they can confide in him or her. For most physicians, the establishment of good rapport with a patient is important. This being said, some medical specialties, such as psychiatry and family medicine, emphasize the doctor-patient relationship more than others, such as pathology or radiology. The doctor-patient relationship forms one of the foundations of contemporary medical ethics. Most medical schools and universities teach medical students from the beginning, even before they set foot in hospitals, to maintain a professional rapport with patients, uphold patients' dignity, and respect their privacy.

With increasing access to computers and published online medical articles, the internet has contributed to expanding patient knowledge of their own health, conditions, and treatment options. Some doctors are fearful of misleading information and being flooded by emails from patients, which take time to read and respond to them.

Perspectives

The four great corner stones of diagnostic medicine are anatomy (structure: what is there), physiology (how the structure/s function), pathology (what goes wrong with the anatomy and physiology) and psychology (mind and behavior). In addition, the physician should consider the patient in their 'well' context rather than simply as a walking medical condition. This means the socio-political context of the patient (family, work, stress, beliefs and other patient's involvement) should be assessed as it often offers vital clues to the patient's condition and further management.

A patient typically presents a set of complaints (the symptoms) to the physician, who then obtains further information about the patient's symptoms, previous state of health, living conditions, and so on and so forth. The physician then makes a review of systems (ROS) or systems inquiry, which is a set of ordered questions about each major body system in order: general (such as weight loss), endocrine, cardio-respiratory, etc. Next comes the actual physical examination and often laboratory tests; the findings are recorded, leading to a list of possible diagnoses. These will be investigated in order of probability.

The next task is to enlist the patient's agreement to a management plan, which will include treatment as well as plans for follow-up. Importantly, during this process the healthcare provider educates the patient about the causes, progression, outcomes, and possible treatments of his ailments, as well as often providing advice for maintaining health. This teaching relationship is the basis of calling the physician doctor [dubious–discuss], which originally meant "teacher" in Latin. The patient-physician relationship is additionally complicated by the patient's suffering (patient derives from the Latin patior, "suffer") and limited ability to relieve it on his/her own. The physician's expertise comes from his knowledge of what is healthy and normal contrasted with knowledge and experience of other people who have suffered similar symptoms (unhealthy and abnormal), and the proven ability to relieve it with medicines (pharmacology) or other therapies about which the patient may initially have little knowledge.

The physician-patient relationship can be analyzed from the perspective of ethical concerns, in terms of how well the goals of non-malfeasance, beneficence, autonomy, and justice are achieved. Many other values and ethical issues can be added to these. In different societies, periods, and cultures, different values may be assigned different priorities. For example, in the last 30 years medical care in the Western World has increasingly emphasized patient autonomy in decision making.

The relationship and process can also be analyzed in terms of social power relationships, or economic transactions. Physicians have been accorded gradually higher status and respect over the last century, and they have been entrusted with control of access to prescription medicines as a public health measure. This represents a concentration of power and carries both advantages and disadvantages to particular kinds of patients with particular kinds of conditions. A further twist has occurred in the last 25 years as costs of medical care have risen, and a third party (an insurance company or government agency) now often insists upon a share of decision-making power for a variety of reasons, reducing freedom of choice of healthcare providers and patients in many ways.

The quality of the patient-physician relationship is important to both parties. The better the relationship in terms of mutual respect, knowledge, trust, shared values and perspectives about disease and life, and time available, the better will be the amount and quality of information about the patient's disease transferred in both directions, enhancing accuracy of diagnosis and increasing the patient's knowledge about the disease. Where such a relationship is poor the physician's ability to make a full assessment is compromised and the patient is more likely to distrust the diagnosis and proposed treatment. In these circumstances and also in cases where there is genuine divergence of medical opinions, a second opinion from another physician may be sought or the patient may choose to go to another doctor.

In some settings, e.g. the hospital ward, the patient-physician relationship is much more complex, and many other people are involved when somebody is ill: relatives, neighbors, rescue specialists, nurses, technical personnel, social workers and others.

In non-Western societies, the physician/patient relationship may be couched in different terms. The illness may be seen as a violation of the spiritual realm and the cure will be seen likewise as having to take place in the spiritual realm. Violation of some spiritual rule can result in illness; persons distant to the patient may have caused illness by maneuver in the spiritual realm, by cursing or causing another practitioner/shaman/healer to place the curse. Powerful faith in these factors can result in serious illness or cure. Spirits can be part of a culture's usual pantheon, ancestor spirits or arbitrary new spirit forces arising independently or as derived from an existing object in the real world: such as an animist spirit coming from a totem animal, mountain or other thing. As in the scientific West, the practitioner is assumed to have special knowledge or power, and is paid by the patient in some form.

Patient Behavior

Behavior may be related to:

- *Physical discomfort*: Illnesses or medication.
- *Overstimulation*: Loud noises or a busy environment.

- *Un-familiar surroundings*: New places or the inability to recognize home.
- *Complicated tasks*: Difficulty with activities or chores.
- *Frustrating interactions*: Inability to communicate effectively.

Aggression

Aggressive behaviors may be verbal (shouting, name-calling) or physical (hitting, pushing). These behaviors can occur suddenly, with no apparent reason, or can result from a frustrating situation. Whatever the case, it is important to try to understand what is causing the person to become angry or upset.

How to Respond

Try to identify the immediate cause. Think about what happened right before the reaction that may have triggered the behavior. Focus on feelings, not facts. Try not to concentrate on specific details; rather, consider the person's emotions. Look for the feelings behind the words.

Do not get angry or upset and be positive and reassuring. Speak slowly in a soft tone. Limit distractions examine the person's surroundings, and adapt them to avoid other similar situations. Try a relaxing activity. Use music, massage or exercise to help soothe the person. Shift the focus to another activity. The immediate situation or activity may have unintentionally caused the aggressive response. Try something different.

Anxiety or Agitation

A person may feel anxious or agitated. He or she may become restless and need to move around or pace. Or the person may become upset in certain places or focused on specific details. He or she may also become over-reliant on a certain caregiver for attention and direction.

How to Respond

Listen to the frustration. Find out what may be causing the anxiety, and try to understand. Provide reassurance. Use calming phrases. Let the individual know you're there for him or her. Involve the person in activities. Try using art, music or other activities to help the person relax. Modifying the environment decrease noise and distractions, or move to another place. Find outlets for the person's energy. He or she may be looking for something to do. Take a walk, or go for a car ride.

Confusion

The person may not recognize familiar people, places or things. He or she may forget relationships, call family members by other names or become confused about where home is. The person may also forget the purpose of common items, such as a pen or fork. These situations are extremely difficult for caregivers and require much patience and understanding.

How to Respond

Stay calm, although being called by a different name or not being recognized can be painful, try not to make your hurt apparent. Respond with a brief explanation. Do not overwhelm the person with lengthy statements and reasons. Instead, clarify with a simple explanation. Show photos and other reminders. Use photographs and other thought-provoking items to remind the person of important relationships and places. Offer corrections as suggestions continue to be appreciated.

Engage the Person in an Activity

The individual may simply be bored and need something to do. Provide structure and engage the person in a pleasant activity. Use memory aids. If the person asks the same questions over and over again, offer reminders by using notes, clocks, calendars or photographs, if these items are still meaningful to the individual. Accept the behavior, and work with it if it isn't harmful, let it be. Find ways to work with it.

10 quick tips: Responding to behaviors:

1. Remain flexible, patient and calm
2. Respond to the emotion, not the behavior
3. Do not argue or try to convince
4. Use memory aids
5. Acknowledge requests, and respond to them
6. Look for the reasons behind each behavior
7. Consult a physician to identify any causes related to medications or illness
8. Explore various solutions
9. Do not take the behavior personally
10. Share your experiences with others

Patient Depression

Depression is an important factor in suicide between both adolescents and the elderly but those with late onset of depression are at a higher risk. Recent advances in the treatment of depression are very relevant for suicide prevention in primary care. Education of the general practitioner in identifying and treating depression was found to reduce suicide risk among the depressed. The full therapeutic dose of medication should be continued for several months. In the elderly it may be necessary to continue treatment for two years after recovery. Patients on regular lithium maintenance therapy have been found to have lower suicide risk.

Mood disorders: All types of mood disorders have been associated with suicide. These include bipolar affective disorder, depressive episode, recurrent depressive disorder and persistent mood disorders (e.g. cyclothymia and dysthymia), suicide is therefore a significant risk in unrecognized and untreated depression. Depression has a high prevalence in the general population and is not recognized by many as a disease. It is estimated that 30% of patients seen by a physician are suffering from depression. Roughly 60% of those who do seek treatment initially contact a general practitioner. It is a special challenge for the physician to work with both physical disease and psychological disorders simultaneously. In many instances, depression is masked and patients present only with somatic complaints.

In typical depressive episodes, the individual usually suffers from:
- Depressed mood (sadness)
- Loss of interest and enjoyment
- Reduced energy (fatigability and diminished activity).

Common presenting symptoms of depression are:
- Tiredness
- Sadness
- Lack of concentration
- Anxiety
- Irritability
- Sleep disturbances
- Pain in different parts of the body.

These symptoms should alert the physician to the presence of depression and lead to an assessment of the suicide risk. Specific clinical features associated with increased risk of suicide in depression are:
- Persistent insomnia
- Self-neglect
- Severe illness (particularly psychotic depression). Collaborating with the psychiatrist and ensuring that adequate and appropriate treatment is given is a crucial function of the physician.

In typical depressive episodes, the individual usually suffers from:
- Depressed mood (sadness)
- Loss of interest and enjoyment
- Reduced energy (fatigability and diminished activity)
- Impaired memory
- Agitation
- Panic attacks.

The following factors increase the risk of suicide in people with depression:
- Age below 25 years in men
- Early phase of the illness
- Abuse of alcohol
- Depressed phase of a bipolar disorder
- Mixed (manic-depressive) state
- Psychotic mania.

Alcoholism

Alcoholism (both alcohol abuse and dependence on alcohol) is a frequent diagnosis in those who have committed suicide, particularly in young people. There are biological, psychological and social explanations for the correlation between suicide and alcoholism.

Specific factors associated with increased suicide risk among alcoholics are:
- Early onset of alcoholism
- Long history of drinking
- High level of dependence
- Depressed mood
- Poor physical health
- Poor work performance
- Family history of alcoholism
- Recent disruption or loss of a major interpersonal relationship.

PATIENT SUICIDE

One of the worst things a physician has to face is the suicide of a patient. The common reactions experienced by physicians who have gone through such an event are disbelief, loss of confidence, anger and shame. The suicide of a patient can trigger feelings of professional inadequacy, doubts about one's competence and fear for one's reputation. In addition, physicians confront the enormous difficulty of dealing with the family and friends of the deceased.

These resources are intended primarily for general physicians. Their objectives are to outline the main disorders and other factors associated with suicide, and to provide information on the identification and management of suicidal patients.

The psychological and social impact of suicide on the family and society is immeasurable. On average, single suicide intimately affects at least six other people. If a suicide occurs in a school or workplace it has an impact on hundreds of people.

However, a substantial proportion of people who commit suicide die without having seen a mental health professional. Hence improved detection, referral and management of psychiatric disorders in primary care is an important step in suicide prevention. A common finding in those who commit suicide is the presence of more than one disorder. The common disorders occurring together are alcoholism and mood disorder (i.e. depression), and personality disorder and other psychiatric disorders.

Suicide is the largest single cause of premature death among schizophrenics. Specific risk factors for suicide are:

- Young unemployed male
- Recurrent relapses
- Fear of deterioration, especially in those of high intellectual ability
- Positive symptoms of suspiciousness and delusions.

Depressive Symptoms

The suicide risk is highest at the following times:

- Early stages of the illness
- Early relapse
- Early recovery.

Suicide risk decreases with increasing duration of the illness.

Personality disorders: Recent studies on young people who committed suicide have shown a high prevalence (20–50%) of personality disorders. The personality disorders that are more frequently associated with suicide are borderline personality and antisocial personality disorders. Histrionic and narcissistic personality disorders and certain psychological traits such as impulsivity and aggression have also been associated with suicide.

Anxiety disorders: Among anxiety disorders, panic disorder has been most frequently associated with suicide, followed by obsessive-compulsive disorder (OCD). Somatoform disorder and eating disorders (anorexia nervosa and bulimia) are also related to suicidal behavior.

Suicide and physical disorder: Suicide risk is increased in chronic physical illness. In addition, there is generally an increased rate of psychiatric disorder, especially depression, in people with physical illness. Chronicity, disability and negative prognosis are correlated with suicide.

Marital status: Divorced, widowed and single people are at increased risk of suicide. Marriage appears to be protective for males in terms of suicide risk but not significantly so for females. Marital separation and living alone increase the risk of suicide.

Occupation: Certain occupational groups such as veterinary surgeons, pharmacists, dentists, farmers and medical practitioners have a higher risk of suicide. There is no obvious explanation for this finding, though access to lethal means, work pressure, social isolation and financial difficulties might be the reasons.

Unemployment: There are fairly strong associations between unemployment rates and suicide rates, but the nature of these associations is complex. The effects of unemployment are probably mediated by factors such as poverty, social deprivation, domestic difficulties and hopelessness. On the other hand, people with mental disorders are more likely to be unemployed than people in good mental health. At any rate, due consideration should be given to the difference in the significance of recent loss of employment and long-term unemployment: greater risk is associated with the former.

Rural/urban residence: In some countries suicides are more frequent in urban areas, whereas in others they occur more frequently in rural areas.

How to identify patients at high risk of suicidal behavior: A number of clinically useful individual and socio-demographic factors are associated with suicide. They include:

- Psychiatric disorders (generally depression, alcoholism and personality disorders)
- Physical illness (terminal, painful or debilitating illness, AIDS)
- Previous suicide attempts
- Family history of suicide, alcoholism and/or other psychiatric disorders
- Divorced, widowed or single status
- Living alone (socially isolated)
- Unemployed or retired
- Bereavement in childhood.

If the patient is under psychiatric treatment, the risk is higher in:

- Those who have recently been discharged from hospital
- Those who have made previous suicide attempts.

In addition, recent life stressors associated with increased risk of suicide include:

- Marital separation
- Bereavement
- Family disturbances
- Change in occupational or financial status
- Rejection by a significant person
- Shame and threat of being found guilty.

There are various scales to assess suicide risk in surveys, but they are less useful than a good clinical interview in identifying the individual who is at immediate risk of committing suicide.

The physician may be confronted with a variety of conditions and situations associated with suicidal behavior. An elderly male, recently widowed, treated for depression, living alone, with a history of attempted suicide, and a young lady with a few scratches on the forearm whose boyfriend has left her are two contrasting examples. In reality, most patients fall between those two extremes and they may fluctuate from one category to the other.

When physicians have a reasonable indication that the patient could be suicidal, they face the dilemma of how to proceed. Some physicians are uncomfortable with suicidal patients. It is important for them to be aware of that feeling and to seek help from colleagues, and possibly mental health professionals, when confronted with such patients. It is essential not to ignore or deny the risk.

Management of Suicidal Patients

If a patient is emotionally disturbed, with vague suicidal thoughts, the opportunity of ventilating thoughts and feelings to a physician who shows concern may be sufficient. Nevertheless, an opportunity for further follow-up should be left open, particularly if the patient has inadequate social support. Whatever the problem, the feelings of the suicidal person are usually a triad of helplessness, hopelessness and despair. The three most common states are:

1. Ambivalence. The majority of suicidal patients are ambivalent till the very end. There is a see-saw battle between the wish to live and the wish to die. If the ambivalence is used by the physician to increase the wish to live, the suicide risk may be reduced.

2. Impulsivity. Suicide is an impulsive phenomenon and impulse by its very nature is transient. If support is provided at the moment of impulse, the crisis may be defused.
3. Rigidity. Suicidal people are constricted in their thinking, mood and action and their reasoning is dichotomized in terms of either/or. By exploring several possible alternatives to death with the suicidal patient, the physician gently makes the patient realize that there are other options, even if they are not ideal.

Enlisting Support

The physician should assess the available support systems, identify a relative, friend, acquaintance or other person who would be supportive to the patient, and solicit that person's help. Entering into a "no suicide" contract is a useful technique in suicide prevention. Other people close to the patient can be included in negotiating the contract. The negotiation of the contract can promote discussion of various relevant issues. In the majority of instances patients respect the promises they give to a physician. Contracting is appropriate only when patients have control over their actions. In the absence of severe psychiatric disorder or suicidal intent, the physician can initiate and arrange pharmacological treatment, generally with antidepressants, an psychological (cognitive behavior) therapy. The majority of people benefit from continuing contacts; these should be structured to meet individual needs.

Except for the treatment of underlying diseases, few persons require support for longer than two or three months and the focus of the support should be providing hope, encouraging independence, and helping the patient to learn different ways of coping with life stressors.

Referral to Specialist Care

Patients should be referred to a psychiatrist when they have:

- A psychiatric disorder
- A history of a previous suicide attempt
- A family history of suicide, alcoholism and psychiatric disorder
- Physical ill-health
- No social support.

How to refer?

After deciding to refer a patient, the physician should:

- Take the time to explain to the patient the reason for the referral
- Allay anxiety about stigma and about psychotropic medication
- Make clear that pharmacological and psychological therapies are effective

- Emphasize that referral does not mean "abandonment"
- Arrange an appointment with the psychiatrist
- Allocate a time for the patient after his or her appointment with the psychiatrist
- Ensure that the relationship with the patient continues.

When to hospitalize a patient?

These are some of the indications for immediate hospitalization:

- Recurrent thoughts of suicide
- High level of intent to die in the immediate future (the next few hours or days)
- Agitation or panic
- Existence of a plan to use a violent and immediate method.

How to hospitalize the patient?

- Do not leave the patient alone
- Arrange for hospitalization
- Arrange for transfer to the hospital by ambulance or the police
- Inform the concerned authorities and family.

22 Patient Safety and Satisfaction

INTRODUCTION

The healthcare is a great challenge to all healthcare organizers and providers in view of wide range of patient safety problems worldwide. Patient safety is now recognized as a priority for any health-care system seeking to assure and improve the quality of patient care. All patients have a right to effective, safe care at all times.

The earliest record of this problem dates from the 17th century BC. The response in those days was clearly and solely punitive for example, cutting off a surgeon's hand. Today's solutions for improving patient safety offer a more constructive approach; one in which safe care is determined by how well caregivers work together as a team, how effectively communicate with one another and with patients, and how carefully the overall patient care plan is designed and executed.

The healthcare policy makers are reforming to improve quality and practice that are known to be unsafe or wasteful to be eliminated. Similarly, patients and their families are becoming increasingly experienced in accessing information to make personal health care decisions about treatments and their choice of providers, and demanding safer care as well. Healthcare providers are also becoming more proficient at incorporating evidence-based knowledge into their clinical decision-making practices by using information technology as a source of support.

BACKGROUND INFORMATION ON ADVERSE OUTCOMES

Studies of adverse outcomes and harm to patients have been carried out for many years. As far back as 1850, Hungarian physician Ignaz Sommeliers linked transmission of infections to poor hand hygiene, but failed to persuade his colleagues to alter their behavior. In the USA at the beginning of the 20th century, Ernest Codman, a Boston surgeon, argued for the routine assessment of outcomes. The Confidential Enquiry into

Maternal Deaths in the UK dates from 1952. Many other examples could be given of isolated studies into errors and iatrogenic effects of drugs and other effects. But it was not until the 1970s that any attempt was made to provide an overview of the scale of harm and adverse outcomes. In 1977, the California medical insurance feasibility study suggested that almost 4% of patients admitted to hospital suffered some kind of adverse event. Ivan Illich's critique Limits to medicine: medical nemesis, the expropriation of health went so far as to argue that health care was in fact a major threat to health.

DEFINITION OF PATIENT SAFETY

The patient safety can be defined "as the condition of being safe, freedom from danger or hazard or risk or injury and adverse effects, exemption from hurt, or loss. Freedom from whatever exposes one to danger or from liability to cause harm, or loss, hence the quality of making safe or secure or giving confidence, justifying trust, insuring against harm or loss etc., happening to a patient as part of systematic relevance of data obtained from incident reports, from any healthcare organization and learning from near miss and adverse events to facilitate in either eradicate or minimize the adverse outcome is called patient safety".

WHERE THE SAFETY OF PATIENT IS AFFECTED?

The health sector is a high-risk area because of adverse events, arising from treatment rather than disease, can lead to death, serious damage, complications and patient suffering. Current data show that almost half of all preventable adverse events are a consequence of medication errors. Most of the current evidence on adverse events comes from hospitals, because the risks associated with hospital care are high, but many adverse events also occur in other health-care settings, such as physicians' offices, nursing homes, pharmacies and patients' homes.

WHY THE PATIENT SAFETY IS AFFECTED?

Today's health-care context is highly complex and care is often delivered in a pressurized and fast-moving environment, involving a vast array of technology and, daily, many individual decisions and judgments by health-care professional staff. In such circumstances, probability of making mistakes or things could go wrong. Sometimes, unintentional harm comes to a patient during a clinical procedure or as a result of a clinical decision. Errors in the process of care can result in injury or permanent disability and sometimes death.

Patient safety is affected by inadequate information, illegible entries lack or change of information, misinterpretations, and in sufficient interoperability. Continuity of care is badly affected by the lack of shareable information among patient care providers. Healthcare economics are adversely affected with information capture and report generation costs, currently estimated to be well over $50 billion annually in USA. Public safety a major component of public health is administered by the inability to collect information in a coordinated, timely manner at the provider level in response to epidemics and threat of terrorism. Clinical research and outcomes analysis is adversely affected by a lack of uniform information capture that is needed to facilitate the derivation of data from routine patient care documentation (MRI, 2004b, p. 2).

Matter of fact, the safety of a person is affected from the time; the person becomes ill or injured, the way he was dealt with taking to appropriate physician, or hospital and then, the treatment in the healthcare institution. Major safety issues that occur; in collection of patient identification data, collection of history and physical examination, request and process of investigations, diagnosis, and treatment including surgical procedures coupled with institutional environmental, infrastructure and human errors. In every level of patient, every point in the process of specimen collection, analysis, or investigation process, care giving contributes a certain inherent lack of safety, side-effects of drugs or drug combinations, hazards posed by a medical device, substandard or faulty products entering the health service, human shortcomings, or system failures.

Adverse events may therefore, result from problems in practice, products, procedures or systems. Immunization, which is given to healthy individuals, poses a particular challenge. The prime responsibility for adverse events on deficiencies in system could be designed, organized and operation rather than on individual providers or individual products. Adverse drug events in the Utah-Colorado Study in the USA provide a dramatic example, 75% of them being attributable to system failures. Similarly, most adverse events are not the result of negligence or lack of training, but rather occur because of latent causes within systems. For example:

Airway fires during surgery: Airway surgeries that involve ignition sources to cut or coagulate tissue (e.g., electrosurgical units, lasers) pose a significant and sometimes deadly risk of fire. Hazards exist when these ignition sources are used in the oxygen-enriched atmospheres (i.e. atmospheres containing more than 23% oxygen [O_2]) that are commonly present in the airway during surgery.

What's new in MRI Hazards? Two issues have recently come to light concerning magnetic resonance imaging (MRI) hazards. The US Food and Drug Administration (FDA) have received reports of patients with second and third degree burns on skin under electrocardiogram (EKG) electrodes attached to cables. These burns were noted after the patients underwent MRI. Some burns were serious enough to require plastic surgery.

RAISING RATE OF LITIGATION AND FINANCE

The rising rate of litigation in the seventies and eighties was another important stimulus to raising awareness of the problem of patient safety. In the USA and later elsewhere, this led to the development of risk-management programmers. Initially, these had an almost exclusively legal and financial focus, aimed at protecting the institutions concerned; they gradually evolved to tackle clinical issues and act as a gateway to the underlying problem of patient safety.

The financial cost of adverse events, in terms of additional treatment and extra days in hospital, is vastly greater than the costs of litigation. In the UK the cost of preventable adverse events is estimated to be £ 1000 million per annum in lost bed days alone. The wider costs of lost working time, disability benefits and the wider economic consequences are greater still. There is also an enormous human cost; as well many patients suffer increased pain.

STUDIES ON PATIENT SAFETY

The Harvard study found that patients were unintentionally harmed by treatment in almost 4% of hospital admissions in New York State. For 70% of these patients the resulting disability was slight or temporary, but in 7% it was permanent and 14% of these patients died, partly as a result of their treatment. Serious harm, therefore, came to about 1% of patients admitted to hospital. Similar findings were reported from Colorado and Utah. A parallel Australian study found a 16.6% adverse events rate, where about half the cases were judged preventable, but with a similar number of serious incidents to that in the USA studies. In the UK a review of patient records indicated a 10.8% adverse events rate, again about half being preventable. Findings in Denmark, New Zealand and Canada also suggest a relatively high rate of adverse events around 10%.

Risk factors for falls: A case control study of patient, medication, and care-related risk factors for inpatient falls was aimed at identifying risk factors in an acute in-patient hospital. In US, patient falls are among the most common adverse events reported in hospitalized patients, and have been attributed to many factors including trauma, debilitating disease, environmental hazards, age, mental status, length of hospital stay and gender.

The Problem of Patient Safety

Various studies have investigated the extent of adverse events. The Institute of Medicine (IOM) report estimated that "medical errors" cause between 44,000 and 98,000 deaths annually in hospitals in the USA—more than car accidents, breast cancer or AIDS. The UK Department of Health, in its 2000 reported, an organization with a memory, estimated that adverse events occur in around 10% of hospital admissions or about 850,000 adverse events a year. The Quality in Australian Health Care Study (QAHCS), released in 1995, found an adverse-event rate of 16.6% among hospital patients. The Hospitals for Europe's Working Party on Quality Care in Hospitals estimated, in 2000, that every tenth patient in hospitals in Europe suffers from preventable harm and adverse effects related to his or her care. The New Zealand and Canadian studies have also suggested relatively high rates of adverse events: around 10%.

World Health Organization (WHO) figures suggest that developing countries account for around 77% of all reported cases of counterfeit and substandard drugs. It is also reported that at least half of all medical equipment in most of these countries is unusable or only partly usable, at any given time, resulting in neglect of patients or increased risk of harm to them and to health workers. In the European countries that have achieved independence in recent years, about 40% of hospital beds are reported to be located in structures originally built for other purposes. Studies have shown that illegible prescriptions, unconfirmed verbal orders, unanswered telephone calls, and lost medical records can all place patients at risk. The problem with poor quality data is not limited to the patient medical record or other data collected and used at the organizational level, but also across organizations and throughout the overall healthcare environment.

TOOLS DESIGN TO PREVENT ERRORS AND ADVERSE EVENTS

The health sector should be designed in a way to capture instantly and the errors and adverse events are prevented, detected or contained so that serious errors are avoided and compliance with safety procedures is enhanced to establish a culture of patient safety throughout the entire health system. Risk management must be introduced as a routine instrument within the running of the entire health sector. A precondition for risk management is an open and trusting working environment with a culture that focuses on learning from near misses and adverse events as opposed to concentrating on "blame and shame" and subsequent punishment.

HOW IT CAN HELP IN PREVENTING ADVERSE EFFECT?

The information technology (IT) plays a vital role in reducing the errors, improving care coordination, enhancing efficiency, dipping duplication, and increasing the amount of time dedicated to direct patient care. Clinical information systems can have a profound impact on patient quality, outcome and safety. Several studies have shown that physicians who had access to clinical practice guidelines and features such as computerized reminders and alerts were far more likely to provide preventive care than were physicians who did not.

A recent report by Bates and Gawande (2003) states that information technology can reduce the rate of medial errors by (i) preventing errors and adverse effects, (ii) facilitating a more rapid response after an adverse events has occurred, and (iii) tracking and providing feedback about adverse effect. Likewise, electronic medical record (EMR)-type systems can improve communication, make knowledge more readily available, required key pieces of information (such as the dose of the drug), assist with calculations, perform checks in real time, assist with monitoring and provide decision support. If effectively incorporated into the care process, of all these features have the potential to improve quality, outcomes, and patient safety. One controlled trial involving hospital inpatients reported a 55 percent reduction in serious medication administration errors following the introduction of Computerized Physician Order Entry (CPOE) system (Bates et al. 1998).

CPOE applications have the opportunity to significantly aid the clinician's decision-making process. Examples of features of CPOE that assist the clinician include providing access to relevant patient data and medical reference information, assuring that the order is specified completely and correctly, performing calculations flawlessly, communicating with other systems in a reliable and timely manner, and providing alerts and reminders that guide the physician through the ordering process. Studies of Errors in medicine have found that the root causes of the majority of problems (e.g., lack of access to patient data, lack of access to knowledge resources, ordering the wrong drug for a given condition or a drug to which the patient is allergic) can be mitigated with CPOE.

Bar codes: In 2003, Federal Drug Administration, (FDA) proposed drug bar code regulations to help reduce medical errors related to prescriptions and medication administration. These regulations would standardize and require the use of bar codes on prescription drugs, over-the-counter drugs packaged for hospital use, and vaccines. The final rule covers blood and blood components. American National Standards Institute (ANSI) has given the Health Industry Business Communications Council (HIBCC) accreditation as the Standard Development Organization (SDO) for bar codes used for human drug products and blood.

Interaction and allergy flags: The biggest improvement in patient safety is when the system flags a drug interaction or allergy," Dr Davis said, "And not just in one practice, but the information is available to all providers in Winona's health community." Patient safety is not just an American health issue. In Italy, the Instituto Nazionale Tumori developed a short questionnaire that patient receive on their mobile phones and fill out based on symptoms such as weight loss, shortness of breath, and sleep loss. This system helps physicians monitor patients with chronic conditions, rather than having them come into the office for monthly checkups.

Patient safety and quality of care standards: In the absence of definitive international standards for patient safety and quality of care; healthcare associations and agencies in the US have developed an array of measures, including quality indicators, datasets, guidelines, and barcodes.

Information is as critical to the providing of safe health care-care that is free of errors of both commission and omission to develop a treatment plan, a doctor must have access to complete patient information (e.g. diagnoses, medications, current test results, and available social supports) and to the most current science base. Errors of commission, such as; prescribing medication that has a potentially fatal interaction with another medication the patients taking. The authors argue that errors of omission are equally important. An example of omission: failing to prescribe a medication from which the patient would likely have benefited [Institute of Medicine (IOM), Committee on Data Standards for Patient Safety, 2004].

Implementation rates, in the inpatient setting, for advanced functionality such as computerized physician order entry (CPOE), clinical decision support systems, and multidisciplinary documentation remains at less than 10%. The Leapfrog Group, an organization composed of employers and other purchasers of health care focused on patient safety and quality indicates that only 4% of hospitals have fully implemented CPOE. CPOE is seen by many as a key element in improving patient safety and quality of care and thus has been a substantial target for many in the industry. For successful CPOE, a partial electronic health record system (EHRS) is a key foundational element.

PATIENT SAFETY SOLUTIONS

"Patient Safety Solution" is defined as: any system design or intervention that has demonstrated the ability to prevent or mitigate patient harm stemming from the processes of health care. In order to observe ensure the following:

- To establish well planned policies, standards and procedures governing the healthcare system that encompasses healthcare safety measures as a must.
- To collaborate between healthcare providers and health professionals at enhancing patient safety at all level during the entire period of care.
- To prioritize patient safety as the main motto of the health institution
- To provide suitable infrastructure with competent healthcare providers and required equipment.
- To create leadership with research facilities exclusively for safety measures.
- To create a friendly situation and mechanism for not happening the adverse events and reporting systems for effective prevention.
- To develop quality and risk management units to improve quality of care including patient safety with cost containment.
- To initiate a system that patients/relatives are made aware of safety measures in collaboration between patients/relatives and health care professionals.
- To implement electronic health records with CPOE and Clinical Decision Support (CDS) support system.
- To facilitate employees training on using of medical devices, tools and appliances manufacturers for safe use of new medical technology and surgical techniques.

SUMMARY

This report presents a consumer recommendations of an international expert panel on indicators for patient safety using structured review process the panel set out to select indicators to cover the five key areas; are as hospital acquired infections, sentinel events, operative and post operative complications, obstetrics, and other care related adverse events. This report proposes 21 indicators as follows:

Area	*Indicator*
Hospital-acquired infection	Ventilator pneumonia
	Wound infection
	Infection due to medical care
	Decubitus ulcer
Operative and post-operative complications	Post-operative pulmonary embolism (PE) or deep vein thrombosis (VDT)
	Post-operative sepsis
	Complications of anesthesia
	Technical difficulty with procedure
Sentinel events	Transfusion reaction
	Wrong blood type
	Wrong site surgery
	Foreign body left in during procedure
	Medical equipment-related adverse events
	Medication errors
Obstetrics	Birth trauma–injury to neonate
	Obstetric trauma–cesarean section
	Obstetric-trauma–vaginal delivery
	Problems with child birth
Other care related adverse events	Patient falls
	In-hospital hip fracture
Change	Change of investigations, medications, diagnosis
	Patient records, site of procedure, organ
	Mother and child, treatment, doctor
	Acquire burns, removal or wounding parts
Increased litigations, overstay	> Number of litigations and > Stay of patients
Financial burden	To care providers and care receivers
The report describes the review process and provides a detailed discussion of scientific soundness and policy importance of the 21 indicators.	

Patient safety is affected by inadequate information; illegible entries lack or change of information, misinterpretations, and in sufficient interoperability and continuity of care is badly affected by the lack of shareable information among patient care providers. Some of major patient safety problems are: medication errors, hospital acquired infections, transfusion reactions, wrong blood type, wrong site surgery, obstetric and birth trauma, anesthesia and post-operative complications, patient falls and in-hospital hip fractures, hospital acquired burns, change of investigations, diagnosis, medications, change of mother and child, change of site procedure and organ.

The IT plays a vital role in reducing the errors, improving care coordination, enhancing efficiency, reducing duplication, and increasing the amount of time dedicated to direct patient care. Clinical information systems can have a profound impact on patient quality, outcome and safety. Several studies have shown that physicians who had access to clinical practice guidelines and features such as computerized reminders and alerts were far more likely to provide preventive care than were physicians who did not.

PATIENT SATISFACTION

The goal of any service organization is to create satisfaction among the customers. There is a famous theory, which says that man wanting animal and his motives go on changing. The fulfilled motive no longer remains a motive; once one's needs are fulfilled the other takes place. The concept of patient satisfaction is rapidly changing to customer's delight which means the patient is not only to be cured of his ailments during the hospital stay but is also pleased with the amenities provided to him by the hospital and its staff during the stay, which he fondly remembers after being discharged. The hospital manpower does play a very important role in patient satisfaction.

The hospital is a complex institution and every person involved directly or indirectly in rendering services that is vital for the patient. The modern treatment based on advance technology and special expertise, which is not only expensive but is full of complexities. Therefore patient satisfaction has a special consideration in treatment. There is no specific tool by which one can gauge quality of services in healthcare field; nevertheless, the level of satisfaction of patient about the hospital services can be considered an important tool of quality services provided. The patients satisfaction is an increasing assessing tool for measurement of quality of services and this can be used a positive feedback methodically to choose between alternative methods for planning, organizing and providing health care to the masses.

RELATIONSHIP WITH THE CARE AND PATIENT SATISFACTION

In order to assess the relationship with the care and patient satisfaction and the Data to test the relative importance of these types of determinants were collected in a general household survey of 400 persons. The patient satisfaction scale developed and tested using non-metric multidimensional scaling was used. Multiple regression analysis was performed on the data. Results show that certain pre-dispositional factors (confidence in the community's medical care system, having a regular source of care, and being satisfied with life in general) are more important predictors of patient satisfaction than patient's age, sex, race, educational attainment, or income.

PATIENT EXPERIENCE WITH CARING HOSPITAL TEAM

Organizations around the world strive to deliver the best clinical, physical and emotional experience to patients and families to deliver with empathy and innovation to demonstrate the care provided is not only comprehensive but with patient centered empathy. How patient experience is evolving from satisfaction surveys into thread throughout quality, safety, access and value. Hospital patient care providers including medical, nursing, and allied healthcare workers, need to know the following:

It is important to ask yourself what is the problem you're actually trying to solve to meet your professional goals. If we evidently understand how patients' feel about their experience in real-time changes and improvements can happen much more frequently and correctly. In real sense, the nursing staffs that are closely activated and engaged with the patient in transforming and sustaining patient experience are real informers of patient satisfaction. In many situations, it is Nursing staff that takes the lead in patient experience that can help in creating a true care coordination model culture in which the medical home should be brought into the hospital, thereby; the patient never likes to be discharged. In order to happen this, we must be tireless in our efforts to advocate for care outside the hospital e.g., ambulatory care or outpatient settings.

Empathy is a vital ingredient in patient care process, it is not being soft, one has to understand customer's needs and application of empathy is a top priority. Hospitals and medical, nursing and other staff are always endeavoring to save the patient's life from disability or death. Empathy was always given a back seat due to limited time of doctors to see more patients, but this could result in bad feeling of patients towards physicians and could lead to bad decision-making in overall care of patient. Where empathy was given priority, have clearly demonstrated that it lead to better outcomes experienced by both care providers and patients. Another most important measure considered to be communication which is the most required common medical practice and procedure, that appears to be small personal connections but makes a significant difference from patient care and satisfaction point of view. The communication gap has to be minimized between what matters to the patient and what doctor thinks patient wants is going. As part of empathy, the doctor has to communicate that he is human first, then a doctor to render possible best care. In doing this, the physician has to be closely associated with patient's needs.

The conventional methods of taking care of patients was measured by the professionals with hard work and good brand, now with global competition is driven by meeting the needs of patient comprehensively.

Empathy is the single biggest missing ingredient in the healthcare space. Take a moment to embrace the emotional impact of what we will do! Empathy is a vital component in the design and execution of healthcare process. Better design can lead to better healthcare outcome. Humanist design can make the patient care provider and the receivers experience is much superior and better. Empathy is the nucleus of healthcare and leads directly to achieving the triple aim; better health, better care and lower cost- humanism in medicine. Success comes from the ability to work together, share best practices and challenge each other. Patients have a right to define their level of engagement in their own treatment. It is refreshing to see physician so engaged in patient experience. Matter of fact, the endeavor of healthcare institution and the staff should be patient good overall experience rather than just patient satisfaction. In the present context, general people have great experience with digital gadgets, and patients are no exception. Therefore, your principal goal to benchmark against patient's expectations instead of comparing with other cares providers.

Patient care is more than just healing- but it is building connection that encompasses mind, body and soul. Empathy is the ability to imagine oneself in another's place and to communicate that understanding back to with the objective.

Recognize care providers (care providers are physicians, nurses, social workers, nurse practitioners, physician assistants) and healthcare professionals, front office staff, social workers, team etc.) who consistently demonstrate an exceptional ability to communicate empathy consistently.

- Recognize those who innovate in their role to deliver empathy constantly.
- Understand the importance of the patient's families and loves ones
- Demonstrate curiosity and openness to know the person not just the disease
- Area of innovation in how they bring empathy and compassion to their work group regardless of their role and position
- Empower the patient to learn and cope effectively with his or her environment
- Create new programs encompassing all aspects of patient's needs to serve effectively.

Discover how the hospital developed a successful and evidence-based music therapy program with the support from hospital and nursing staff. Music therapy has demonstrated positive patient outcomes in difficult patient situations. Nursing and patient stories will be shared in addition to information regarding data that was collected.

Cultivating resilience and managing stress and burn out in medical professionals is challenging imperative in the current healthcare climate. High quality patient care requires providers of all disciplines to bring their best expertise and empathetic approaches to the bedside of patient each day. One has to explore how individuals, teams, and institutions can cultivate flexibility by being present, respectful and vulnerable with one another. More than ever, the healthcare arena today, necessitates looking access from a patient perspective. Receiving care, when and where the patient wants it especially when coupled with care coordination, has been shown to drive patient satisfaction and improve outcomes.

Primary care physicians reporting high levels of distress, which is linked to burnout, attrition, and poorer quality of care. The studies made have demonstrated that primary care physicians participating in a Continuing Medical Education (CME) program that focused on self-awareness experienced improved personal well being, including burnout (emotional exhaustion, and fatigue). They also experienced positive changes in empathy and psychological beliefs, both indicators for a patient-centered orientation to medical care that has been associated with the patient centered behaviors, e.g. attending to the patient's experience of illness and its psychological context and promoting patient participation in care. Furthermore, these patients centered behaviors have been associated with improved patient trust, appropriate prescribing, reaction in healthcare disparities and lower healthcare costs.

Though much work has been done by healthcare organizations to prevent patient falls, and many other incidences against the interest of patient and staff, they continue to occur, resulting in injury, disability, and at times death too. Healthcare organizations have to be committed to transform healthcare into high-reliability industry by developing effective solutions to healthcare's most critical safety and quality problems. Patient and families' stories are powerful in inspiring leaders and staff to improve patient experience. Their perspectives provide meaningful and tangible ways that any staff, no matter what position or department, can have a role in providing best care to patients.

FREQUENTLY ASKED QUESTIONS (FAQ)

Transforming care by delivering care with curiosity, communication and compassion, the empathy we convey to our patients, families and to each other create the culture of caring and we continually work toward that goal.

The medical and other professionals involved in healing the suffering patients is not just about fixing, it is serving ones heart and state of mind is essential to a patient's recovery by embracing and promoting well-being through complementary practice. In every stage of patient care process, it is necessary to understand and hear the perception of the care that they received. As medical and nursing team would be doing many activities related to improving the patient's condition, (status), and patient do not understand how these staff are connected with care delivery system, but timely communication with patient, the process of care will make patient feel much better and healing would be much faster.

COMMUNICATION SKILLS

Relationship centered communication skills are essential in healthcare maintaining process that in turn gives the confidence and satisfaction to healthcare provider. Effective communication impacts patient safety, provider liability, and quality and is at a more basic level, the right thing to do. Hence, the medical colleges, nursing colleges and allied health sciences institutes have to introduce relationship-centered communication knowledge and skills in their program of application of practice.

This course is grounded in educational theory, evidence-based best practices and experiential learning. Effective teaching of communication skills has not been consistently included either in the medical teaching curriculum or continuing medical education courses. It is high time to incorporate in the medical, nursing and other allied health science fields that has been discussed in the aforesaid paragraphs for the benefit of future students to provide comprehensive and satisfactory care.

Various creative methods, including improve action methods, and dynamic small group facilitation, will get everyone out of their seats and into a safe space to practice this and superbly difficult work of communicating effectively. The goal for the course is generate awareness of impersonal and communication skills that clinicians already possesses, and to practice additional skills that can enhance their ability to build meaningful connections with objective to accomplish the following:

- Review the evidence on the value of effective communication skills in healthcare
- Establish rapport and plan an encounter with the patient and their family members
- Elicit the patient prospective using different tools and methods
- Apply a variety of methods to convey empathy
- Incorporate the patient into decision-making and education process
- Practice applying these communication skills in challenging clinical classes.

Mental Health at the heart of public health and disease management, David Woodlock Studies have proven that people with mental illness die 25 years earlier than the rest of us. Let us begin to appreciate mental health as a dimension of one's overall health, as opposed to character flow mental deficiency.

THE YOUNG PROFESSIONALS

It is generally observed, that young professionals lack confidence, and may not aware besides just medical care related attention, other issues such as empathy, personal touch, good regularly and timely communication would keep the patient's spirit high. The senior team to lead group with value-based care must be concerted efforts along with all the colleague or team members. This way of practice and care that gets physician's recognition much easily and outcome of care but not by the big titles or being a leader of a team not having good relationship with staff and patients. All our efforts should be revolve around the patients by not only educating them, but making priority goals to help them in recovering swiftly and get back to their normal routine life or work environment. To be more precise, leaving the suffering episode behind and to have normal style of life without any fear.

CONCLUSION

Some of major patient safety problems are: medication errors, hospital acquired infections, transfusion reactions, wrong blood type, wrong site surgery, obstetric and birth trauma, anesthesia and post-operative complications, patient falls and in-hospital hip fractures, hospital acquired burns, change of investigations, diagnosis, medications, change of mother and child, change of site procedure and organ.

Patient safety is a great challenge that needs to be tackled methodically, to ensure as far as possible that patients receive the highest possible quality of care throughout their journey through the healthcare system. It is important to acknowledge that despite our best efforts, medicine will never be a risk-free enterprise. What we must do in our efforts to make the system as safe as possible for patients and staff is to ensure that we have the right checks and balances in place to detect errant practices, identify and re-train clinicians whose competence falls below appropriate standards, provide the means by which to analyze and learn from mistakes when they do occur and develop standards against which to measure the competence of healthcare providers who seek to provide services to the public in clinical work.

As patient satisfaction has been demonstrated to influence certain health-related behaviors (e.g., compliance with medical regimens and use of medical services), research has attempted to identify its key determinants. Although the influence of patient characteristics often has been studied, attention has been focused on socio-demographic characteristics (e.g., age and sex) rather than attitudinal or situational factors (e.g., confidence in the medical care system including the process of services rendered and service providers and their way of providing the care that may predispose one toward satisfaction with care received.

The hospital administrators should be aware of the needs and expectations of the public besides providing conventional and routine patient care. Patient's expectations have gone up and they wanted swift, safe and improved quality and cost contained care without having any hurdles and problems. This necessitated have a virtual feedback of patient and their families satisfaction prior, during and after care in the hospital or healthcare organizations. Another essential measure that plays a significant role in patient's satisfaction is good communication between the patient and provider of health care is vital factor and there should not be any communication gap between the healthcare providers and the patient.

ACKNOWLEDGMENTS

The information furnished in this chapter is a combination of various authors, and to create a significant value to the text content of this chapter 'Patient safety and Satisfaction,' the information related to different authors were mixed up, yet, not losing the individual author's intrinsic value of their presentation. Thus, it has become hard to quote individual reference serial number of authors as specified in the references list. Nonetheless, the author acknowledges the due credit they deserve for their excellent work in the subject concern and profusely thanks for their contribution as vital information in this book title "Hospital Patient Care Relations Coordinator".

BIBLIOGRAPHY

1. Balas, Weingarten, Garb, Blumenthal, Boren & Brown, 2000; Bates, Kuperman, et al. 1999 Kuperman. Teich, Gandhi, & Bates, 2001; Teich, Merchia, Schmiz, Kuperman, Spurr, & Bates, 2000; Ornstein Garr, Jenkins, Rust, & Arnon, 1991).
2. Bates DW, Kuperman GZJ, Jha A, et at. Does the computerized display of charges affect inpatient ancillary test utilization? Arch Intern Med. 1997:157 (21).
3. Blair J, Cohn S. Critical areas of standardization. In: Demetriades JE, Kolodner RM, Christopherson GA, (Eds). Toward HealthPeople. New York: Springer; 2005.
4. Building a Culture of Patient Safety-Report of the Commission on Patient Safety and Quality Assurance-Department of Health and children.
5. California healthcare Foundation. Program would allow physicians to monitor patients via cell phone. iHealthBeat. June 16, 2004. Available at http://ihelthbeat.org.
6. Carolyn P. Hartley et al. "EHRR Implementation"-2005. pp. 22-23.
7. FDA. Bar Code Label Requirements for Human Drug Products and Biological Products; Final Rule. 21 CFR Parts 201, 606, et al. Federal Register. 2004;69(38):p9120ff.
8. Gonzales R. Steiner JF, Lum A, Barrett PH Jr. Decreasing antibiotics in ambulatory practice impact of a multidimensional intervention on the treatment of uncomplicated acute bronchitis in adults. JAMA. 1999; 281(16):1512-19
9. Harold P. Lehmann, et al. Aspects of Electronic Health Record Systems". 2006. pp. 110-11, 115-40, 275-6, 416.
10. HIBACC: Healthcare's B2B Standards Development Organization, Phoenix AZ; HIBCC; 2005. Available at: http://www.hibcc.org/. Accessed December 17, 2005.
11. Karen A Wager, Frances Wickham Lee, John P Glasser published a book Health Care Information System: A Practical Approach for Health Care Management, 3rd edition. Pp 47, 105-106, 119-120 & 126.

12. KLAS Enterprises, CPOE Digest. Orem Utah. February 2003:5.
13. Krauss M, Evanoff B, Hitcho E, et al. A case-control study of patient medication, and care related risk factors for inpatient falls. J Gen Intern Med. 2005; 20:116-122.
14. Leapfrog Group Survey, Press Release November 16, 2004. Available at: http://www.leapfroggroup.or/media/file/Leapfrog. Survey_Release-11-1604.pdf. Accessed December 20.
15. Miller John, et al. «DELSA/ELSA/WD/http(2004)18, Selecting Indicators for Patient Safety at the Health System Level in OECD Countries»
16. Norman DA. The Invisible Computer: Why Good Product Can Fail, the Personal Computer Is So Complex, and Information Appliances Are the Solution. Cambridge, MA: MIT Press; 1999.
17. Overhage JM, Tierrney WM, Zhou XH, McDonald CJ. A randomized trial of "corollary orders" to prevent errors of omission. J Am Med Inform Assoc. 1997;4(5):364-75.
18. Patel VL, Kushniruk AW, Yang S, Yale JF. Impact of a computer-based patient record system on data collection, knowledge organization, and reasoning. J Am Med Inform Assoc. 2000;7(6):569-85.
19. Schoenfeld MH, Compton SJ, Mead RH, et al. Remote monitoring of implantable cardioverter defibrillators: a prospective analysis. Pacing Clin Electrophysiol. 2004;27(6 pt 1):757-63.
20. Tierney WM, Miller ME, McDonald CJ. The effect on test ordering of informing physicians of the charges for outpatient diagnostic tests. N Engl J Med. 1990;322(21):1499-1504.
21. World Alliance for Patient Safety–Forward Programme-2005. pp. 1-5. www.who.int/patietsafety.
22. "Patient Safety Advisory" PA PSRS (Pennsylvania Patient Safety Reporting System) produced by ECRI Institute & ISMP under control to the Patient Safety Authority. 2007;4(1)1-10.
23. "The Joint Commission & Joint Commission International & WHO". WHO Collaboration Center for Patient Safety Solutions; (Preamble-May 2007).

23 Communication Skills

INTRODUCTION

Despite the vast number of devices, methods, and alternatives for communicating information, the telephone remains the most popular means of communication. It allows for communication between two or more persons, and it is the key instrument in initiating telecommunication networks worldwide.

Since the telephone is such an important communication device. It is essential that the secretary use it to its maximum effectiveness and be familiar with its peripheral equipment.

TELEPHONE TECHNIQUES

The secretary is expected to be knowledgeable in the use of the telephone. It is also important to keep up with the constantly expanding and changing services available from the telephone company, as well as the many and varied pieces of equipment that can add to the efficient operation of the business office. The telephone is the most frequently used audio-communication medium in the business world. The dependence upon this instrument has grown so that currently over a billion telephone calls is made daily.

The reputation and goodwill of the employer and the firm may depend upon the secretary's approach and skill in using the telephone. Although most people in our society begin to use the telephone in early childhood, perhaps the majority of them still need to be trained in proper telephone techniques. An impressive way to point out defects in techniques, and one that results in a rapid and desirable change is to make a recording or tape of a telephone conversation. Such a recording emphasizes the faults in telephone techniques and vividly points out areas needing improvement. Many organizations, even though they are efficiently organized, lose customers, money, and goodwill simply because employees answering calls are incoherent, curt, or impolite.

Speaking Clearly and Pleasantly

The caller at the other end of the phone cannot see the person who is talking. This should be remembered at all times, for it means that the caller has no visual image on which to base impressions. The telephone caller's attention is focused entirely upon the audio impressions coming over the wires. If these sounds are jarring or unpleasant, a busy executive may quickly lose patience and discontinue association with the firm in question. On the other hand, a pleasant and understanding voice coming over an inanimate instrument can accomplish wonders. The power of the spoken word can and does exert a great impact upon the listener.

The telephone is not a nuisance instrument designed to interrupt the secretary in the midst of some important or complicated task. It is rather, a vital business communication facility that assists the employee in carrying out duties and responsibilities owed to the employer.

In order to enhance one's telephone personality, it is necessary to inject variety and flexibility into the voice, so as to convey mood and attitude in telephone conversations. These qualities can be obtained through pitch, inflection, and emphasis. The development of these qualities is individual. A high-pitched voice may convey an impression of childishness and immaturity or of impatience and irritability. On the other hand, a voice that is well modulated carries the impression of culture and polish. "Pitch" in speaking, like "pitch" in music, refers to the key in which one speaks. Everyone has a range of lone within which a pleasant speaking voice is possible, and it can be consciously controlled. Each person must be conscious of his or her own range and practice utilizing it effectively. An individual is said to speak in a "modulated" voice when the pitch is in the lower half of the possible range. This tonal range carries best and is easiest to hear over the telephone.

In cultivating an interesting individual telephone personality, voice development alone is insufficient; it is essential also that the speaker enunciate clearly and distinctly. A garbled and indistinct speech pattern will annoy the listener who cannot understand what is being said. Do not be afraid to move the lips. One cannot form rounded vowel sounds or distinct consonants unless the lips accomplish their function. It is not necessary to exaggerate or to become stilted; clear enunciation and pronunciation should be made a part of the secretary's natural, daily speech pattern, because it is just as important in face-to-face conversations as in telephone conversations. Above all, be sure that your voice reflects your personality, that it transmits alertness and pleasantness, and that it is natural, distinct, and expressive, and neither too loud nor too soft. Avoid repetitious, mechanical words and phrases, and try to enunciate in a manner that is neither too fast nor too slow.

Answering Promptly

Answering a business telephone call is similar to welcoming a visitor. Therefore, it is essential that each call be greeted by a prompt, effective, and pleasing answer.

The telephone should be placed on the secretary's desk so that it is readily accessible. A pad and pencil or pen should be kept handy in order to jot down necessary information. These should not be used for doodling when speaking on the phone: this habit distracts the secretary from the business at hand and interferes with giving the caller undivided attention.

When the telephone rings, answer it promptly—at the first ring, if possible. Try not to put incoming calls immediately on "hold"; many callers find this practice infuriating. If it becomes increasingly necessary to do this, the employer should be alerted, it may be desirable to install another telephone line and to hire another person, if only for the busiest hours of the day, to help handle incoming calls.

If the secretary finds it necessary to leave the desk, arrangements should be made to have someone else answer the telephone and take the messages during that interval. The instrument should not be left unattended. An unanswered telephone becomes an instrument of failure—failure to the company because of the loss of customers and failure of the individuals responsible. It is well to inform the person who covers the telephone why the secretary will be away from the desk and for how long. Armed with this information, the one who answers the telephone can be more helpful to the caller.

This courtesy, of course, should be extended in both directions. Each secretary should reciprocally cover the calls of colleagues when it becomes necessary for them to be away from their desks so that telephones are never unattended for any period of time.

In many businesses, if the telephone is unattended, an answering unit is used. This machine will record a message after a "beep" usually preceded by a message.

Identifying Who is Answering

For efficiency, the office should be identified immediately when the phone is answered. The secretary's name may also be given, it is correct to say, "Mr Wright's office; Miss Dubrowski speaking", or the firm name may be used, as, "Smith and Grey; this is Mr Lopez". The identification formula depends upon the size and structure of the organization. When the telephone is answered in this fashion, the caller is assured that the proper office has been reached. Avoid answering the business telephone by saying, "Hello". Using this form of greeting is much like saying, "Guess who this is", and is un-businesslike. Business people have no time to play guessing games, and this form of address can become irritating, particularly if it is necessary to call the office frequently.

In answering calls for others, identify yourself and the office of the person whose calls are being taken. To quote an example: "Miss Laya' office; Mr James speaking." Unless this is done, the caller will not know whether the right person has been reached at all. If the caller expects to hear the voice of Miss Jones' secretary, he or she may be taken aback when an unfamiliar voice comes over the wire. The fact that the correct office has been reached is made clear at once.

Identifying Who is Calling

The wise secretary develops a keen ear and learns to recognize the voices of important or frequent callers. However, a word of caution does not become too sure of an infallible ear, for voices may sound different over the telephone. If the voice is known beyond a doubt, use the caller's name when speaking. If the voice has been identified correctly, the caller will be pleased to be recognized and addressed by name. Then speak to the person at the other end of the wire, not at the telephone. If the secretary was incorrect in identifying the voice before divulging any information, little harm was done. Since the caller will make the correction. Apologize tactfully and take up the business at hand. However, when the name of the caller is not revealed and/or the nature of the business is not identified, the secretary's skill at diplomacy comes into play.

Many executives prefer their secretaries to screen incoming calls. This must be done with tact and discretion. In some cases the executive will speak with anyone who calls but would like to know beforehand who is calling and the nature of the business. It is the secretary's duty to obtain this information before transferring the call to the executive. Curtness and rudeness must be avoided in doing so. It is correct to say, for example, "May I tell Mr Brown who is calling?" or "Mrs Winslow is talking on another line. Would you care to wait, or may I have her call you? I believe her other call may take some time." or "Mr Zobkiw is in conference. May I help you?" Be sincere and courteous in your explanation, but do not divulge information unnecessarily. Your goal is simply to find out tactfully who is calling if you can.

Screening Calls

Although some executives answer the telephone themselves, many depend upon their secretaries to answer all incoming calls. The secretary must, therefore, be familiar with the executive's preferences. It is important to learn which calls the secretary is expected to handle, which are to be referred to the executive, and which should be transferred to someone else. Consequently, the secretary must classify telephone callers accurately and quickly. Every call is important. Enough information must be ascertained to classify the call. A caller cannot be allowed to get to the end of a long inquiry before being referred to the proper person. In order to forestall this, the secretary may make a discreet vocal sound that may cause the caller to pause slightly so that the secretary may say, "Mr Chan in the shipping department should be able to help you with this. Please let me transfer your call to him".

Handling the Call

Generally the calls that can be handled by the secretary are as follows:
Requests for information: The secretary can handle this type of call if the information is not confidential and if there is no doubt concerning the facts. Sometimes it may be necessary to check with the employer before imparting information. If any complications arise, it is always wiser to turn the call over to the executive, in certain situations; the secretary may ask for a letter of request and, upon its receipt and approval, respond.

Requests for appointments: The secretary is sometimes authorized to make appointments for the employer. However, both the executive's and the secretary's diary should be checked before any appointments are made in order to avoid conflicts. If the employer is out of the office, the appointment should be verified immediately upon return. Commitments could easily have been made about which the executive had either forgotten to inform the secretary or the opportunity had not yet arisen to have had them entered in the desk calendars.

Receiving information: Often the secretary can conserve the employer's time by taking down telephone information. If the message is taken in shorthand, this must be transcribed as soon as possible and placed on the employer's desk.

Transferring calls: If the call cannot be handled by the secretary or the employer, it should be transferred to the office that can give the caller the information sought. This should be done only with the caller's permission, however. If transferal is refused, obtain the information and call hack. If the caller agrees to a transfer, make sure that the right office is reached before hanging up and give the person in that office sufficient information so that the caller will not need to repeat it.

Secretary should know where the executive will be when away from the office, whether urgent messages can be relayed, and the expected time of return to the office.

Also, in taking calls for other persons in the office, as suggested above, it is helpful if one can state when the person called will return or whether the call can be transferred somewhere else. It is best to offer whatever information possible; otherwise the caller may get the impression of being put off with an excuse. Be courteous, and use discretion in explaining an absence from the office. It is less offensive to say, Miss Jones is away from her desk just now. May I have her call you, or would you prefer to leave a message?" than to say bluntly, "She's out", or "This is her coffee break", or "I don't know where she is". The secretary must always use tact in dealing with callers, whether it is for one's own executive or for another secretary whose calls are being taken.

Taking Action

The secretary should promise the caller some definite action and see to it that the promise is kept. If the caller is told that the executive will call back, then this information must be conveyed to the employer so that the call can be made. A broken promise can result in a canceled order or a lost customer, and it may take many months to regain lost goodwill.

On some calls that the secretary can handle, more information may be needed than is within immediate reach. Therefore, it may become necessary to leave the telephone to look up the necessary information and to inform the caller of this fact and of the length of time it may take to obtain the material. Offer the caller a choice of waiting or of being called back. The customer should never be left waiting for an unreasonable amount of time at the other end of the wire. If a promise is made to call back with the needed information, this promise must be honored.

If the caller is waiting to speak to the executive, the secretary should reassure the caller periodically that the call will be connected as soon as the employer is free. Otherwise the caller will be uncertain as to whether the call is still connected, and a minute's silent delay will seem like a half-hour's wait. When the secretary is ready to transfer the call, thank the customer for waiting.

Completing the Incoming Call

At the completion of the call, indicate readiness to terminate the conversation by summing up the details. Use the caller's name when saying a pleasant "Goodbye". It is courteous to wait for the caller to terminate the call first; the secretary who is too hasty in hanging up the receiver may cost the firm money. The impression may be given that the caller's business is of little importance to the organization because the call is cut short. Permitting the caller to say "Goodbye" first also allows time for last-minute orders or special instructions. The receiver should be replaced gently in its cradle, for the pleasantest "Goodbye" can be spoiled by the jarring sound of a receiver dropped into position. It is like slamming the door after a visitor. The abruptness may not be intentional, but the effect is the same. Do not hang up until your caller has done so first.

Limiting Personal Calls

Because of the secretary's status and the prestige of that position, an example should be set for the office personnel by refraining from making and accepting personal calls during business hours except those that stay strictly within the rules set by the employer. The policy of the company or executive should be determined by the secretary at the very beginning of employment.

Telephone Dictation

Frequently the secretary is called upon to take dictation over the telephone. For this reason a shorthand notebook and pen should be placed near the telephone and ready for use. The caller is always informed of the fact that the conversation will be taken by the secretary. The secretary picks up the receiver and indicates readiness to record the proceedings. In the case of telephone dictation, unlike dictation taken at the employer's desk, the dictator cannot tell whether the secretary is getting all the information. Therefore it is necessary for the secretary to repeat the material phrase by phrase as it is taken down in shorthand.

This informs the dictator as to the rate of dictation, clarity of reception, and errors in grammar or facts. Corrections can then be made immediately instead of waiting until the end of the dictation, which may lead to confusion. If the dictation is too fast, it is best to indicate this immediately. It is a good practice to read back the notes at the termination of the dictation to ensure that the correct information was received and recorded and to correct any misinterpretations. The notes should be transcribed as soon as possible, and a copy should be sent to the telephone dictator. Of course, if the transcription equipment is used is of the type that can be utilized for recording telephoned dictation, the caller will be able to complete the dictation far more rapidly.

Telephone Reference Materials

The efficient secretary must be aware of the available sources of information that will be of help in placing a call expeditiously, skillfully, and economically. Directories and booklets published by the telephone company provide much information. A desk file for frequently used numbers should also be maintained. In the modern automated office, a secretary with a computer terminal at his or her desk may create a database for telephone reference materials and retrieve information from it in a matter of seconds.

Telephone Directories

Telephone directories contain three general sections—the introductory pages, the alphabetical listing of subscribers (which may be divided into subsections), and the classified section, familiarly known as "the Yellow Pages." In many areas of the country, all three sections appear in one volume of the telephone directory. However, in metropolitan areas where the listings are voluminous, the classified section is a separate book.

The introductory section gives instructions on what numbers to call in various types of emergencies, where to place service calls, how to ask for directory assistance, how to make mobile and marine calls, and the different types of calls that can be made. It lists area codes for faster calling and sample rates for long-distance and person-to- person calls. It explains how to make collect calls; how to call overseas; how to call the telephone company's business office and the operators who handle customer information; where to pay bills and transact business in person; and what modern telephone services are available to the customer. A map illustrates area code zones.

The subscriber section lists in alphabetical sequence the names, addresses, and telephone numbers of all the telephone subscribers in a locality, borough, town, village, city, or county. Sometimes the kind of business or the occupation of a subscriber is also shown. In some large directories, business, professional, and organizational listings are given in a separate section from that for residences. Government offices may also be listed in still another section.

At the top outside corner of each page guide, names, or "telltales", indicate the first and last listings on the page for quick location of the page on which a particular name appears. If a name might be spelled in several ways, a cross-reference spelling directs the user to additional listings. The divisions, departments, or branch offices of an organization with separate telephone listings are usually indented under the firm name. Alternate call listings can likewise be found in the telephone directory. These listings indicate telephone numbers to be called when no one answers the regular numbers. Governmental agencies and state, county, and municipal offices are shown with major headings for the principal listing and indented entries for subordinate departments and divisions.

The local alphabetical and classified directories are usually distributed to all subscribers. Out-of-town directories may be purchased by calling the telephone business office.

Street-address Directories

In some cities, street-address directories are available and may be rented from the telephone company. These directories list telephone numbers according to the alphabetical and numerical arrangements of streets in that city. They are of special value and usefulness to credit and collection agencies and for companies or organizations who desire to make up mailing lists.

Desk Telephone Files

For efficiency and expediency, a desk telephone file of numbers and area codes should be compiled. This list consists of:

1. Business numbers the employer calls frequently and, possibly, taxi, railroad terminal, and airline numbers
2. Emergency numbers for ambulance service, fire department, police department, and so on
3. Personal numbers of the employer's family
4. Extension numbers in other offices
5. Frequently called long-distance numbers, with notations indicating the difference in time zones.

Unlisted numbers should be added to this list, with an identifying mark indicating the nature of such a number. Unlisted numbers are never revealed without specific instructions from the executive to do so. They were given to the employer for personal use, and this fact should be respected.

It is a good idea when compiling a desk telephone list to make it as informative as possible. The secretary should identify individual names by noting title and company affiliation in addition to the address and telephone number and area code. In entering the name, address and telephone number of an organization, also indicate the name and title or department of the person or persons with whom the secretary or the employer talks most frequently.

The placement of the desk telephone list depends upon its size, it may be taped neatly to the top or the slide panel of the desk; if long, it may be kept in a book or on a rotary file attached to or near the telephone.

Database Files

Because electronic communication is used in today's automated office, you may have access to or use a terminal at your desk or workstation. To automate telephonic communications, create databases for telephone reference materials and desk telephone files. Then, you can easily retrieve complete citations for easy reference as well as make changes and additions within seconds. The advantage is that you don't have to handle a book and check via a system to find the data needed. You simply key the data to initiate retrieval. Such databases help speed up directory assistance inquiries. Instead of paging through phone books, operators input a name, and a list of possibilities appears on the screen. Through scrolling, the desired number, if listed, is revealed.

Assembling Data for Outgoing Calls

In order to place outgoing calls quickly for the employer, the secretary should master all the telephone techniques that enable one to do this skillfully. Be absolutely certain of the telephone number before calling. It will save time, trouble, and irritation if the number is checked with the desk list, telephone directory, or correspondence file before calling.

Then assemble all the information that may be necessary to conduct the business transaction when the call is put through. It may be necessary to obtain materials from the files to refresh the executive's memory on previous business or other information that will be of help in making a successful call. All pertinent material should be placed on the executive's desk before the call is made.

It is also a good practice to be sure the executive will be free and available to take the call as soon as it goes through. No one likes to be called and then find that it is necessary to wait because the caller is talking on another line or is otherwise not ready to take the call immediately. Delay may not only lower the prestige of the company and the executive and cause annoyance but also prove costly to the firm making the call.

The question frequently arises as to which executive should answer first. Courtesy prescribes that the caller should be on the line, ready to talk, when the person called is put on the line by his or her own secretary, particularly if the person called outranks the caller. The secretary should put the executive on the line immediately, if possible. This can be done readily if the secretary identifies the employer when the call is answered. The secretary at the other end will then be able to transfer the call to the person called without delay or immediately inform the caller of how to reach that individual.

Telephone Services

In addition to business calls within the local community or surrounding areas, it frequently becomes necessary to place calls to more distant points. The ability to handle long-distance calls capably will enhance the secretary's value to the employer.

Toll Calls

Long-distance calls are those made from one town or city to another town or city outside of a local calling area. A charge is made for such calls in addition to the charge for the regular telephone service. The amount of the charge depends upon the distance, the type of service requested, the time of day or night the call is made, and the time taken for the conversation.

There are two classes of long-distance calls—station-to-station and person-to-person.

Station-to-station calls: Any state in the United States can be reached by direct dialing today. The telephone directory carries a listing of cities and states and their area codes. In order to place a call to any of these localities, dial "I" first, the area code second, and then the local telephone number of the individual. If the city or town is not listed at the front of the telephone directory, refer to the area code directory; then call the directory assistance operator in that area and give the name and address of the party you want to reach. A station-to-station call is made to a particular telephone number, and the caller speaks to anyone who answers the telephone. Therefore, if someone answers the ring, the individual making the call is charged for it, and the charges start as soon as the call is answered. However, this type of call is less costly, is more frequently made, and is usually faster than the person-to-person call.

Person-to-person calls: To place a person-to-person call, the secretary dials zero, the three-digit area code, and then the telephone number; at this point the operator intercepts and the secretary gives the name of the individual being called. When the call is put through the person called may not be present or available to take the call. Then a decision may have to be made as to whether the call can be diverted to someone else who can handle the call transaction. A person-to-person call is made to a particular person only, and the caller is not charged for the call unless the person called is reached or the caller consents to speak to some other specifically identified individual. Charges start as soon as the caller consents to the call and begin speaking; therefore, the secretary should not start a conversation, but must make sure that the employer is ready to take the call immediately. It is advisable to avoid using "I" where telephone operator is involved and especially in person-to-person calls.

Direct distance dialing: Almost all calls in the United States and abroad may be put through by means of direct distance dialing. A "1" must precede the area code. A list of the area codes one must use for direct dialing is found at the beginning of the telephone directory or in the expanded area code directory available from the telephone company. The direct dialing system works by dialing "1" and a three-digit area code, followed by the local telephone number. There are no two areas that have the same area code, nor are there two identical telephone numbers in an area. The numbers of adjacent geographical area codes are widely different numerically to help avoid confusion and error.

It is a quick and accurate system. If a wrong number is reached, the secretary, before disconnecting, should ascertain the name of the city that was reached. He or she should then dial the operator, or in some cases the credit bureau, and promptly report that an incorrect destination was reached, so that the telephone bill will not reflect a charge for the wrong number. Also, if the transmission was poor or the call was cut off, the operator or the credit bureau should be called in order that the appropriate adjustment may be made. The phone directory also explains how to use direct dialing for credit-card and collect calls and for overseas calls. A "1" must also precede the area code.

Time differences: It is vital to check the differences in time when planning to place a long-distance call. One must be aware not only that this country is divided into time zones, but also that certain regions change to daylight saving time during the summer months and that difference in time exist in all countries. For example, the United States (excluding Alaska and Hawaii) is divided into four standard-time zones: Eastern, Central, Mountain, and Pacific. Each zone is one hour earlier than the zone immediately to the east of it: when it is 12 noon Eastern Standard Time, it is 11 AM in the Central zone, 10 AM in the Mountain zone, and 9 AM Pacific time. Greenwich Mean Time, which is the mean solar time of the meridian at Greenwich, England, is used as the basis for standard time throughout most of the world.

Appointment Calls

The telephone operator is asked to put through a person-to-person call at a specified hour. Contact is established at the time indicated and the caller is then notified that the connection has been made. The charge for such a call is the same as that for an ordinary person-to-person call. This service is not available for international calls.

Sequence Calls

The sequence-calls service is of value when a number of calls are to be made to out-of-town points. Much time is saved by furnishing the operator with a list, oral or written, of the calls to be made at the specified times. The secretary should supply the names of the individuals to be called, the cities and states where they are located, their telephone numbers, if known, and the hour at which the executive wishes to speak to each person on the list. However, it should be noted that this is an expensive procedure, as each call is charged at the "operator-assisted call" rate. If the secretary makes the calls by direct dialing, money is saved.

Conference Calls

Another instance of the various accommodations that the telephone company offers its subscribers is the conference service. It is of particular value to executives of organizations with branches and/or plants located over a wide area who find it necessary to confer speedily with those at the different branches. The telephone company provides two methods for setting up a telephone conference.

1. An arrangement can be made with the conference operator to connect several people in various cities simultaneously for a conference or discussion. No special equipment is required for this hookup.
2. An arrangement can be made with the conference operator whereby a conference call can be placed to a large group of employees. This type of call requires setting up a loudspeaker at the called point in a different city, so that the executive can talk by phone to the entire group at one time.

When placing such a call, the secretary should signal the operator; ask for the conference operator describe the setup desired; and furnish the names of the people to be called, their telephone numbers, if known, the city and slate where each is located, and the time of the conference.

Collect Calls

Calls can be charged to the phone of the person who is being called. The individual called may either accept the call and be charged for it or refuse the call and, of course, not be charged. Collect call rates are higher than direct-dialed station-to-station rates. A subscriber can also charge to his or her own phone long-distance calls placed from other phones. It behooves the efficient secretary to discuss with the employer when collect charges should be accepted. Determine from whom collect charges will be honored. If in doubt, ask the operator to wait while the matter is checked with the executive.

Overseas Calls

You can direct-dial many overseas points. Information on such calls can be obtained from the front pages of the directory, the International Dial brochures, or from the long-distance operator. For person-to-person overseas calls, the secretary must dial the long-distance operator and ask for an overseas operator. The name of the person to be called and the telephone number, if known, must be provided. The charges for this service are higher than those for domestic calls. There are reduced rates for evenings and for nights and weekends. (See section on "Telephoning a Telegram".)

Calls to Ships, Planes, Trains, and Automobiles

Telephone calls to mobile conveyances by way of radio telephone are similarly made by the operator. Such service is not available without the installation of special equipment by the telephone company in the car, plane, or ship, of course. Calls can then be placed directly from the office telephone to the destination desired. (See section on "Satellite Communications Network".)

Returning Long-distance Calls

Frequently a long-distance call is received when the executive is not in the office to take it. In such a case, the long-distance operator will give the secretary the operator's number, the city calling, and the name and telephone number of the person calling. To return the call, the secretary must dial the operator, ask by number for the operator who placed the call, and identify the city from which the call originated. When the connection is made with the proper operator, the secretary should tell the employer the name and telephone number of the person who placed the call. Collect calls are excluded from this service.

Telephone Record-keeping

Many organizations require that a record be kept of all long-distance calls made, in order to verify the telephone bill, and have special printed forms for this purpose. The secretary may ask the telephone operator, when placing such calls, to provide the charges when the call is completed. However, the request for charges must be made in advance, not after the call is completed. If you log long-distance calls, record the following: date, time, and caller.

Special Telephone Equipment and Systems

A good secretary should be familiar with the various types of telephone equipment available, in order to meet the needs of the company and those of the executive. Tremendous strides have been made in the field of telephone research. Not only business but also the world in general benefits from the discoveries made by telephone technicians and telephone researchers.

Call director: A push-button telephone that provides the capacity of several ordinary push-button phones in one compact, attractive unit is known as the Call Director. It can handle up to 29 lines and is available in 18- to 30-button models, which can be adjusted as needs change. The Call Director can be combined with the speakerphone feature (see below), which makes it possible to telephone with the hands free when needed. A plug-in headset model is also available; this frees the hands so that the secretary can take notes, consult records, and so forth.

The telephone company has also added the conference feature to the Call Director. This permits an executive to set up an intercom conference by merely dialing a code or pushing a button.

Speakerphone set: The speakerphone consists of a microphone and a loudspeaker and permits the user to convey on a telephone conversation clearly from anywhere in an office without lifting the receiver from its rest. The microphone picks up the user's voice, and the loudspeaker, with an adjustable volume control, broadcasts it to the party at the other end of the line. By sitting around the microphone all members of a group can engage in a telephone conversation at one time. Everybody can talk and offer a viewpoint, and everybody can hear and understand fully what is being discussed.

Direct inward dialing: A setup is available whereby an outside caller can dial the central office designation, followed by the extension needed, and thereby put the call directly to the office desired instead of to the switchboard operator.

Data phone: The data phone is a telephone-computer setup which, after activation by human hands, enables office machines to talk to one another and transmit data at tremendous speeds in various machine-usable forms.

AT & T's Merlin: This system is equipped with a microprocessor and has its own internal software. Programming features are possible. These include automatic dialing, privacy, and "do not disturb" mechanisms. Expansion is possible with other custom features and outside lines.

AT&T's Key 416: The key system links a group of key telephones. Each telephone permits the user to select an intercom or outside line. Paging is possible. The ultimate capacity is 16 stations, 4 central office lines, and 2 intercom paths. It is also possible to set up multilane conferences. Other systems include:

	System		*Lines*	*Stations*
Com	Key	718	7	18
Com	Key	1434	14	34
Com	Key	2152	21	52

The Com Key system offers many standard and optional features and a choice of telephone sets in various colors.

Custom calling services: These services are available on individual and auxiliary lines for both business and residence telephones. These features can be provided if a customer is served by the central office of ESS (Electronic Switching System). Custom calling services will operate in connection with rotary or touch-tone service. There are four custom calling services.

Call waiting: This service is designed to let the called party know that someone is trying to call while the telephone is in use.

Call forwarding: This service transfers calls to another number when the called party is not at the office or at home.

Three-way calling: A third party may be cut into an existing conversation.

Speed calling: One or two digits can be dialed in order to reach local or long-distance numbers more quickly.

To obtain custom calling services, it is not necessary to install extra equipment or to have an installer visit. These services are available with the regular telephone setup and may be attained by request at the central telephone office.

Dimension PBX: This electronic system uses stored program control, a time division switching network, and switched loop consoles. It is modular in design and has a solid-state system; therefore it saves space, speeds operation, and simplifies installation and maintenance.

There are two types of systems that are available to customers:
1. Dimension 400 has an approximate capacity of 400 lines and 90 trunks.
2. Dimension 2000 has an approximate capacity of 2000 lines and 350 trunks.

However, the capacity of lines and trunks for both dimension 400 and 2000 may change depending upon the line and trunk combinations and how they are used. Information on dimension PBX or any other type PBX telephone system or service may be obtained by calling the local telephone company.

Data speed 40 service: This communication service transmits the written word. It is available for private-line and expanded switched networks. The data speed 40 selective calling system is designed for use with private-line applications in both half duplex and full duplex. ("Full duplex" pertains to a simultaneous two-way and independent transmission in both directions. "Half duplex" service permits communication alternately in either direction or in one direction only.) Data is always prepared on a typewriter prior to transmission. All transmissions are fast, because the data proceeds at a maximum speed rather than the slower keyboard speed. The transmission accuracy is high, since the data is displayed on a monitor in its entirety before it is sent. This permits editing of data before transmission if necessary.

Horizon communications system: This is a microprocessor-controlled system that utilizes stored programs and multi-button electronic telephone (MET) sets. It has a capacity of 32 lines and 79 stations (excluding bridged, not MET, stations). A customer access unit (CAU) provides the ability to make feature changes or telephone-set rearrangements. There are further standard and optional features for both the stations and the system that are too numerous to mention. Local telephone companies can be called for further detailed information.

Picture phone meeting service: With this service a videophone, which is a telephone combined with a television receiver and transmitter, enables users to see, as well as speak to, one another. The service is offered in color in a limited area and in black and white between several large cities.

It brings people together for an important meeting so that everyone can participate. It makes it possible to conduct monthly or quarterly administrative reviews, to introduce new products to the sales force, to screen applicants for employment, to resolve production or distribution conflicts, to handle emergencies, etc. Visual aids such as slides, charts, artwork, or graphs may be used to illustrate or clarify facts discussed. Hard copies of information can be transmitted and videotapes can be sent or received. This service has now advanced to video-conferencing, a new technology.

Portable conference telephone set: This permits individuals from an audience to speak directly to the speaker, to ask or answer questions, by means of a standard telephone receiver that may be carried anywhere; it connects to a standard telephone jack.

Computerized Branch Exchange (CBX): This system is used lot large offices. This type of exchange can handle up to 800 stations. It is controlled by a microcomputer that automatically chooses the circuits to use and determines holding times.

Touch-tone telephones: These telephones have buttons. All numbers are used; the symbols and * are for special services. The "tone" permits the transmission of data to computers, similar to voice communications, a new technology. They are much easier to use than rotary-dial telephones.

Touch-automatic: This automatic telephone dialer "remembers" up to 15 (or 31, depending on the type) numbers. It dials them at the touch of a button. Numbers may be added or changed at will.

Wide area telecommunications service (WATS): This service allows subscribers to contract for station-to-station calls within a specified service area at a fixed monthly rate, in lieu of individual call billing. It includes a listing in the National information center records (800-555-1212); by calling this number a subscriber can obtain the number of any other WATS-line subscriber.

Outward WATS provides outgoing direct-distance dialing of long-distance calls by means of a WATS line from the customer's premises to other telephones within a specified service area. Each WATS line has its own WATS number.

Inward WATS allows a subscriber to receive calls over a WATS line without charge to the originating party. The call is automatically charged to the called number without the announcement and acceptance necessary with a collect call.

Service areas number 1 through 7 indicates interstate service. Included within the range of WATS service is all of the United States including Alaska, Hawaii, Puerto Rico, and the US Virgin Islands (St Thomas, St Croix, and St John). The purchase of one service area, 2 through 7, includes the area or areas in the lower numbered service area or areas. Service area "0" is an intrastate service available only in some states. WATS service is available in either of two forms.

Full business day: The initial period allows 240 hours including up to 14,400 completed incoming station-to-station calls a month from any telephone within the specified service area.

Measured: The initial period allows 10 hours including up to 600 completed station-to-station calls a month from any telephone within the specified service area.

Card dialers: A plastic card is inserted in an automatic dialing telephone. The cards are coded with frequently called numbers. The number is dialed rapidly and accurately by the telephone mechanism. In a business that makes a great many calls to the same numbers, the amount of time saved by these cards can be considerable. The telephone that takes the cards may be used in a normal way.

Bellboy: This is a signaling device that may be kept in the pocket, purse, or briefcase. When the user is within a certain range of the office, the Bellboy will beep when the secretary dials its number. The user then goes to the nearest telephone and calls the office to receive the message. Another name for Bellboy is "Beeper". Due to the advances in electronic communication, beepers may be activated up to 30 miles. Specially manufactured, "high-tech" beepers may range 30 miles plus. These are now common communication devices for top executives.

Telephone Answering Services

Many offices maintain contact with customers or others in the business world through an answering service that takes calls at night and on weekends and holidays. For a small office that closes entirely for vacations, an answering service is valuable.

The answering service may transfer the messages taken by calling at the beginning of the next business day. However, it is more common for the secretary to call in periodically and take the messages that have been received.

Trial and error may be necessary in finding a reliable answering service. If the service does not have enough lines or operators and callers are put on "hold" for unreasonable lengths of time, much good will can be lost. Then again, it is important to have a service that can be trusted to take messages accurately. The secretary planning to engage an answering service will do well to consult other secretaries and take their recommendations. Once the system is in operation, the secretary should check response time regularly.

When it comes time to take the messages from an answering service, the secretary should have pen and paper on hand and be scrupulously accurate in transcribing any messages given and especially so if the answering device does not have playback equipment. A set of priorities may be set up in advance with the employer as to which messages call for immediate action and which may be delayed for a shorter or greater length of time.

A sophisticated service available through the telephone company has an apparatus by which the subscriber can dial a two-digit code and have incoming calls transferred to an answering service. This does not "tie-up" the line, as the subscriber may still make outgoing calls. When the subscriber wishes to disengage the service, a second two digit code will restore the incoming calls to the client's own telephone line. Telephone answering services also provide "wake-up" calls, courtesy calls, and reminder-of-appointment calls at an additional cost.

Telephone Answering Devices

A great variety of telephones answering devices, usually activating a cassette tape recorder, are available. The simplest of these give a recorded message, as for example a statement telling the caller when the person called will be available, telling hours when the business is open, or the like. An equally common type is the recorder in which the person called has prerecorded a message that invites the caller to leave a message. When a tone sounds, the caller can talk for varying lengths of time, depending upon the way in which the recorder is set to operate.

Messages recorded by such a device should be transcribed by the secretary as early as possible at the start of a business day. If it is not possible to understand clearly any portion of a message, a notation should be placed on the transcript to alert the employer that the secretary was not sure of the message given.

A remote-control feature on such devices as the Phonemate allows the user to call the device on any telephone from anyplace in the world and hear whatever messages have been recorded. One phone call plays all messages, and a special feature allows the user to replay any given message without waiting for the entire tape to rewind and replay.

- Assembling data for outgoing calls
- Telephone services
- Telephone record-keeping
- Special telephone equipment and systems
- Telephone answering services
- Telephone answering devices.

Effective and efficient communication is an essential for any business and is required of all employees. Some basic methods of communication have remained largely unchanged; others have changed greatly with technological developments and increasing sophistication. The secretary must be familiar with all communications techniques and how and when to use them. This chapter briefly discusses the major communications techniques: mail, telegrams, cables, radio messages, and the telephone.

OFFICE MAIL

The processing and handling of mail constitutes the most important method of communication between a company and its contacts in the business world. The way in which mail is handled by the secretary affects every phase of a company and its external and internal procedures of information processing. A secretary who can effectively deal with office mail is indeed a valuable asset to an employer.

Electronic Mail Transmission

Electronic mail is the popular term for many of the new forms of communication that use computer and telecommunications technology. Also sometimes called electronic data communication, it is the non-interactive communication of text, data, voice, and image messages between a sender and a recipient using system links.

There are two advantages to electronic mail. One is the high speed with which large amounts of data can be sent from one place to another. The second is that data can be distributed to a specific location and stored in electronic form until it is needed by the recipient.

Electronic mail is rapidly becoming an indispensable tool in communications. Not only do companies use electronic mail for in-house communication but also for many employees who work at home from computer work stations and terminals. With the use of public access networks, such as Tymnet, Telenet, and other digital systems, it is possible to link host computer facilities simply, through a local phone call from almost anywhere in the world.

Electronic mail is implemented with several different technologies, among them facsimile transmission, telex, communicating word processors, microcomputers and other computer-based networks, electronic document distribution systems, and voice technologies. We shall discuss briefly a few of these means.

Telecommunications is the process of transmitting information over a distance, or "at a distance", by electromagnetic or electrical systems. (The prefix tele is derived from a Greek root meaning "at a distance".) Telecommunicated information may be in several forms, including voice, data, image, or message. The transmission systems include telephone lines, cables, microwaves, satellite transmission, and light beams.

Message systems: Message systems send information in data form. Telegrams and teletypewriter messages transmitted through systems as TWX and Telex are examples of message systems. These systems which the secretary may use frequently provide for faster transmission of information than does the postal system.

International electronic postal service: Various networks and services are available for rapid telecommunications. The secretary in an automated office should be familiar with the various network services, know which is best suited for particular purposes, and be able to use them. One such service is the International Electronic Postal Service, usually known as Intelpost.

Intelpost is a computerized network designed for high acceleration of information. The service links the United States, Canada, and Europe. Messages are transmitted by satellites, which use electronic and microwave technology. Documents such as charts, graphs, and photographs, as well as any type of printed text, can be transmitted.

Facsimile Transmission (Table 23.1)

Facsimile transmission is perhaps the oldest form of electronic mail and also a rapidly advancing telecommunications technology. Often known as fax, facsimile transmission is a proven method for sending information in the form of image replication (facsimile). It is flexible, inexpensive, and easy to do. Fax machines are now in many business offices and all secretaries should know how to use them effectively.

A fax unit can send a variety of documents—photographs, diagrams, drawings, statistical information, and handwritten or typewritten

Table 23.1 Facsimile standards		
Group	*Minutes per page*	*Technology*
1	6	Low resolution; analogs*
2	2–3	Low resolution; mostly analog
3	Fraction of a minute	Higher resolution; digital**
*Conversion to electric signals **Conversion to binary signals		

language messages—to any location that has a telephone line. The telephone line is the connection; without the telephone the system cannot work. The distance between two fax units is irrelevant. Information can be sent to another office in the same building or across the continent.

Fax units can store and forward information. They also have delay features that permit automatic dialing of one or more stations so that unattended transmission to multiple locations is possible on a 24-hour basis.

In 1980 the Consultative Committee on International Telephone & Telegraph (CCITT) set facsimile standards and groupings. The groupings refer to the amount of time it takes to send or receive a standard message over the telephone.

Incoming Mail

A new secretary may find a well-established system of handling mail within an organization. Changes may need to be suggested tactfully. The size of the organization has a great bearing on the system that evolves, in a small office one person may sort and open all mail except that marked "Personal" or "Confidential." (Letters so marked are delivered unopened to the person to whom they are addressed.) A large organization usually has a mailing department, where both incoming and outgoing mail are handled according to a fixed system. In an office where the secretary is assigned the responsibility for opening the mail for the employer, a routine procedure will permit rapid handling of each day's mail.

Necessary Supplies

The secretary will need supplies to open the mail. The following items and others you will need on your desk or work station should be placed there before the mail is processed. You may arrange the items in a circular fashion or another configuration for convenient and easy access. The suggested items are:

- Envelope opener
- Stapler or clips
- Date or time stamp
- Routing slips
- Transparent tape
- Pencils/pens (at least two different colors)
- Memo pad
- Mail register or log, if needed
- Staple remover.

If electric equipment, such as a mail opener or lime stamp, is available, use it. It will save two-thirds of the time as compared to manual equipment.

Opening the Mail

The mail should be opened as soon as it is delivered to the secretary's desk, and an orderly procedure should be followed to ensure that nothing is misplaced or lost, that time is not wasted, and that the executive receives the information needed.

Opening of the envelopes: All the envelopes should be opened before the contents are removed from any of them. To ensure that the contents will not be torn while the letter is being opened, tap the envelope firmly on the edge of the desk so that the contents will slip away from the top. Slit the upper edge of the envelope with a letter opener. If the contents of a letter are cut by the opener, use transparent tape to paste the parts together.

Checking tile contents: After removing the contents of an envelope, check the letter for a return address. If there is none, staple the envelope containing the return address to the contents. (Caution: If the contents include a punched card, use a paper clip for fastening rather than a staple.) The envelope should also be retained if the signature on the letter is not easily distinguishable.

Another check should be made to determine that all enclosures stipulated in the letter are accounted for. If not, a notation should be made immediately on the face of the letter, indicating what is missing.

Even though annotating a letter is one of the procedures encouraged, some companies do not like correspondence marked up, especially legal or business firms that might have to submit a piece of correspondence as evidence in a court of law. Always follow company policy. Some companies prefer that you place a buck slip (adhesive) with the notation on the face of the letter. In theory, it serves the same purpose.

Dating the mail: It is always wise to affix each day's date on incoming mail. The easiest procedure is to use a rubber stamp. Such a procedure is helpful if the letter has arrived too late to meet a deadline requested, has been in transit longer than it should have been, or is undated. In either of the latter two cases, it is well to staple the envelope to the letter in addition to dating the letter. This will give evidence of the date of mailing as well as the date of receipt.

Envelopes: Generally the envelope may be destroyed after it has been ascertained that everything has been removed and that there are no problems concerned with the names, addresses, or dates. However, in certain situations, especially legal matters, envelopes sometimes serve as evidence of date and time received (from the precanceled postage stamp). In such situations, envelopes may be kept and clipped or stapled to the back of the letter.

Preparation of Mail for Employer

In order to save the employer's time, the efficient secretary should take the time to prepare the mail. This involves two basic steps:

1. Read each letter, underlining important points that will aid you and your employer in answering the letter. Underline only those things that are of significance, such as publications, dates, and names of people.
2. Make annotations on each letter. This involves writing notes in the margins. Generally, annotations fall into three categories, namely, a note indicating:
   a. Action required by the letter—date of appointment for correspondent, reservations for a trip the employer may have to make as a result of the correspondence, etc.
   b. Procedures to be followed. These may depend upon former correspondence with the same person or related correspondence, which will have to be sought in the files.
   c. The priority the letter should receive, symbolized by a code. In an agreement with the employer a given place on each letter should be established for this code. For example, a red number may be written in the upper left corner. Such a code might be:
   Code 1: Mail and Reports with high priority and requiring a decision, these should be answered the same day they are

received. (It is assumed that personal or confidential mail is delivered unopened to the addressee as soon as it arrives on the secretary's desk.)

Code 2: Mail for which additional information must be procured, for which answering may have to be deferred for a day or two while data are being collected. All mail should be answered within 48 hours of receipt, except under very unusual circumstances.

Code 3: Routine mail that the secretary may be able to handle, many employers want to see all mail; it is wise to determine an employer's preference in this regard. After the relationship is well established, many secretaries have their employers' permission to reply to routine letters. In such instances it is usually good procedure to supply the employer with carbons of the letters sent and the original letter.

Code 4: Letters that require notations but no reply.

As the secretary reads and annotates the mail, it becomes a simple matter to encode and sort the mail as it is prepared for the employer. A fifth or even a sixth category may be added as needed. Usually important reports require a special category, while weekly, monthly, or semimonthly periodicals may require no encoding. Most employers prefer to examine the periodicals before they are made available to others in the office.

Preparing supplementary material. As the letters are being annotated, an efficient secretary will also make a list of files or pieces of correspondence and other information to be looked up before presenting the correspondence to the employer.

Some employers wish to see the mail as soon as it has been opened. In that case the secretary may bring the mail in as soon as it has been annotated. While the mail is being read, the secretary may take the compiled list and seek the necessary files, reports, and other information for acting upon the urgent mail. To keep all papers pertaining to each piece of correspondence together, use file folders or small clips.

Arranging the mail. After the sorting process has been completed, the secretary may arrange the mail either in one pile with the high priority mail on top or in any other arrangement that has been agreed upon. Whenever the mail is placed on the desk of the employer, some provision should be made to prevent others from reading the top letter. Some secretaries simply place the top letter face down.

Absence of the employer. When the employer is away from the office, letters requiring immediate replies may be handled in either of two ways. First, if a decision must be made immediately, it may be necessary to give the mail to the person in charge during the employer's absence.

Second, if the employer will be in the office within a day or two and the decision can wait, the secretary should write the sender immediately and explain when a reply may be expected and the reason for the delay. The efficient secretary to whom the employer has entrusted routine correspondence will maintain a file of materials handled during an absence of the employer. The folder should be readily at hand upon the employer's return.

Outgoing Mail

If the secretary is responsible for the preparation of outgoing mail, as the case may well be in a firm too small to have a separate mailing and shipping department, time and expense can be saved by learning about the various postal and shipping services available and the general regulations and normal charges pertinent to these services. It is important to be alert to frequent changes.

An accurate scale for weighing postal matter is a worthwhile piece of office equipment. It saves time and eliminates guesswork.

Sources of Mail Information

To obtain correct information on postal procedures and rates, which are subject to change, consult the local postal authorities. From them, or from the Superintendent of Document, Government Printing Office, Washington, DC 20402, may be obtained a number of useful pamphlets which are periodically brought up to date. These are some of them:

- Mailers guide
- Packaging pointers
- Domestic postage rates, fees, and information
- How to prepare second- and third-class mailings
- Mailing permits
- International postage rates and fees.

Some of the information in these pamphlets is taken from the Postal Manual, which contains complete data on postal regulations and procedures. Chapters 1 and 2 of this manual, which deal with domestic postal service and international mail, respectively, may be purchased separately.

A monthly publication called memo to mailers is available to business mailers without charge. It tells of rate and classification changes, along with other news of postal matters.

24 Leadership

INTRODUCTION

A leader is "a person who influences a group of people towards the achievement of a goal". A leader by its meaning is one who goes first and leads by example, so that others are motivated to follow him. This is a basic requirement. To be a leader, a person must have a deep-rooted commitment to the goal that he will strive to achieve it even if nobody follows him. Thus a leader is a person who steers the organization to a very high level alongside maintaining the harmony in the organization such that every individual is motivated towards the purpose with his unique qualities.

It is a proven technique that has stood the test of time. Although terminology and external environments may change, the concept is the same, people are a valuable resource and they can be influenced.

Hospitals face very dynamic environments and must meet diverse needs in the communities they serve and respond to multiple expectations imposed by their stakeholders. Coupled with these variables, the fact that leadership in these organizations is a shared phenomenon makes organizational leadership in them very complicated. An integrative overview of the organizational leadership role of CEOs in hospitals is presented, and determinants of success in playing this role are discussed.

Leaders will always be required to make the right decisions and manage dilemmas. They must also take risks and at times withstand the ridicule from others. Courage is the strength to choose and stand for the right course of action. Leaders will experience failure (the great teacher), and leaders must respond courageously to failure and take responsibility. Owning up to a failed action, learning from it, and adjusting your course is a courageous act.

In today's highly competitive world, there is a lot of pressure on leaders to create highly productive organizations. To be successful with this task, leaders will need all of the talent, skills, techniques, and experience they can master through leadership development. The pressure to succeed can create a real dilemma: whether to "manage" people or to "lead" people.

Leaders clearly must understand a great deal about the company and industry as a whole. It is this knowledge that enables them to understand the business landscape and communicate a clear vision, mission, and objectives. Knowledge can be classified into strategic knowledge and technical knowledge a leader at various levels should have a good balance among the two types of knowledge.

Strategic knowledge is that of the industry, the company, and business units. It understands evolving trends, emerging technologies, business principles, organizational roles and responsibilities, organizational culture, corporate and business unit visions, missions, and objectives, and how to lead, manage, and motivate people among other things.

Technical knowledge is that of particular business processes and technologies. It is understanding each step of the process, how that step is executed, what systems and screens are used, what details are included on those screens, and what logic the system uses in support of that step among other things.

	Strategic knowledge	*Technical knowledge*
Senior leader	High	Low
Midlevel leader	Moderate	Moderate
Technicians	Low	High

If you know too little, learn from those that really know, If you already know the details, do not try to unlearn. Just be aware and make sure that you are not getting in the way.

Knowledge of the details for a leader is a wonderful thing so long as it is knowledge of the right stuff and at the right level and used in the right way.

The humble leader assumes they do not know all the answers and allows people to explain things to them. They look for the opportunity to learn something new and they use every opportunity to make others feel valued. The humble leader knows the world around them is changing faster than they can keep up and is grateful for the opportunity to learn something new or reinforce knowledge they might already possess.

This is not to say that you need to act stupid to be humble. There is no harm in someone walking away knowing you are knowledgeable so long as the process did not leave them feeling "less than you." Sharing your wisdom is important, but must be done in a way that "lifts the other person up."

The vast majority of leadership training available to managers focuses primarily on skill and behaviors: how to delegate, how to communicate, how to manage conflict. These skills are unquestionably important and necessary. However, we maintain there is another important ingredient that has been severely neglected in leadership training, that ingredient is character.

A leader can never achieve greatness and success on the outside unless he or she has developed fundamental qualities on the inside. Behavior decisions and choices are all a reflection of our inner world.

Leadership training that focuses on character, values, and principles help bring balance to the practice of leadership. It helps leaders build lasting and productive relationships that unleash employee motivation and help leaders who want to bust down the status quo and build an innovative culture. It helps leaders build lasting and productive relationships that unleash employee motivation and help leaders who want to bust down the status quo and build an innovative culture. The real leader is one who willingly guide and build team to accomplish set goals of an organization **(Fig. 24.1)**.

This is a time when we need leaders and members alike who can move forward, think positively, and act creatively. Character based leadership provides the foundation for building skills and confidence.

There are certain important aspects a leader should follow to improve his relationship with his colleagues to maintain a smooth and efficient work flow.

We believe that sound character has the greatest impact on leadership success. Leaders simply attract people, ideas, circumstances,

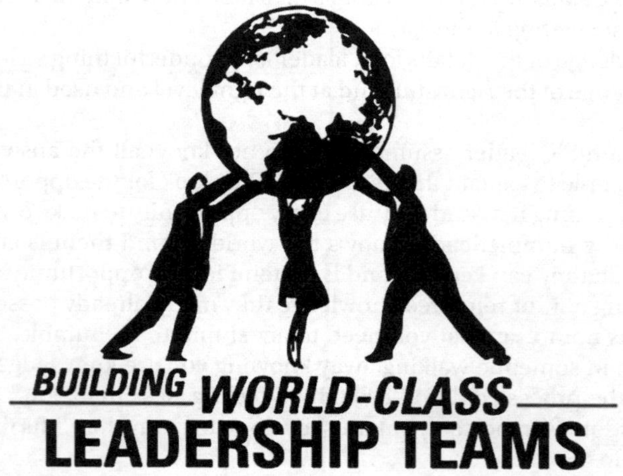

Fig. 24.1 Leadership is to guide and build team to accomplish set goals (*For color version, see Plate 5*)

opportunities, and resources that are in harmony with their core thoughts and being.

TRUST BUILDING

"Trust is the emotional glue that binds followers and leaders together."

—Warren Bennis and Bert Nanus

Trust is the foundation for every successful leader's accomplishments. When people do not trust the leader, they will not follow very far.

Creating an environment of trust is a tricky issue. People carry past hurts with them. Some people expect more from their leaders than they are willing to give themselves. We hear people say that they want to perform at a higher level, but they do not trust that they will be recognized or rewarded.

It is not always fair, and it is not always easy for a leader to give in to gain the trust but it is always the leader's responsibility to build trust among his colleagues.

Two tips have been advised to the leader in his way of working to gain trust of his colleagues:

1. Do what you say you are going to do.
   This will create a positive feeling among the people that the leader is clear in his thought about what to achieve and is really serious in implementing them.
2. Show people you trust them if you want them to trust you.
   This principle is known as the principle of reciprocity. The principle of reciprocity states that we tend to feel obligated to repay in kind what someone else has given to us. In a nutshell, it says that if you want trust, you must first give trust.

EFFECTIVE LISTENING

No matter what role you play in your company, becoming a more effective listener will help you get ahead in your position. It means fewer errors, improved accuracy, and enhanced working relationships. And, listening to your customers and referral sources will definitely help you in your marketing efforts. You will solicit better information from other people whether interviewing job candidates, solving work problems, or working to make a sale.

Contrary to what many people think, being an effective listener is not a passive activity. It takes concentration, effort, and active attention.

When listening, you are giving a gift of your time and attention to the other person. Work to respond both verbally and nonverbally to the person who is speaking. This lets the speaker know that you are listening and that you understand what he or she is trying to communicate. Here are some ideas to help you hone your listening.

1. Do not talk. Be courteous and give your listener your full attention. Avoid offering solutions if the speaker is expressing a problem. Just listen.
2. Listen fully. A good listener looks interested in what the speaker is saying. Your body language speaks volumes. Maintain eye contact, sit still, lean slightly toward the speaker, and nod your head (but not too vigorously or you will look like a chicken!).
3. Ask clarifying questions. Wait for the speaker to pause, and ask clarifying questions. It is a good idea to paraphrase what the speaker has said and to ask questions such as, "Did you mean..." or "If I understand correctly, you said..."
4. Provide feedback. Remain engaged in what the speaker is saying and show this verbally. He or she will appreciate the occasional "I see..." or "Really?" or "I know!"
5. Keep your mind open. The point of listening is to gain new information. Do not just search for a point that supports your own opinions. Be willing to gain new insights and learn about someone else's ideas.
6. Be on the same level. Make sure you are at eye level with the other person. Avoid having an employee or customer stand in front of your desk. Have comfortable chairs available so that a desk is not a barrier between you.
7. Respect your speaker. If the conversation involves criticism from either party or contains personal information, go to a private room for the discussion. Make sure other people cannot listen to your discussion. This will help the speaker feel more at ease and demonstrate your respect for what he or she has to say.
8. Pay attention to cues. What is not being said is often as important as what is being said. Body language speaks volumes. Watch the speaker's facial expressions, posture, eyes, gestures, and other nonverbal cues.
9. Avoid invalidating language. While you may not agree with what the speaker is saying, avoid defensive statements or phrases that argue with his or her points. Later, you can take time to review what was said and formulate a response. As an active and effective listener, your role is to allow the person the time and space to fully express his or her feelings.
10. Express appreciation. Thank the listener for sharing his or her thoughts and feelings. It takes courage to speak up. True sharing builds trust and encourages further dialog.

It takes time and energy to become a better listener. Be patient. As you begin to improve your listening skills, you may be surprised to find people will seek you out to share their thoughts and feelings. You will also find yourself involved in fewer conflicts and be perceived as a more positive and trustworthy person. Attentive listening is a rare skill that people respect and welcome.

LEADERSHIP TALK

The most important point to be observed here is leadership talk does not drive purpose. Purpose drives the leadership talk. There is one and only one purpose of the leadership talk: that is to motivate people to be your cause leaders in meeting the challenges you face.

But the point here is that applying leadership to a task changes the expectations of the task. It even changes the task itself. Think of it, when we ourselves are challenged to lead and not simply do, our world is, I submit, changed.

Furthermore, though you may order people to do a job, you cannot order anybody to take leadership of it. It is their choice whether they take it or not. This is where the leadership talk comes in. Using it, you set up the environment in which they make that choice.

The leadership talk is not only the most important way to get cause leaders; it is the only way to get them on a consistent basis.

The leadership talk not only communicates information. It does something much more. It has you establish a deep, human, emotional connection with people—so important in motivating them to achieve results.

Once you understand the leadership talk, you will find it is indispensable to your leadership. You will never go back to giving presentations/speeches again.

Leadership talks can be formal ways of communicating but mostly they are informal. Unlike a speech, they are usually interactive. They can be delivered anywhere: at a conference table, over lunch, at a water cooler, across a desk. (One of the best Leadership Talks as the author says witnessed was given by a plant supervisor to one of his team members at a company picnic while they sat on the back of a truck, sipping beers).

Qualities of a Leader

As per David Hakala the definition of leadership is "Ones ability to get others to willingly follow top ten leadership qualities" **(Fig. 24.2)**.

1. *Vision*: Dream, hallucination, apparition, idea, mental picture, image, visualization, revelation.

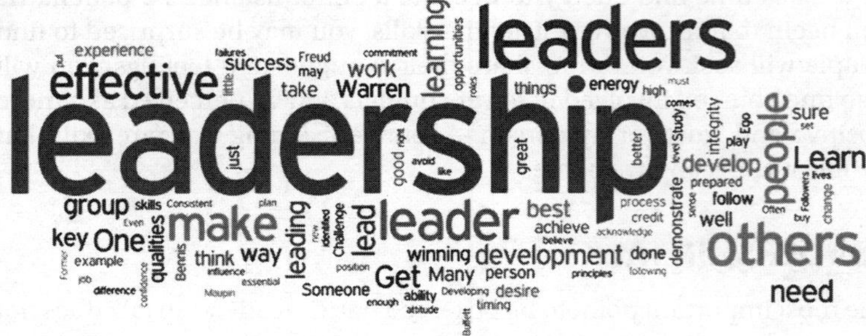

Fig. 24.2 Qualities of a leader (*For color version, see Plate 6*)

2. *Integrity:* Honesty, truth, truthfulness, honor, veracity, reliability, uprightness.
3. *Dedication:* Devotion, commitment, enthusiasm, keenness, perseverance, allegiance, ardor, loyalty.
4. *Magnanimity:* Nobility, generosity of spirit, high mindedness, fairness.
5. *Humility:* Humbleness, modesty, unassuming nature, meekness.
6. *Openness:* Honesty, directness, frankness, sincerity, candidness, ingenuousness
7. *Creativity:* Originality, imagination, inspiration, ingenuity, innovativeness, resourcefulness.
8. *Fairness:* Justice, equality, even-handedness, Sprite
9. *Assertiveness:* Not aggressiveness, boldness, brazenness, forcefulness, insolence
10. Sense of humor.

What is Your Leadership Style?

High Efficiency

Do it.
Do it then tell me what you did.
Tell me what you are going to do and do it.
Tell me what you want to do and wait for a decision.
Do not do anything without my approval.
Do not do anything until I tell you.

Low Efficiency

25 Motivation

Motivation is an internal state or condition (sometimes described as a need, desire, or want) that serves to activate or energize behavior and give it direction (see Kleinginna and Kleinginna, 1981a).

- Internal state or condition that activates behavior and gives it direction
- Desire or want that energizes and directs goal-oriented behavior
- Influence of needs and desires on the intensity and direction of behavior.

Motivation comes from a complex of words beginning with "mo." Motion, motor, momentum, etc. all denote physical action. The word *motivation* derives from the Latin root "to move." Motivation involves movement; yet the Latin root indicates it's not just movement but also "that which triggers movement."

The job of a manager at work place is to get things done through employees, to do this the manager should be able to motivate employees but that is easier said than done.

Motivation is inducing others in a specific way towards goals specifically stated by the motivator.

It is more effective to have people want to go from point A to point B instead of to be ordered to go from A to B.

The ability to instill "want to" in others, to motivate them, marks the difference between average leaders and great leaders. But many leaders misunderstand the true meaning of motivation. And if you misunderstand its meaning, you can't make it happen. Break the laws, and you'll fail to motivate people. Or you may motivate them—but motivate them against you.

Getting people to not simply be inspired but motivated to take physical action may seem like a simple, even simplistic, approach to leadership. However, once you begin to see your leadership interactions in terms of physical action, you'll see your leadership, and the way you get results, in fresh ways.

Sources of motivational needs: The **Table 25.1** furnishes some important motivational sources due to which, people tend to get motivated to do some work.

Table 25.1 Sources of motivational needs	
Behavioral/ External	• Elicited by stimulus associated/connected to innately connected stimulus • Obtain desired, pleasant consequences (rewards) or escape/ avoid undesired, unpleasant consequences
Social	• Imitate positive models • Be a part of a group or a valued member
Biological	• Increase/decrease stimulation (arousal) • Activate senses (taste, touch, smell, etc.) • Decrease hunger, thirst, discomfort, etc. • Maintain homeostasis, balance
Cognitive	• Maintain attention to something interesting or threatening • Develop meaning or understanding • Increase/decrease cognitive disequilibrium; uncertainty • Solve a problem or make a decision • Figure something out • Eliminate threat or risk
Affective	• Increase/decrease affective dissonance • Increase feeling good • Decrease feeling bad • Increase security of or decrease threats to self-esteem • Maintain levels of optimism and enthusiasm
Cognizant	• Meet individually developed/selected goal • Obtain personal dream • Develop or maintain self-efficacy • Take control of one's life • Eliminate threats to meeting goal, obtaining dream • Reduce others' control of one's life
Spiritual	• Understand purpose of one's life • Connect self to ultimate unknowns

Here are four "laws" of motivation that you must adhere to if you want to consistently motivate people to get great results.

Law 1. Motivation is physical action. Motivation is not about what people think or feel but about what they physically do. In leadership, you should understand the difference between inspiration and motivation.

Remember, people who simply take some action are useless to the organization. The useful ones are those who take action for results. For the end of all action in an organization are results. Therefore, the best action is freely chosen action directed toward specific results.

Law 2. Motivation is their choice. When you face a particularly tough challenge, avoid meeting that challenge by ordering people; instead, have people make the choices to meet the challenges.

An effective way to have them make the right choices is to ask them questions.

Some of the most powerful questions a leader can ask are: "What is our challenge here? Why is it worth tackling? How do we feel about it? Do we have the facts we need? Are we asking the right questions? What results are we really seeking? What's the worst thing that can happen? Why are we having this problem? Can you explain that further? What if we do nothing? Have we explored creative approaches? What do you propose? And what can I do to help?"

Law 3. Emotion drives motivation. The words "emotion" and "motivation" come from the same Latin root meaning to move. When you want to move people to take action, you must engage their emotions.

Emotion (an indefinite subjective sensation experienced as a state of arousal) is different from motivation in that there is not necessarily a goal orientation affiliated with it.

The point here is not about getting people emotional but about having people make strong emotional commitments to what you're challenging them to achieve.

Law 4. Face-to-face speech is generally the best way to motivate people (i.e. have those people choose to be motivated) A middle-manager told me, "Where is our new CEO? We call him 'Elvis.' We seldom see him in person. There is only purported sightings of him. Maybe I'll see a blurry photo of him in one of those supermarket check-out tabloids."

Isolation may be good for monks but it's an affliction with leaders. When you want to motivate people, relationship is the name of the game; and you can't have a relationship, at least a productive one, as an absentee leader.

Get out and about. This is more than MBWA (Management By Walking Around). The key is what you do when walking around. Don't be about simply sharing information but also creating the environment for motivation. People hunger to be motivated. Even more: people are ALWAYS motivated. And if they won't be motivated for your cause, they will be motivated for their cause—a cause that may be at cross purposes with yours.

In your interactions, strengthen the relationships by keeping the laws of motivation in mind. When interacting with people, challenge them to take physical action, understand that motivation is their free choice, their HEARTFELT free choice, give Leadership Talks to develop deep, human, emotional relationships; and take opportunities to speak with them face-to-face.

A thorough understanding of these ideas enables a leader to think and act with greater clarity and effectiveness causing people to voluntarily follow the leader's direction and example.

Heighten Your Curiosity, Jump Start Your Personal Brilliance with Your Inquisitiveness

Curiosity helps you clarify problems, ideas, and situations, and it encourages you to explore how they could be different. Actively exploring the environment, asking questions, investigating possibilities, and possessing a sense of wonder are all part of being curious.

Questioning takes you to deeper levels of knowing and helps you relate to others. When you develop heightened curiosity, you improve the quality of your life by asking better questions and being receptive to new ideas. Albert Einstein, one of the most innovative thinkers in history, said, "The important thing is not to stop questioning. Curiosity has its own reason for existing." Your outcomes are greatly determined by the quality of the questions that you ask yourself and others. Heightening your curiosity improves the quality of your life. People who are curious are open to thousands of potentialities and therefore increase their power to find the best solutions, the most lucrative offers, and the most creative ideas. Rather than being entrenched in their current beliefs, they withhold judgment, knowing that the last chapter has yet to be written.

You learn more because you have a desire to know more. When you approach an idea, person, or situation with a heightened sense of curiosity, your natural tendency is to "quest" for additional information. Even when you can't immediately apply what you learn, you are training to keep your curiosity muscles "buff." Another advantage of being curious is that your brain is designed to reward you for exploring fresh ideas and trying new activities. When you experience novelty, your brain produces more dopamine—an important brain chemical that lifts your mood and increases your sense of well-being.

Motivation to heighten curiosity: The power that heightening your curiosity can create in your life is truly unlimited. When you put past judgments aside, you come up with some of your most innovative ideas. For example, when Henry Ford made a commitment to develop an "unbreakable" glass for car windshields his highly educated engineers reported that it was "impossible." Undaunted, Ford directed them to find someone who did not know it was impossible. The plant recruited some

MOTIVATION
" I am better today than yesterday, but not as good as tomorrow."

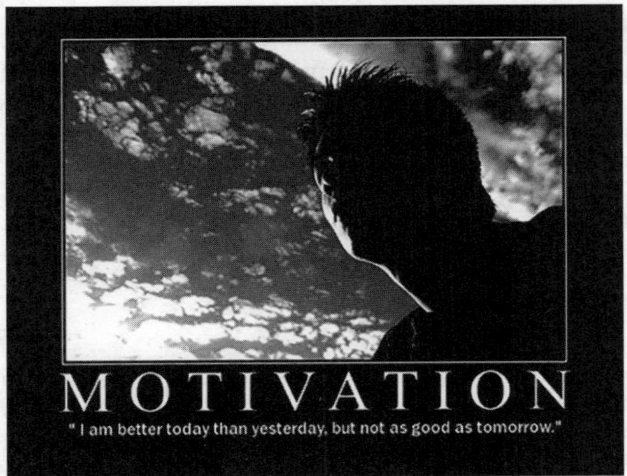

Fig. 25.1 Motivation comes within to heighten your curiosity to achieve set objectives (*For color version, see Plate 6*)

curious engineers who had not yet accumulated a mass of limitations based on what they "knew" and this group came up with the formula to manufacture shatterproof glass. A commitment to curiosity solved a seemingly impossible problem and has saved scores of lives in the decades since this innovation was introduced **(Fig. 25.1)**.

Neutralizing Situations Causing Worry

Your job is to organize your work so as to minimize surprises and problems. However, this is not always possible, in spite of your best efforts. If you are already facing a fear - or worry-inducing situation, here are the four steps of what we refer to as the "worry buster."

Clarity is Everything

Step number one: Define the worry situation clearly in writing-fully half of all problems can be solved just by clearly defining them. Remember, "Accurate diagnosis is half the cure."

Determine the Worst

Step number two: Determine the worst possible outcome of the situation. What is the absolute worst that can happen?

Be Willing to Have It So

Step number three: Resolve to accept the worst should it occur. The first step in dealing with any negative situation is to be willing to have it so. Once you resolve to accept the worst, your mind will become calm and clear and you'll be ready to take some constructive action.

Take Action

Step number four: The final step is to immediately begin doing everything you possibly can to improve upon the worst.

—Brain Tracy

Remember, worry is merely a sustained form of fear caused by indecision. The only real antidote to worry is purposeful action. Get so busy doing something about your situation that you do not have time to worry. As you take action, your confidence, courage and sense of control will return and wipe away your fears.

Mistakes and Failures are Learning Experience

Mistakes and failures of today are learning experience of tomorrow that motivates and leads to success **(Fig. 25.2)**.

Mistakes are painful when they happen.
But year's later collection of mistakes is called experience, which leads to success.

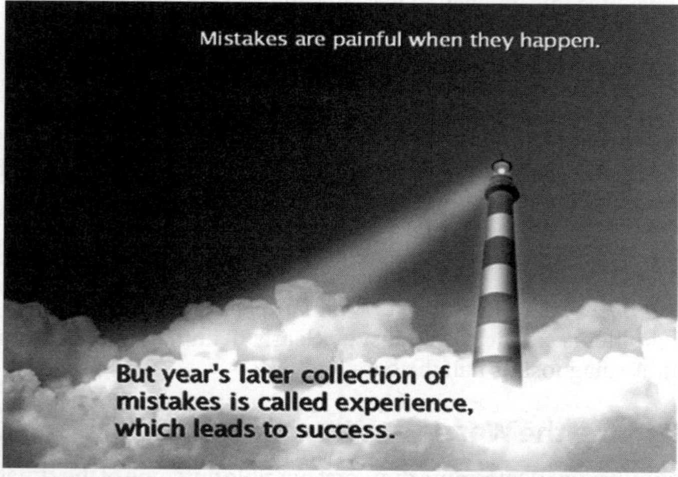

Fig. 25.2 Mistakes and failures of today are learning experience of tomorrow that motivates and leads to success (*For color version, see Plate 7*)

26 Terms and Definitions

The following are some of the important terms and definitions which are required for those practicing the healthcare profession including healthcare providers directly and indirectly.

Accident and emergency record: It is used for emergency (casualty) patients in the A/E department. This term is commonly used as A/E record, or casualty record or emergency room record or emergency file. These records are kept in the Casualty Department for one year and later transferred to Medical Record Department.

Admission waiting list: A list of names of patients maintained by the admission office waiting for a vacant bed and room for admission to the hospital.

Adult patient: A patient 12–14 years of age or older.

Etiology: A science dealing with the causation of disease.

Allergy: A condition of unusual or exaggerated specific susceptibility to a substance which is harmless in similar amounts for other members of same species. This term embraces all types of human hypersensitiveness.

Allied health personnel: Those not involved in the direct care of the patient but are vital in providing healthcare (such as dietary, social services, and medical records personnel).

Amalgamation of records: Bringing together of two or more files and numbers of one single patient created at different times under one hospital number and one file.

Anesthesia: Loss of feeling or sensation.

Analysis of hospital service: A gross appraisal of the efficiency of the hospital and medical staff primarily for benefit of, and use by, the patient and hospital. It is intended to give a picture of the type of illnesses cared for by the hospital and their end results.

Anatomy: The study of different organs which make up the body, their arrangements, and relationships to each other, and the different types of cells recognizable on microscopic examination.

Anomaly: It is a structure or organ which is irregular in formation (malformation). Examples of congenital anomalies are missing fingers or toes and heart defects.

Angiocardiography: A diagnostic procedure involving an X-ray dye into the blood stream, followed by chest X-rays to show the dimensions of the heart and the large blood vessels.

Arthroscopy: Visual examination of the inside of a joint with an endoscope.

Assembling of records: Arrangement of different forms in a standard order, e.g. outpatient file and inpatient file as recommended in the work procedures.

Assistant medical record technician (AMRT): It is a trained employee of the Medical Record Department who works under the supervision of a Medical Record Technician (MRT).

Audiometric: An instrument (audiometer) which delivers acoustic stimuli of specific frequencies to determine the patient's hearing for each frequency. The results are plotted on a graph called an audiogram.

Authorized personnel: Are employees of the hospital and are directly involved with the medical care of the patient, e.g. medical, nursing, and paramedical staff.

Autopsy: Examination of organs of a dead body (autopsy) to determine the cause of death. Also called a postmortem examination.

Autopsy rate: The ratio during any given period of time of all autopsies to all deaths.

Average daily census: The total number of inpatients days (exclusive of newborn) care rendered for a period is computed and divided by the total number of days in that period.

Average length of stay: The total number of inpatient day's care rendered to discharged patients (exclusive of newborn) in a given fiscal period divided by the total number of patients (exclusive of newborn) who were discharged or who died during the same period. In computing the length of stay, the day of admission should be counted but not the day of discharge.

Bacteriology: The study of bacteria and diseases caused by them.

Bassinet: For the use of infant other than newborns. Bassinets used for newborn infants are not considered to be hospital beds and should not be included in the bed complement of a hospital.

Bed complement: It is the total number of hospital beds, exclusive of newborn bassinets, normally available for 24 hours service to inpatients in the hospital.

Bed occupancy board: This board is maintained by the admission office, is also termed as the "bed control board" or the "bed utilization board" for keeping the account of occupied and vacant beds in different wards of the hospital.

Benign tumor: A benign tumor is a slow growing neoplasm and does not metastasize. Benign tumors are limited in extent and often are surrounded by a capsule.

Biochemistry: The science which deals with the chemistry of life.

Biopsy: Excision of tissue from a living body for microscopic examination to establish a diagnosis.

Birth: It is the acceptance of an infant patient newly born in the hospital for inpatient service. This involves occupancy of a newborn infant bassinet and maintenance of a hospital chart during the period of care.

Birth weight: The first weight of the fetus or newborn obtained after birth. This weight should be measured preferably within the first hour of life before significant postnatal weight has occurred.

Burn: A lesion of the tissues due to chemicals, dry heat, electricity, flame, friction, or radiation. They are usually classified into three types:

1. *First degree burns:* No blisters; superficial lesions mainly in the epidermis; hyperesthesia; and erythema.
2. *Second degree burns:* Damage to the epidermis and corium; blister; erythema; and hyperesthesia.
3. *Third degree burns:* Both the epidermis and corium are destroyed and subcutaneous layer is damaged, leaving charred, white tissue.

Cesarean section: Delivery of the fetus by an incision through the abdominal and uterine wall.

Cesarean section rate: The ratio of cesarean sections performed to viable births.

Carcinomas: The largest group of solid tumors which are derived from epithelial tissue.

Cardiac catheterization: A thin flexible tube (catheter) is introduced into a vein or artery and is guided into the heart for detecting pressure and pattern of blood flow. Dye can also be injected and X-rays taken.

Cardiology: The study of the structure, function, and disease of the heart.

Casualty: This term is synonymous to "Accident and Emergency" or "Emergency".

Causes of death: The causes of death to be entered on the medical certificate of cause of death are all those diseases, morbid conditions, or injuries which either resulted in or contributed to the death and the circumstances of the accident or violence which produced any such injuries.

Cauterization: Burning a part of tissue.

Census: The number of inpatients present in a hospital or healthcare facility at any one time. Ward clerk (AMRT) will prepare a daily ward census report and send it to the Medical Record Department.

Centralized filing system: A system in which all information is filed in one central location. Outpatient and inpatient files are kept in medical record folder and filed in the Medical Record Department.

Central processing unit (CPU): The part of a computer system that contains the circuits which control the interpretation and execution of instructions, including arithmetic, logic, and control functions.

Central registration: This section works around the clock to register new patients for outpatient and inpatient services. This section also maintains patient master index filing to enable verification of previous registration numbers.

Chart (Record) analysis: Careful review of the entire record (patient file); identification of specific areas that are incomplete or deficient.

Chemotherapy: It is the administration of a drug which destroys microorganisms, parasites, or malignant cells within the body and is utilized in the treatment of infectious diseases.

Child patient: Any patient less than 12–14 years is called a child patient, excluding newborn infants (born in the hospital).

Coding: A numerical assignment that provides an organized approach to data retrieval. The term coding for disease and operation classification as per International Classification of Diseases and Operations. The medical record staffs are responsible for coding of diseases and operations.

Color coding: It is used in terminal digit filing system, in which ten different color strips or labels are used for numerals 0–9 to facilitate and to identify the numbers of records filed by color.

Communicable disease: Causative agents which transfer disease from one person to another directly or indirectly.

Completion of records: Completing the records (patient files) which are deficient in number of forms or content as per the established standards. The medical record staff reviews each case and notes the deficiencies of physician and other documentation.

Complication: A disturbance occurring in the course of a disease and arising wholly or in part separate from the disease itself.

Comprehensive record: It is the one which has all the required forms with detailed and complete clinical and other information in a patient file as per established criteria.

Computer: An electronic device which stores, transmits, and manipulates information according to predetermined instructions known as a program.

Confidential information: A statement made to a physician, an attorney, or a clergyman in confidence with the implicit understanding that it should remain confidential. Patient health records are confidential documents.

Confidentiality: Status accorded to data or information which is sensitive for some reason and therefore must be protected against theft or improper use, and disseminated only to authorized individuals or organizations.

Consent: Concurrence of Wills; voluntary yielding of one's will to the proposition of another; acquiescence or compliance. This is obtained in the hospital generally for rendering treatment and performing surgical procedures to patients.

Consultation: A meeting of two or more physicians at the request of the attending physician or other authorized persons or body for study of a problem case, with necessary examinations to arrive at an accurate diagnosis and a written opinion as to prognosis, therapeutic measures, and recommendations proposed.

Contagious disease: One communicable by contact with an individual suffering from it or by contact with an object touched by that person.

Convalescent patient: A patient who is recovering from disease and who is preparing for normal activity.

Cribs: Equipped with sides or guards, for the use of young children (i.e., below 12–14 years of age).

Criteria: Predetermined elements against which aspects of the quality of medical service may be measured; for instance, two criteria for care of urinary tract infection might be the obtaining of a urinalysis and a urine culture.

Cross index: Cross indexing of diseases and operations may be defined as listing on a card for a specific disease or operation entity, according to recognized classification, all essential data of each patient having that particular condition, with a cross reference on other cards to every other entity involved in the particular case.

Cryosurgery: Using cold temperature to destroy tissue. The cold is usually produced by a probe containing liquid nitrogen.

Data bank: Computer term for storage of information.

Death rate: The ratio of total number of deaths in the hospital during any given period of time to the total number of discharges and deaths during that same time.

Deficiency: A non-justifiable variation from expected standards.

Deficiency check: Reviewing of outpatient and inpatient files for deficiencies by the Medical Record Department staff.

Dermatology: The science which deals with the skin, its structure, function, disease, and treatment.

Detrimental: Harmful; damaging; undesirable.

Diagnosis: It is made on the basis of extensive knowledge about the patient such as family history, physical examination, and investigation including X-rays and laboratory tests. The following are some of different kinds:

- *Clinical diagnosis:* Based upon symptoms shown during life, irrespective of the morbid changes producing them.

- *Final diagnosis:* A statement of opinion arrived at after extensive study, which is complete and accurate and is in conformity with the accepted medical terminology.
- *Pathological diagnosis:* Based on gross and microscopic examinations of the structural lesions present.
- *Differential diagnosis:* Based on symptoms and physical signs of two contrasting diseases.
- *Provisional diagnosis:* Based upon the availability of sources of information but subject to change.
- *Tentative diagnosis:* as above (provisional).
- *Preoperative diagnosis:* Made before operation and based on clinical findings.
- *Post-operative diagnosis:* Based upon findings observed during the operation.

Dialysis: Literally means "complete separation". A dialysis machine (artificial kidney) can completely separate out from the blood the harmful waste products of the body which are normally removed in the urine.

Dilatation and curettage: Dilatation (widening) of the cervical opening is accomplished by inserting a series of probes of increasing size. Curettage (scraping) is accomplished by using a curette (metal loop at the end of along, thin handle) to remove the lining of the uterus.

Direct admission: A patient admitted onto a ward and occupying a bed without processing through the admission office. This is permitted in emergency and obstetrics cases.

Discharge analysis: The tabulation of data on discharged hospital patients to reflect the professional services provided in a hospital.

Disease: Any deviation from or interruption of the normal structure and function of any part of the body. It is manifested by a characteristic set of signs and symptoms and in most instances the etiology, pathology, and prognosis is known.

Disease and operation Index: A numerical index of patient problems, diagnoses, and surgical procedures by individual categories. This work is performed by the Medical Record Department.

Dividers: Heavy-weight fabric forms of pressboard, used to designate different sections, e.g. "outpatient", "correspondence", "investigations", and "inpatient" records of the patient folder. Also used to designate alphabetical breaks in the Patient Master Index or numerical divisions of the Disease or Operation Index.

Doctor's conference room: Area in the Medical Record Department allocated exclusively for doctors to periodically complete deficient records.

Doubtful cases: Are those in which either hospital number or the name of the patient is recorded wrongly.

Echocardiography: A diagnostic procedure in which pulses of high frequency sound waves (ultrasound) are transmitted into the chest and echoes returning from the surfaces of the heart are electronically plotted and recorded. This can show the structure and movement of the heart over time and may be useful in determining structural defects in the heart.

Elective surgery: A surgical procedure is planned or performed which is subject to the choice or decision of the patient or physician; applied to procedures that are advantageous to the patient but not urgent.

Electrocardiography (ECG or EKG): The record of the electrical activity flowing through the heart.

Electrocochleography: A direct recording of the action potential generated following stimulation of the cochlear nerve.

Electro convulsive therapy (ECT): A form of physical treatment occasionally used by psychiatrists mainly in the management of depression.

Electroencephalography (EEG): Ultrasonic waves are beamed through the head and echoes coming from brain structures are recorded as a image. This procedure is useful in detecting brain tumors, and hydrocephalus.

Electromyography (EMG): The use of an instrument which records electrical current generated by inactive muscle.

Electrooculography (EOG): The use of an instrument which records eye position and movement.

Emergency: Any condition which could result in serious permanent harm to a patient or aggravation of injury or disease, or in which the life of a patient is in immediate danger, and any delay in administering treatment could add to the danger. Casualty or accident & emergency (A/E) or emergency is synonymous terms.

Emergency record: Patient file of an emergency or casualty or A/E patient. If the patient is transferred to outpatient or inpatient care, then the emergency record also becomes part of main patient file.

Emergency treatment: Treatment immediately necessary to save life. For example: treatment of a fracture case is not, whereas the treatment of a shock and hemorrhage case is.

Endemiology: The special study of endemic disease (recurring in an area, e.g. tuberculosis).

Endocrinology: The study of the ductless glands and their internal secretions (hormones).

Endoscopy: An instrument used for visualization of body cavities or organs.

Epidemiology: A branch of medical science that deals with the incidence, distribution, and control of disease in a group of people (population).

Eponym: A name or phrase formed from or including the name of a person such as Brigit's disease or Paget's disease.

Evaluation of medical Record Service: This evaluation should provide information on how effectively medical record services are being performed; e.g. how accurate is the filing of records or index cards, or how accurate is the disease index, etc.

Fetal death: A death prior to the complete expulsion or extraction of the product of conception from the mother irrespective of the duration of pregnancy. Death is indicated by the fact that, after such separation, the fetus does not breathe or show any other evidence of life such as beating of heart, pulsation of the umbilical cord, or definite movement of voluntary muscle.

- *Early fetal death or abortion:* Completed less than 20 weeks gestation (500 gram or less).
- *Intermediate death:* Completed 20 or more week's gestation but less than 28 weeks gestation (501 to 1000 gram).
- *Late fetal death or stillbirth:* Completed 28 weeks gestation and over 1001 gram.

Filing: Placing a collection of records or cards in a methodical manner so that they may be instantly available:

- *Alphabetical filing:* The method of filing charts or cards in strict alphabetical (dictionary style) sequence.
- *Serial number filing:* The method of filing charts or cards in strict numerical sequence.
- *Centralized serial:* The method of issuing one series of numbers to both the outpatient department and the inpatient department, and

storing all records in one place. In addition, a patient is given a new number on each admission either in the outpatient department or in the inpatient department.

- *Centralized serial unit:* Same as centralized serial, but the earlier records of the patient are brought to the folder of the latest admission.
- *Unit numbering system:* Whereby only one serial number is given to the patient irrespective of the number of admissions either in the outpatient department or in the inpatient department and all records of the patient are available in one folder.

File folders: Solid, two sided binders of Kraft, manila, press-board or patent composition used to store paper records. This term relates to a patient file (folder).

Follow-up: The periodic examination of a patient following disease or injury to determine the progress was being made toward complete recovery and normal health, and to study the end results of treatment.

Follow-up appointment: Giving an appointment for an existing patient to attend the relevant clinic on a particular date and time. All referral hospitals have to observe a follow-up appointment system in collaboration with the related health centers and hospitals.

Forensic medicine: Also called "legal medicine". The application of medical knowledge to legal proceedings.

Format: The arrangement of a form, or an organization of forms in a permanent folder, which directs the type of entries, the way entries are made, and the future use of those entries.

Fracture: The breaking of a bone due to injury or disease; some terms describing fractures and related injuries are:

- *Closed fracture:* A bone is broken but there is no open wound in the skin (simple fracture).
- *Open fracture:* A broken bone with an open wound in the skin (compound fracture).
- *Comminuted fracture:* The bone is splintered or crushed.
- *Impacted fracture:* The bone is broken, and one end is wedged into the anterior portion of the other.
- *Greenstick fracture:* The bone is partially bent and partially broken as when a greenstick breaks.

Gastroenterology: The study of the digestive tract, including the liver, biliary tract, pancreas and the accompanying diseases.

Gerontology: The scientific study of the problems of aging in all their aspects: e.g., clinical, biological, historical, and sociological.

Gestational age: The duration of gestation is measured from the first day of the last normal menstrual period. Gestational age is expressed in completed days or weeks (e.g. events occurring 280–286 days after the onset of the last normal menstrual period are considered to have occurred at 40 weeks of gestation).

Gynecology: Study of the female reproductive system (organs, hormones, and diseases).

Health center: Generally provides primary care and, if requiring further special care, refers the patient with a referral letter to an appropriate hospital.

Health information: Any data pertaining to the physical, mental, or social well-being of an individual or group of individuals.

Health record: Documentation of direct or indirect healthcare services to patients or clients by providers and users of the data in any type of health-related institution.

Hematology: The science dealing with formation, composition, function, and disease of the blood.

Homonyms: Word of same forms as another word but with different meaning (different spelling but pronounced alike).

Hospital bed: A bed installed for regular 24 hours use by an inpatient (other than newborn infant) during his or her period of hospitalization.

Hospital inpatient: A hospital patient who is provided with a bed, a room, board, medical care, and continuous general nursing service in an area of the hospital where patients generally stay at least overnight.

Hospital number: It is a unit number allocated to a new patient who visits the hospital for outpatient or inpatient service for the first time. This is a permanent number used for all episodes and subsequent admissions. Patient files including relevant forms are represented by this number.

Hospital record: A written account of all the services provided to the patient as an outpatient, emergency, or inpatient from the time of the visit or admission until discharge. This identifies the dates, the ward, the bed, and the room where the patient was physically located, the names of the physicians, the nurses, and the other health professionals who provided care, and the results of that care.

Immature infant: It is a live born infant with a recorded birth weight of 2500 grams or less.

Immunology: The study of the immune system of lymphocytes, inflammatory cells, associated cells, and protein which affect the individuals response to antigens.

Implied consent: That which is given by mutual understanding.

Incident report: In the event of occurrence of an incident in which the patient has suffered during hospitalization that was recorded and intimated to the concerned officials.

Incomplete record: Any hospital record of an outpatient or a discharged patient was lacking essential data.

Index: An organized and condensed list of data selected and recorded on a designed index for easy and quick retrieval of information.

Infectious disease: A disease due to organisms ranging in size from viruses to parasitic worms; it may be contagious in origin, result from nosocomial organisms, or be due to endogenous microflora from the nose, throat, skin, or bowel.

Information: Knowledge or intelligence; facts and data.

Informed consent: That which is documented to show the following: all procedures and treatment explained (including advantages and disadvantages) signed by a person giving consent as a result of their own decision.

Inpatient: A person who occupies a hospital bed, crib, or bassinet while housed in a hospital, for observation, care, diagnosis, or treatment.

Inpatient census: The number of inpatients present at any one time in all of the hospital wards.

Inpatient discharge: The release of a hospitalized inpatient from the hospital by the admitting physician after providing necessary medical care for a period deemed necessary.

Institutional deaths: Are those which occur 48 hours or more after admission.

International classification of diseases (ICD): A basic system of three-digit categories with four-and five-digit subcategories in some areas as recommended by the World Health Organization.

Job description: A document containing information about a position such as required education, training, and experience, as well as lines of authority and designation of supervisor, with a description of general duties and responsibilities and major job functions.

Laparoscopy: Endoscopic examination of the interior of the abdomen by means of a laparoscope.

Legal liability: Accepting responsibility before the court of law for reasonable care of the patients with reasonable maintenance of facilities for that purpose.

Length of stay: The number of days a patient remains in a facility (the day of admission should be counted but not the day of discharge unless the patient was admitted the same day).

Live birth: The complete expulsion or extraction from the mother of a product of conception, which, after such separation, breaths or shows any other evidence of life such as beating of heart, pulsation of the umbilical cord, or definite movements of voluntary muscles, whether or not the umbilical cord has been cut or the placenta is attached; each product of such birth is considered a live birth.

Low birth weight: Less than 2500 grams (up to, and including 2499 grams).

Malignant tumor: One that has the properties of invasion and metastasis and that shows a greater degree of anaplasia than do benign tumors.

Malpractice: Improper, careless, or ignorant treatment.

Maternal mortality: The death of a woman while pregnant or within 42 days of termination of pregnancy irrespective of the duration and the site of the pregnancy, from any cause related to or aggravated by the pregnancy or its management but not from accidental or incidental causes.

Medical audit: An evaluation system in which established standards are used to measure performance. Once corrective action has been taken on problems identified through this review process, performance is remeasured after an appropriate time period.

Medical board: A meeting or conference of the medical staff of the hospital held for the purpose of reviewing and analyzing the clinical work of the hospital. This board deals with death cases, unimproved cases, infection, complications, or performance not conforming with the standard. The board also deals with problems concerning organization and management of the various medical services of the hospital.

Medical care evaluation: A structured program to measure the quality of care given to patients. It is a global term that encompasses methods used to carry out such measurement functions as audit, appraisal, peer review, quality assurance, and assessment in various specific forms.

Medical certificate: It is a document containing disease and injury specifications and duration of treatment of a patient in the emergency, outpatient, or inpatient areas of a hospital and attested to by the treating physician.

Medical consultation: The response by one member of the medical staff to a request for consultation by another member of the medical staff, characterized by review of the patient's history, examination of the patient, and completion of a consultation report presenting recommendations and opinions.

Medical file: Or medical record or patient record or patient file all are synonymous terms. This file contains both outpatient and inpatient records.

Medical record: An orderly written report of the patient's history, physical, laboratory findings, treatment, and hospital course. When complete, it should contain sufficient data to justify the diagnosis and also describe the result of the care rendered.

Medical record committee: A committee which ensures that accurate and complete medical records are developed and retained for every patient treated. Also evaluates the work of the Medical Record Department to ensure that the department is functioning efficiently.

Medical record department (MRD): One of the important departments in the hospital responsible for proper custody of the medical records of the patients, for conducting medical audits, for preparing reports necessary to demonstrate the quantity and quality of medical practice, and for assisting in the advancement of medical science through assuring accurately recorded data.

Medical record form: A piece of paper or card, which is a formal arrangement of information (usually with spaces for the entry of additional information). A set of 90 basic medical record forms are recommended for adequate patient care in the hospital.

Medical record officer (MRO): An individual responsible for establishing, organizing, and controlling a Medical Record Department which initiates medical records for patient care. The MRO is also responsible for developing a good information system to compile and distribute patient or client data. He or she is the chief administrator of the Medical Record Department (MRD).

Medical record technician (MRT): A trained person who works under the supervision of a medical record officer. He or she is an intermediate supervisory staff person and performs most of the technical jobs in the department and supervises the work of the assistant medical record technicians.

Medical report: It is a document containing medical information such as history, physical examination, investigations, diagnosis, and treatment including surgical procedures, end results, duration of treatment, and recommendations about a patient treated in the hospital.

Medical social service: The sociological investigation of a patient and his environment to ascertain any factors which might have a bearing on the diagnosis, treatment, and aftercare of the patient, followed in close collaboration with the physician with respect to the findings.

Medico legal case (MLC): Case which is either accidental, suicidal, or homicidal. The casualty medical officer (CMO) determines a case as medicolegal or not. Except in minor injury cases, all cases of traffic accidents, burns, poisonings, and quarrels have to be treated as medicolegal cases.

Metastasis: Tumor spreading from its primary location to secondary sites throughout the body.

Medicine: (1) The science or art of healing, especially as distinguished from surgery and obstetrics. (2) A therapeutic substance such as a drug.

Microbiology: The science which deals microorganisms.

Microfilming: A process of photographing and reducing a given report to a miniature of the original on film. The Medical Record Department may microfilm certain old records as per the "record retention schedule" as recommended by regulations.

MoH: Ministry of Health.

Morbidity: The incidence of disease or proportion of diseases in a given population; statistical data that represents rates or ratios of disease.

Morphology: The science which deals with the structure and form of living things.

Mortality: The incidence of deaths or the proportion of deaths in a given population; statistical data that represents rates or ratios of deaths.

Mounting of investigation (diagnostic) reports: Reports of laboratory, X-ray and other investigations mounted on laboratory mount sheets, and X-ray mount sheets or EKG strips. All inpatient reports are received on the ward and mounted by the ward nurse or clerk (AMRT). Reports of outpatient are received and mounted by the Medical Record Department. The reports of A/E department are received by casualty staff and inserted with the relevant casualty record. If patient is transferred to outpatient or inpatient services, the casualty record along with all associated reports become part of the main patient file.

Necropsy (autopsy): Post-mortem examination; see "Autopsy".

Neonatal death: An infant's death occurring less than 28 completed days after delivery.

Neoplasm: New growth; tumor.

Nephrology: The special study of the kidneys and the diseases which affect them.

Neurology: (1) The science and study of the nerves, their structure, function, and pathology. (2) The branch of medicine dealing with diseases of the nervous system.

Newborn: Any infant newly born in the hospital.

New patient: A new patient is one who visits the hospital for the first time, for whom a new hospital number has to be allocated, or an outpatient record has to be created after obtaining accurate and complete identification data.

Non-institutional deaths: Are those which occur under 48 hours after admission.

Numbering system: An identifying method that utilizes assigned numbers to label each record for filing in a systematic manner to facilitate easy retention and retrieval.

Obstetrics: It is a specialty concerned with pregnancy and delivery of the fetus.

Odontology (dentistry): The science which deals with the structure, function, and diseases of the teeth.

Old medical records: Those records which are inactive and kept for a certain duration or period as per the retention schedule for administrative, educational, research, and legal purposes. These include patient files, X-rays, medical registers, reports, index cards, etc.

Old (Follow-up) patient: One who has been treated in the hospital either as an outpatient or inpatient for whom a patient file with hospital number exists.

Oncology: The scientific study of tumors.

On-line: A device that currently is an operating part of the computer system. A terminal is on-line if it is logged into the system. An idle service is on-line if it may be activated by the computer.

Operation index: It is a card possessing patient information about particular surgical operation undergone by different patients. Operation indexing is performed by the medical record staff.

Ophthalmology: The science which deals with the structure, function, and diseases of the eye.

Oral surgery: Pertaining to structures found in the mouth.

Orthopedics: Branch of study dealing with all conditions affecting the loco motor system.

Otorhinolaryngology (ENT): The science which deals with the structure, function, and diseases of the ear, nose, and throat.

Outguide card: This is also known as the "tracer card" or "locator". This card contains patient identification information which indicates the movement of the patient file.

Outpatient: It is a person who makes use of the diagnostic or therapeutic services of a hospital but does not occupy a regular bed.

Outpatient clinic schedule: It is the list of patients new and established to be seen in the clinic. Each unit in consultation with the administration and medical record officer decides upon the number of patients (new and established) to be seen in the clinic and the appointments are booked accordingly.

Outpatient record: It is a patient file created with a hospital number for treatment as an outpatient and generally comprises: the medical record folder, the outpatient form, the history and physical examination report, the outpatient follow-up form, laboratory and X-ray mount sheets, and other special forms added wherever required.

Paramedical: Are those personnel who are qualified to render treatment or assist in patient care under the supervision of the medical staff, e.g. occupational therapists, radiographers, laboratory technicians, and so on.

Pathology: The science which deals with the cause and nature of disease.

Patient day: A unit of measure for the service rendered an inpatient between the census-taking hours on two successive days, the day of discharge being counted only if the patient was admitted the same day. Only patients admitted, assigned abed, and having a medical record initiated should be counted in the census. When a patient is admitted and discharged the same day, the length of stay should be considered as one patient day.

Patient file: Medical record.

Patient Master Index (PMI): A 5″ × 3″ card containing patient identification information with hospital number; this card is filed in the central registration section in strict alphabetical order. This process assists in tracing out whether a patient has registered previously or not. This is also known as "master patient index".

Pediatrics: Any patient less than 12–14 years of age, treated by a pediatrician on a pediatric unit is considered as a pediatric patient or child patient.

Pharmacology: The science that deals with the origin, nature, chemistry, and uses of drugs, as well as their effects on the body.

Physiology: The science which deals with the normal functions of the body.

Policy: A basic guide of action which prescribes the boundaries within which activities are to take place.

Pregnancy: The condition of having a developing embryo or fetus in the body after union of an ovum and a spermatozoon. In normal pregnancy, the embryos develop within the uterus. In an ectopic pregnancy, the embryo is implanted outside the uterus, it is most commonly found in the fallopian tubes, and sometimes in the ovary or in the abdominal cavity.

Premature infant: A live born infant with a period of gestation of less than 37 completed weeks, or specified by the obstetrician as "premature".

Pre-numbered folder: Patient files with required forms numbered well in advance and kept ready for registration of new cases.

Presentation (obstetrical): The relationship of the long axis of the fetus to that of the mother. There are two divisions, the longitudinal, in which the head or breech may be present, and the transverse in which the shoulder is the presenting part and may include shoulder, arm, or any other part of the trunk.

- *Breech:* Presentation of buttocks or feet of the fetus in labor; breech presentation complete mean presentation of the buttocks in labor, with the feet alongside of the buttocks, the feet being in the same position as in vertex presentation, but with polarity reversed.
- *Cephalic (Head):* Presentation of any part of the fetal head in labor, including occiput, brow, or face.
- *Transverse:* Shoulder; scapula is the point of direction.

Preservation of records: Patient files and related documents are preserved in a safe location and well protected area for the period recommended in a "record retention schedule" furnished by regulations.

Privacy: A right to declare information confidential and to recognize formally the patient's inherent right to privacy.

Privileged communication: Any information acquired by a physician or surgeon in attending a patient which was necessary to enable him or her to prescribe or act for the patient and which cannot be revealed in a civil action without the consent of the patient.

Procedure: An act or manner of proceeding or method of conducting a business proceeding. A procedure is a series of tasks designed to accomplish work in a given time.

Processing of records: Reviewing of records (files) to determine whether the records are quantitatively and qualitatively complete. This also refers to effective documentation of the details of the patient's history and physical examination, other diagnostic measures, specific treatment procedures, etc.

Prodrome: Symptoms of disease (such as rash or fever) which appear before and signal the onset of an approaching more severe illness.

Prognosis: A prognosis made by a doctor after diagnosis about the nature of the patient's illness. It is a prediction about the disease.

Psychiatry: The branch of medical study devoted to the diagnosis and treatment of mental illness.

Qualitative analysis: Retrospective review program by the organized medical staff. It assesses the quality of care as compared to locally or internally developed standards and verifies that the standards or exceptions are met, that deficiencies are corrected, and that the original problem is reassessed on a planned program basis.

Quality assurance: Activities performed to determine the extent to which a phenomenon fulfills certain values and standards, and to assure changes in practice that fulfill the highest of a predetermined level of values.

Quality assurance program (QAP): A comprehensive and coordinated network of formal mechanisms that provide ongoing objective assessment of patient care services and the correction of identified problems.

Quality control: It is defined as those evaluation procedures that are performed systematically to ensure that established policies and standards are being met.

Quantitative analysis: The responsibility the Medical Record Department to check and analyze the component parts of the medical record to ensure that it is complete, adequate, and accurate, and is available at all times for legitimate needs of the patients, the hospital, and the physician.

Radiology: The study of the diagnosis of disease by using X-rays and other allied imaging techniques.

Record control: The supply of records (patient files) for patient care, administrative, and other reasons and the collection and accounting for that effective control, as well as the safeguarding of the confidentiality of information.

Referral: There are of two types: (i) from outside, e.g. from health centers and other hospitals or (ii) from inside, e.g. within the hospital from one department to another. Any referral of a patient must be on a written prescribed document. Referral forms are in triplicate. When a health center refers a patient, two copies are given to the patient to be forwarded to the hospital, and the third copy is retained by the patient. After treatment, the hospital returns one copy with details as feedback information to the health center and retains one copy in the hospital.

Relapse: A relapse is the reappearance of symptoms of disease.

Remission: A remission is the lessening or disappearance of disease symptoms.

Reports: Relating to statistics: daily, monthly, and yearly. Daily report is the analysis of hospital services which include the work performed by the different departments such as outpatient, accident/emergency, inpatient, and allied departments. Monthly report is a cumulative daily report for calendar months with ratios (or percentage rates) of service facilities used, and other statistical data and rates. Annual report is a compilation of the twelve monthly reports. The figures are cumulated monthly, just as the monthly report figures are cumulated from daily analysis.

Responsibility for medical certificates of cause of death: Medical certification of cause of death should normally be the responsibility of the attending physician. In the case of deaths certified by coroners or other legal authorities, the medical evidence supplied to the certifier should be stated on the certificate in addition to any legal findings.

Retention of records: Keeping information for a specific period so that it may be used in the future. Planning, implementation, and control of a system that safeguards physical and information characteristics of medical or health data for future use. The patient files and other documents are retained in accordance with the "record retention schedule" as suggested per regulations.

Review: Examination of a medical record by a physician to determine if continued hospitalization is medically necessary.

Sarcomas: Rare types of cancer which are derived from supportive and connective tissue, such as bone, fat, muscle, cartilage, bone marrow, lymphatic tissue, or blood cells.

Serial numbering: A system of numbering in which the patient is assigned a new number each time treatment is received.

Sphygmomanometer: Instrument to measure blood pressure.

Stages of Labor: The act of giving birth to a child. The following three stages are recognized.

First stage: From beginning of labor to complete dilatation.

Second stage: From complete dilatation to birth of infant.

Third stage: From birth of infant to expulsion of placenta.

Standard: Generally, a measure set by a competent authority as the rule for measuring quantity or quality. Conformity with standards is usually a condition of licensing, accreditation, or payment of service.

Sterilization: The act or process of rendering sterile; the process of freeing from germ life. Any procedure by which an individual is made incapable of reproduction such as a vasectomy or a tubectomy.

Stethoscope: An instrument used for listening to the various body sounds, especially those of the heart and chest.

Stillbirth: Fetal death

Suit: An action or process in a court of law for the recovery of right or claim.

Summons: A process (document) served on a defendant in civil court action to secure his or her appearance in the action.

Surgery: The branch of medicine which treats diseases, deformities, and injuries wholly or partly, by manual or operative procedures.

Symbiosis: Refers to the living together in close association of two organisms, either for mutual benefit or not. The bacteria which normally lie in the digestive tract of humans are an example of symbiosis.

Syndrome: It is a group of signs or symptoms which commonly occur together and indicate a particular disease or abnormal condition. An example of a syndrome is Homer's syndrome, characterized by ptosis of the eyelid, enophthalmos, and cool, dry face on the affected side due to nerve damage.

System: Related elements that are coordinated to form a unified result, specifically people, activities, equipment, materials, plans, and controls, working together to achieve a unified objective or whole; an array of components that interact to achieve some objective through a network of procedures that are integrated and designed to carry out a major activity.

Terminal digit filing: A method of filing by the last digits of a number instead of by the first digits. The entire number is broken into groups of two or three, with the last group being filed first. This system is suggested to all the referral hospitals.

Topography: A description of the regions of the body.

Toxicology: It is the study of harmful chemicals and their dangerous effects on the body.

Transfer of patient: If a patient is transferred within the hospital (except from casualty) from one unit to another, the same patient file will be continued for the duration of treatment except for change of ward census. In the case of a patient transferred from other hospitals, the case has to be registered and a record has to be created (if he or she is not an established patient).

Traumatology: The branch of surgery dealing with injury caused by accident.

Treating physician: One under whose care the treatment to the patient is rendered. Physician can be a Surgeon, a Pediatrician or an Obstetrician or Gynecologist. This term is synonymous to a medical doctor.

Treatment: The application of any measure to assist in bringing about the cure of disease or relief of symptoms or to correct the disturbances of the function was arising from an infection. Therapeutics or therapy is the general term for all forms of treatment of disease. The kinds of treatment are:

- *Symptomatic:* Directed towards the removal of the cause based on the treatment of symptoms as they are manifested.
- *Prophylactic:* Aimed to prevent the occurrence of disease.
- *Palliative:* Designed to check or to reduce symptoms.
- *Specific:* Assigned treatment devised for specific action.

Underlying cause of death: The underlying cause of death is the disease or injury which initiated the chain of events leading directly to death or the circumstances of the accident or violence which produced the fatal injury.

Unit numbering: A system in which only one number is assigned to the patient's record and is retained permanently.

Unit record system: A method that compiles all information on a single patient or subject and records it in one document and file folder.

Urology: The branch of medicine which deals with disorders of the female urinary tract and with disorders the male genital urinary tract.

Utilization review: The evaluation of the necessity, appropriateness, and efficiency of the use of medical services, procedures, and facilities. In a hospital, this includes review of the appropriateness of admissions, services ordered and provided, length of stay, and discharge practices on a concurrent and retrospective basis. This can be done by a utilization review committee, by peer review, or by any other assigned committee.

Venereology (sexually transmitted disease): The study and treatment of diseases transmitted during sexual intercourse.

Viable Infant: A fetus that has reached a stage of development that has enabled itself to live outside the uterus, usually consider and as 28 completed weeks of gestation or more.

Virology: The study of viruses and the diseases caused by them.

27 Electronic Health Record Terminology

GLOSSARY OF TERMS

The following glossary discusses terms and acronyms that you may find on our website, or during your search for the proper electronic health record (EHR).

Addendum	Text that is added to a document after it has been finalized.
Alerts	Pop-ups or reminders. An automated warning system such a clinical alerts, preventive health maintenance, medication interactions, etc.
Ambulatory care	Medical care provided on an outpatient basis.
Annotator	A system function that allows an explanatory note or diagram to be added to an image.
ASP application service provider	An application service provider (ASP) is a third party entity that deploys hosts and manages software from a centrally managed host facility (offsite). Applications are delivered over networks (WAN, Internet) on a subscription fee/rental basis. This model is also been referred to as "software-as-a-service".
Audit trail	Security system that tracks a user's access, deletion or modification of data. The term used in healthcare information security refers to a chronological record of system resource usage. This includes user login, file access, other various activities, and whether any actual or attempted security violations occurred, legitimate or unauthorized.
Authentication	The verification of the identity of a person or process.

Bandwidth A data transmission rate; the maximum amount of information (bits/second) that can be transmitted along a channel.

Bar code A printed horizontal strip of vertical bars which represent decimal digits used for identification. Bar codes must be read by a bar code reader.

Biometrics Biometrics are automated methods of recognizing a person based on a physiological characteristic such as fingerprints, retina, voice, etc.

Browser Short for Web browser, a software application used to locate and display Web pages.

Case management A process of identifying individuals at high risk for problems associated with complex healthcare needs and assessing opportunities to coordinate care to optimize the outcome.

Chart Medical record

Chart note A document, written by the clinician or provider, which describes the details of a patient's encounter. Sometimes referred to as a progress note.

Client/Server architecture An information-transmission arrangement, in which a client program sends a request to a server. When the server receives the request, it disconnects from the client and processes the request. When the request is processed, the server reconnects to the client program and the information is transferred to the client. This usually implies that the server is located on site as opposed to the ASP (Application Server Provider) architecture.

Clinical data repository (CDR) A real-time database that consolidates data from a variety of clinical sources to present a unified view of a single patient. It is optimized to allow clinicians to retrieve data for a single patient rather than to identify a population of patients with common characteristics or to facilitate the management of a specific clinical department.

Clinical decision support system (CDSS)	A clinical decision support system (CDSS) is software designed to aid clinicians in decision making by matching individual patient characteristics to computerized knowledge bases for the purpose of generating patient-specific assessments or recommendations.
Clinical guidelines (protocols)	Clinical guidelines are recommendations based on the latest available evidence for the appropriate treatment and care of a patient's condition.
Clinical messaging	Communication of clinical information within the electronic medical record to other healthcare personnel.
CPG	Clinical Practice Guidelines
CPM	Clinical Performance Measures
CPOE (computerized provider order entry)	CPOE refers to the act of a clinician entering an order for patient services into an information system.
CPR (computerized patient record), (computer-based patient record)	Electronically maintained information about an individual's lifetime health status and healthcare from all specialties.
CPT (current procedural terminology)	The purpose of CPT codes is to provide a uniform language that accurately describes medical, surgical, and diagnostic services.
Data conversion	The conversion of data from one software to another.
Data encryption standard (DES)	Data encryption standard (DES) is a widely-used method of data encryption using a private (secret) key.
Data integrity	Refers to the validity of data. A condition in which data has not been altered or destroyed in an unauthorized manner.
Data mining	The process of analyzing or extracting data from a database to identify patterns or relationships.

Data set	A group of data elements relevant for a particular use.
Data structure	A way to store and organize data in order to facilitate access and modifications.
Data base	A collection of information organized in such a way that a computer program can quickly select desired pieces of data.
Database management system (DBMS)	A set of computer programs for organizing the information in a database. A DBMS supports the structuring of the database in a standard format and provides tools for data input, verification, storage, retrieval, query, and manipulation.
DICOM (digital imaging and communications in medicine)	Digital imaging and communications in medicine (DICOM) is a standard to aid the distribution and viewing of medical images, such as CT scans, MRIs, and ultrasound.
Dictation	The process by which a physician records his/her notes about a patient. This recording is intended for reproduction in written word (Transcription).
Digital signature	Sometimes referred to as advanced electronic signature. Digital signature takes the traditional hand-written signature and creates a digital image of the signature to eliminate the need to print and sign documents.
Discrete data	A set of data is said to be discrete if the values belonging to it are distinct and separate, (i.e. they can be counted). Discrete data is more easily reportable as opposed to nondiscrete or unstructured data.
Document imaging	Converting paper documents into an electronic format usually through a scanning process.
Documentation	The process of recording information.
Document management	Is a system involving scanning, categorizing and storing vital patient documents.

DOQ-IT Doctors office Quality information technology	DOQ-IT is a two-year special study that is designed to improve quality of care, patient safety, and efficiency for services provided to medicare beneficiaries by promoting the adoption of EHR's and Information technology (IT) in primary care physician offices.
E&M coding evaluation and management coding	Documentation guidelines for evaluation and management (E&M) CPT codes from the center for medicare and medicaid services (formerly HCFA).
EDI	Electronic data interchange.
EHR (electronic health record)	An electronic repository of information regarding the health of an individual. It is also a generic term for all electronic patient care systems. EHR's imply a level of interoperability beyond the capability of an EMR (electronic medical record).
Electronic super bill	An electronic encounter form used for coding and billing.
EMR (electronic medical record)	Electronic medical record has a level of sophistication beyond a document management system. An EMR is a provider-based medical record that includes all health documentation for one person covering all services provided within an enterprise.
EOE (electronic order entry)	The function of this program is to move from hand-written and verbal orders to computer-based entry.
EPR (electronic patient record)	Same as a CPR—computerized patient record.
Encryption	Process of converting messages or data into a form that cannot be read without decrypting or deciphering it.
e-prescribing	Prescribing medication through an automated data-entry process and transmitting the information to participating pharmacies.

Evidence based medicine	Evidence-based medicine (EBM) is the integration of best research evidence with clinical expertise to aid in the diagnosis and management of patients.
Face sheet	Also called a summary screen or patient dashboard. This screen includes a summary of patient relevant information on one screen.
Fat client	A fat client is a network computer with a hard disc drive, as opposed to a thin client which has no disc drive.
Firewall	A system designed to prevent unauthorized access to or from a private computer network.
Formulary	A listing of prescription drugs established by a particular health plan which includes both brand name and generic drugs. It serves to suggest covered, preferred and lower cost drugs.
FTP	File transfer program

Index

Page numbers followed by *f* refer to figure and *t* refer to table

L

M

Q

R

S